COMPREHENSIVE
REHABILITATION
OF BURNS

This volume is one of the series,
Rehabilitation Medicine Library,
edited by John V. Basmajian.

New books and new editions published, in press or in preparation for this series:

BANERJEE: Rehabilitation Management of Amputees

BASMAJIAN: Therapeutic Exercise, fourth edition*

BASMAJIAN (ROGOFF): Manipulation, Traction and Massage, second edition*

BISHOP: Behavioral Problems and the Disabled: Assessment and Management

BLOCH AND BASBAUM: Management of Spinal Cord Injuries

BRANDSTATER: Stroke Rehabilitation

BROWNE, KIRLIN AND WATT: Rehabilitation Services and the Social Work Role: Challenge for Change

CHYATTE: Rehabilitation in Chronic Renal Failure

EHRLICH: Rehabilitation Management of Rheumatic Conditions, second edition

GRANGER AND GRESHAM: Functional Assessment in Rehabilitation Medicine

HAAS ET AL.: Pulmonary Therapy and Rehabilitation: Principles and Practice

INCE: Behavioral Psychology in Rehabilitation Medicine: Clinical Applications

JOHNSON: Practical Electromyography, second edition

LEHMANN: Therapeutic Heat and Cold, third edition*

LONG: Prevention and Rehabilitation in Ischemic Heart Disease

MOLNAR: Pediatric Rehabilitation

REDFORD: Orthotics Etcetera, third edition*

ROY AND TUNKS: Chronic Pain: Psychosocial Factors in Rehabilitation

SHA'KED: Human Sexuality and Rehabilitation Medicine: Sexual Functioning Following Spinal Cord Injury

STILLWELL: Therapeutic Electricity and Ultraviolet Radiation, third edition*

Originally published as part of the Physical Medicine Library, edited by Sidney Licht.

COMPREHENSIVE REHABILITATION OF BURNS

Edited by

Steven V. Fisher, M.D.

Assistant Professor
Department of Physical Medicine and Rehabilitation
University of Minnesota
Burn Center Consultant and Staff Physician
St. Paul-Ramsey Medical Center
St. Paul, Minnesota

Phala A. Helm, M.D.

Professor and Chairman
Department of Physical Medicine and Rehabilitation
The University of Texas Health Science Center at Dallas
Chief, Department of Physical Medicine and Rehabilitation
Parkland Memorial Hospital
Dallas, Texas

WILLIAMS & WILKINS
Baltimore/London

Editor: George Stamathis
Editorial Assistant: Victoria M. Vaughn
Copy Editor: Shelley C. Potler
Design: Bert Smith
Illustration Planning: Lorraine Wrzosek
Production: Carol L. Eckhart

Accurate indications, adverse reactions, and dosage schedules for drugs are provided in this book, but it is possible that they may change. The reader is urged to review the package information data of the manufacturers of the medications mentioned.

Made in the United States of America

Library of Congress Cataloging in Publication Data

Main entry under title:
Comprehensive rehabilitation of burns.

(Rehabilitation medicine library)
Includes index.
1. Burns and scalds—Patients—Rehabilitation.
I. Fisher, Steven V. II. Helm, Phala A. III. Series.
[DNLM: 1. Burns—Rehabilitation.
WO 704 C737]
RD96.4.C67 1984   617'.1106   83-16805
ISBN 0-683-03242-9

Composed and printed at the
Waverly Press, Inc.
Mt. Royal & Guilford Aves.
Baltimore, MD 21202, U.S.A.

Dedication

To those who have suffered burn injuries and from whom we have gained knowledge through clinical and research activities.

Series Editor's Foreword

From the first moment I concluded that a volume in the *Rehabilitation Medicine Library* series should be devoted to burn rehabilitation, I have been in a state of suspense. My excitement and hopes have been well repaid: Steve Fisher and Phala Helm have put together an outstanding book of which all of us can be proud.

This book bridges like a Colossus the two overlapping fields where clinicians and their associates have received incomplete messages for several decades. Here, considerations of rehabilitation and of acute burn care are carefully woven together into one text.

Having decided on the scope of the book, Doctors Fisher and Helm chose their authors carefully and wisely. Looking on anxiously and not being an expert in burn management, I could not be as sure then as I am now of that care and wisdom. After seeing a few and then all of the manuscripts, my early sense of relief has expanded to exhilaration. We have a fine book in our hands, written by well-informed experts. It will bring credit to the *Rehabilitation Medicine Library*, and the editors and their chosen authors deserve the thanks of both the professionals and the patients who are the subject of this book.

JOHN V. BASMAJIAN, M.D.

Preface

Because the burn trauma victim may suffer contractures, disfiguring scars, amputation, and subsequent disability, physical medicine and rehabilitation should be an integral part of the care of these patients. Burn care requires a team concept with the involvement of the entire physical medicine and rehabilitation team. Burn rehabilitation is a somewhat unique and specialized area of care of which physical medicine and rehabilitation has become increasingly involved.

There are over 200,000 patients hospitalized each year because of burn trauma. A greater percentage of these patients survive extensive burns than a decade ago. Although the mortality figures have improved, the morbidity from burns is still very significant. Physical medicine and rehabilitation can play an extremely important role in reducing this morbidity.

Unfortunately, little has been published in any detail regarding the overall rehabilitation approach to the burn patient. This volume of the *Rehabilitation Medicine Library* deals in detail with important aspects of this comprehensive care. The authors were selected from members of the burn team. The objective of the volume is to give an in depth approach to the rehabilitative care of the burn patient as it is perceived nationally. It is hoped this manuscript will not only be useful to neophytes but will also be a working handbook for those dealing with burns on a day to day basis.

Acknowledgments

We cite John Basmajian who envisioned this book and encouraged us in our efforts. We wish to sincerely thank Amelia (Mimi) Rinks and Trudy Evans for their unselfish efforts and their skilled organizational and administrative assistance. Finally, we thank the contributors, without whom this book would have been impossible.

STEVEN V. FISHER, M.D.
PHALA A. HELM, M.D.

Contributors

Verna Cain, R.N.
Head Nurse, Burn/Plastic Surgery Clinic, Burn/Plastic Operating Room, University of Washingrton, Harborview Medical Center, Seattle, Washington

G. Fred Cromes, Jr., Ph.D.
Chairman, Division of Rehabilitation Psychology; Assistant Professor of Clinical Physical Medicine and Rehabilitation, Department of Physical Medicine and Rehabilitation; The University of Texas Health Science Center at Dallas, Dallas, Texas

Alan R. Dimick, M.D.
Associate Professor of Surgery, Director of Burn Center, University of Alabama Hospital, Birmingham, Alabama

Irving Feller, M.D.
Clinical Professor of Surgery, Director of Burn Program, Chief Division of Burn Surgery, University of Michigan Medical Center, Ann Arbor, Michigan

Steven V. Fisher, M.D.
Assistant Professor, Department of Physical Medicine and Rehabilitation, University of Minnesota; Burn Center Consultant and Staff Physician at St. Paul-Ramsey Medical Center, St. Paul, Minnesota

Charles E. Hartford, M.D.
Director Burn Treatment Center, Crozer-Chester Medical Center, Chester, Pennsylvania

Marjorie D. Head, L.P.T.
Chief Physical Therapist, Department of Physical Medicine and Rehabilitation, Parkland Memorial Hospital of Dallas; Clinical Assistant Professor, Department of Physical Medicine and Rehabilitation, The University of Texas Health Science Center at Dallas, Dallas, Texas

David M. Heimback, M.D.
Professor of Surgery, University of Washington, Director of Burn Center, Harborview Medical Center, Seattle, Washington

Phala A. Helm, M.D.
Professor and Chairman, Department of Physical Medicine and Rehabilitation, The University of Texas Health Science Center at Dallas, Chief, Department of Physical Therapy, School of Allied Health Sciences; Chief, Department of Physical Medicine and Rehabilitation, Parkland Memorial Hospital, Dallas, Texas

John L. Hunt, M.D.
Associate Professor, Department of Surgery, The University of Texas Health Science Center at Dallas, Chief of Burn Service, Parkland Memorial Hospital, Dallas, Texas

Claudella A. Jones, R.N.
Director of Education, Administrator, National Institute for Burn Medicine, Ann Arbor, Michigan

Jean E. LeMaster, R.P.T.
Burn Unit, University of Iowa Burn Center, Iowa City, Iowa

Janet A. Marvin, R.N., M.N.
Associate Professor, Associate Director, Burn Center, University of Washington, Seattle, Washington

Robert H. Meier, III, M.D.
Director, Houston Center for Amputee Services at the Institute for Rehabilitation and Research; Assistant Professor, Department of Rehabilitation, Physical Medicine and Orthopedic Surgery, Baylor College of Medicine, Houston, Texas

Donna Nothdurft, O.T.R.
Occupational Therapist II, Department of Physical Medicine and Rehabilitation, The University of Texas Health Science Center at Dallas, Dallas, Texas

Gerry Pullium, O.T.R.
Chief Occupational Therapist, Department of Physical Medicine and Rehabilitation, Parkland Memorial Hospital at Dallas; Clinical Assistant Professor, Department of Physical Medicine and Rehabilitation, The University of Texas Health Science Center at Dallas, Dallas, Texas

Elizabeth A. Rivers, R.N., O.T.R.
Burn Rehabilitation Specialist, St. Paul-Ramsey Medical Center, St. Paul, Minnesota

Roger E. Salisbury, M.D.
Director, Burn Center, Chief, Plastic and Reconstructive Surgery, Westchester Burn Center, Westchester County Medical Center, New York Medical College, Valhalla, New York

Patricia S. Smith, L.P.T.
Chief Physical Therapist, Department of Physical Medicine and Rehabilitation, The University of Texas Health Science Center at Dallas, Dallas, Texas

Lynn D. Solem, M.D.
Assistant Professor, Department of Surgery, University of Minnesota; Burn Center Director, St. Paul-Ramsey Medical Center, St. Paul, Minnesota

Suzanne C. Tate-Henderson, M.S.
Rehabilitation Specialist Tate-Henderson Associates Overland Park, Kansas

George Varghese, M.D.
Associate Professor, Department of Physical Medicine and Rehabilitation, University of Kansas, College of Health Sciences and Hospital, Kansas City, Kansas

Contents

1

Introduction—Statement of the Problem

IRVING FELLER
CLAUDELLA A. JONES

History of Burn Care

Throughout history, burn care has been remarkable in its variety but limited in its progress. Ancient formulas, found on Egyptian papyri over 5000 years old, told how to "feed" the wound. Hippocrates, called the Father of Medicine (400 B.C.), recommended old swine's fat mixed with resin and bitumin, spread on a piece of cloth, warmed in a fire and applied as a bandage to the burn. Byzantines in the 7th century advocated soaks using bull's gall dissolved in much water, with the brine of pickled olives and pounded leeks. This same nutritional approach continued through the Renaissance. Ambroise Paré, a famous French surgeon of the 15th century, upon the recommendation of a country lady, advised treating the burn wound with salted onion; this was perpetuated in medical literature for three centuries. Once the germ theory was accepted (late 19th century), physicians soaked burn dressings in 10% silver nitrate to eliminate "beasties", which it did, along with any surrounding tissue. Today, as in the past, a variety of topical agents are used to control the bacteria in the wound. Because the burn wound is clearly visible to all, it is not surprising that doctors in the past concentrated their efforts on applying the medication of the times.

Full-thickness burns (third degree) cannot heal without skin grafting, a technique known to ancient Hindus and the first form of tissue transplant used in man. Skin grafting was seldom attempted until the late 19th century. Not until Reverdin's success with tiny epidermal grafts in 1869 did this procedure become common practice. Shortly after, others reported success with larger pieces of skin, then with deep slashes, and finally with full-thickness grafts. In 1939, Padgett invented the dermatome (a device to cut a layer of skin) and eliminated the roadblock to freehand slicing. We now know that topical therapy of the wound and skin grafting must be combined with meticulous systemic therapy if the severely burned patient is to survive.

Many years ago, blood-letting was the most popular form of systemic therapy. David Cleghorn, an English brewer during the Renaissance era, is credited with recognizing that purging was harmful to the burned victim. Cleghorn gained a great deal of clinical experience through treating burns among his employees. Contrary to prevailing antiphlogistic theories, he advocated a supportive regimen; allowing his employees to drink the brew during their recovery provided them with fluids and nutritional replacement. It was noted in 1831 that cholera victims seemed to share a fluid depletion similar to that of burn victims, and saline solution was occasionally given to patients with major burns. In 1857, Passavant introduced continuous saline baths—using them to treat survivors of an explosion and fire in Frankfurt am Main. Twenty-five years later, autopsy studies in Munich revealed that the water content of the blood was reduced in severe burn victims. In 1905, an article in the *Journal of the American Medical Association (JAMA)* addressed the importance of treating burn victims with parenteral saline as well as early skin grafting. Hardor Sneve of St. Paul is credited with recognizing the need for combining fluid therapy with appropriate wound care and pain control, and introducing common sense to burn care (1905). Not until World War II was attention directed to complete systemic therapy.

One of the first organized approaches to managing the severely burned individual was initiated by Sir Archibald McIndoe, a plastic surgeon. Sir Archibald took an interest in resolving the problems encountered by pilots burned during the Battle of Britain. (The survivors of his efforts formed a club calling themselves the Guinea Pigs.) He not only pioneered a system of resolving their many-faceted problems, but trained plastic surgeons in the intricacies of débridement and grafting, and set up one of the world's first specialized burn care facilities in East Grinstead, Sussex, England.

Even after the 1940's, few physicians specialized in burn patient care, and they were slow to adopt advances being made in general medicine and surgery. The tragedy and magnitude of the Coconut Grove fire in Boston in 1940 focused a great deal of attention on solving the acute medical problems of the burn-injured. Oliver Cope, M.D., is credited with leading the care after this disaster. The burns today considered moderate were then viewed as critical. The cosmetic changes that occur with scarring, especially of the face and limbs, led to a morbid cultural response perpetuating the stigma associated with recovery from a burn. Doctors and nurses avoided the burn patient not only for these reasons, but also because of the excessive physical and emotional energy required to care for even minor burns without a system of care and an adequate facility. Attention to the rehabilitation of burned victims was only an afterthought and lagged behind progress in other medical specialties. Major advances in burn care have been relatively recent, virtually all have occurred since 1940.

In the 1950's, based on a concern for a possible atomic catastrophe involving large numbers of burn casualties, the military supported an interest in burns. The Surgical Research Unit of Brooke Army Medical Center at Fort Sam Houston, Texas, was the site of an early burn conference. In December 1959, the first National Burn Seminar was also held there. Nine burn facilities were represented. These meetings continued yearly and the attendance had grown to 82 in 1966. Based on the burgeoning interest in burn care, by not only physicians, but by nurses, occupational therapists, physical therapists, and others, a committee was formed to offer membership to the entire spectrum of the burn care team. At the Eighth National Burn Seminar, bylaws for the American Burn Association (ABA) were drafted and the ABA came into formal existence in 1968.

The Progress of Burn Care to Date

Today, advances in burn care have not only kept pace with, but in many instances, have led the way for other medical specialties in problem solving.

Over the past 20 years there has been a dramatic increase in interest in burn patient care. Professionals are increasingly participating in burn care and burn care facilities are proliferating. At the present time, there are about 175 hospitals providing specialized burn care. Naturally, of interest is whether this has led to any improvements in the quality of care.

The National Burn Information Exchange (NBIE), established in 1964, collects and analyzes data on the burn problem, including etiology, mortality, morbidity, acute treatment, reconstruction, and cost. Over 50 specialized burn care facilities add uniform patient data on approximately 6000 new cases each year. At present, the data files contain over 70,000 case reports on patients treated at 125 burn care facilities.

The large volume of data accumulated by the NBIE allows a quality care assessment. Two outcomes are of primary interest in examining the quality of burn care: survival and, for survivors, the length of hospitalization. Figures 1.1 and 1.2 show, for all cases reported to the NBIE between 1965 and 1978, changes in survival rates and hospitalization time for survivors. Survival curves, modeled by probit analysis for the time periods 1965–1971, 1972–1975, and 1976–1978, show a steady increase in survival at all levels of burn severity (Fig. 1.1). Analysis of the data grouped by age and size of total body area (TBA) burned shows that improvements in survival are statistically significant for all but the most minor and most critical burns (tested at $\alpha < .05$). Especially dramatic are the survival increases in burns of 20–70% TBA. Improvements in survival are difficult to detect with minor burns because survival has been high since 1965, and in patients over age 50 with the very largest burns (80–100% TBA) because of the relatively

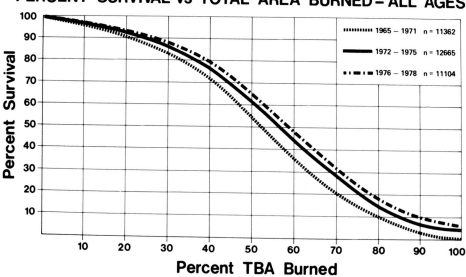

PERCENT SURVIVAL vs TOTAL AREA BURNED – ALL AGES

Legend:
- ⋯⋯ 1965 – 1971 n = 11362
- ▬▬ 1972 – 1975 n = 12665
- ▪ ▬ ▪ ▬ 1976 – 1978 n = 11104

Figure 1.1. Improvements in burn patient survival in NBIE hospitals. (© National Burn Information Exchange, I. Feller, M.D.—Director, Ann Arbor, MI.)

small number of cases. The improvements noted here were not due to a change in patient population, they persisted after controlling for such important severity factors as age, area of full-thickness burn, and changing referral patterns.

Of the 125 hospitals that have submitted data, 58 hospitals submitted enough cases in at least two time periods to make valid comparisons of survival records. The Standardized Mortality Ratio (SMR) (1) allows for comparisons after correcting for effects of size of full- and partial-thickness burns, age, sex, part of body burned, and time from the burn to admission in a burn facility. These comparisons showed 15 hospitals to have definite survival improvement, 22 with slight improvement, 16 with a slight decline, and five with a definite decline in survival results. Overall care has been improved despite the fact that several hospitals have declined.

Figure 1.2 shows the average length of hospitalization for survivors of severe burns. Again, the improvements are consistent across the three year groupings, and these improvements persist after controlling for group differences in severity factors. The shortened average hospitalization is statistically significant at all levels of burn severity, and is greatest for the most critical burns. Averages for patients with burns greater than 80% TBA are not shown; the figures would be unreliable because of the small number

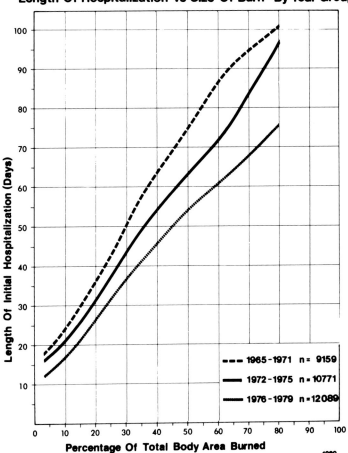

Figure 1.2. Decrease in length of stay of burned patients in NBIE hospitals. (© National Burn Information Exchange, I. Feller, M.D.—Director, Ann Arbor, MI.)

of such survivors. The specific reasons for these improvements are not addressed here. The increasing survival rates and decreasing hospitalization times are evidence that the majority of professionals who have shown an interest in burn patient care are improving the quality of care. With the reduced mortality and reduced length of hospitalization, rehabilitation takes on added importance.

Preventing Burn Accidents

Burns and fires are the third leading cause of accidental death in the United States. Each year an estimated two million people are burned.

Approximately 70,000 people are hospitalized, and more than 9000 die from their injuries. For children in the age group 1–14 years, burns are the leading cause of accidental death in the home. The National Institute for Burn Medicine estimates that one-half of these accidents could be prevented. To plan an effective prevention program three questions must be answered: Who gets burned? Where do they get burned? How do they get burned?

One way of identifying the WHO of the (burn) accident population is by analyzing risk factor. Risk is calculated by taking the percentage of burn victims in a given age group and dividing it by the percentage of that age

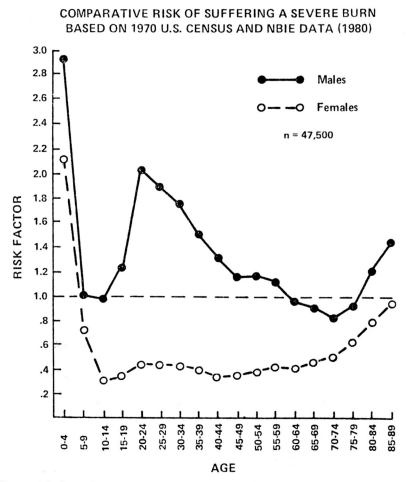

Figure 1.3. Comparative risk of suffering a severe burn. Risk factor analysis tells us that at the 1.0 level, risk is average, about 1.0 is greater, below 1.0 is less. (© National Burn Information Exchange, I. Feller, M.D.—Director, Ann Arbor, MI.)

Table 1.1.
Measures to Prevent Burns (© 1980, National Institute for Burn Medicine, Ann Arbor, MI)

IN THE KITCHEN
Cooking:
Keep an eye on youngsters when you are cooking!

Keep handles of pots and pans turned in so children can't "pull" them off the edge of the stove or countertop; better yet, cook on back burners.

Supervise children, when they are ready to learn to cook.

Don't squirt barbecue lighter fluid on fires.

Don't reach across a lit gas or electric burner. Don't store foods, especially cereal, over the stove—children could climb onto the stove to reach it.

Use only proper lighter fluid to light a barbecue, not gasoline or any other flammable fluid.

Keep children away from barbecue fires.

Electrical Appliances:
Use only UL approved electrical appliances.

Coil electrical appliance cords so children can't pull on dangling cords!

Unplug electrical appliances when not in use.

Keep electrical appliances away from water.

Don't misuse or overload extension cords; if a toddler is in the home, don't use extension cords.

IN THE BATHROOM
Set the temperature of hot water heater at 124 degrees (F); a water temperature of 140 degrees can scald.

Test the temperature of baby's bath water. Never bathe a baby or youngster in hot water—their skin is too tender.

Supervise toddlers and youngsters in the bathtub.

IN THE BEDROOM
Use fire-retardant sleepware for infants, toddlers, and young children.

Be careful when using heating pads—follow directions provided.

Don't let cords from vaporizers dangle!

Keep the baby's or toddler's crib a safe distance from radiators.

Table 1.1—Continued

No smoking in bed.

Keep space heaters and vaporizers away from cribs, beds, and curtains.

IN GENERAL
If you smell gas or suspect a gas leak, call the gas company or fire department for help. Do not light a match or turn on the electric lights.

Install heat and smoke detectors and keep them operating properly.

HAVE A FIRE ESCAPE PLAN for all family members with a place to meet outside the home. PRACTICE IT. Instruct babysitters of the plan.

Keep fire and police numbers by the phone.

Do not allow candles to burn unattended.

Keep the fireplace screened.

Matches:
Keep matches and lighters out of reach of toddlers and youngsters.

Teach children (when they are ready to learn) that MATCHES ARE A TOOL and teach them proper use.

Gasoline and Other Chemicals:
Don't misuse gasoline! Gasoline should only be used in proper engines.

Store gasoline, other combustibles, and cleaning or toxic chemicals in special closed containers, out of reach of children. Better yet, don't store them. Buy a one-time-use quantity and replenish as needed. Never store in the home.

Use combustible liquids ONLY with proper ventilation. Do not pour from any container when inside of any building.

Don't refill a hot lawn mower or snow blower. Let it cool.

---

group in the U.S. population. Once the risk factor for varying age groups is known one asks WHERE the victim was at the time of the accident (Fig. 1.3). WHERE is where people usually spend the most time: overall, 74% of accidents in the NBIE database occurred in the home. HOW do accidents occur? Of all the burn cases from the NBIE, the majority (76%) are victims of their actions; 15% are innocent bystanders, 5% are victims of their medical condition, 4% are intended victims, and 1% are rescue workers. Simple measures that cost little and result in no change in lifestyle could reduce these injuries to one-half (Table 1.1).

REFERENCE

1. Cornell RG, Feller I, et al.: Evaluation of burn care utliizing a national burn registry. *Emerg Med Serv* 7:107–117, 1978.

2

Classification

LYNN D. SOLEM

Classification of Burns

Burns may be classified in several different ways including etiology of burn or burning agent, depth of injury, severity of injury, and surface area of skin involved. Classification of burns is important prognostically, allows comparison of injuries of similar etiology, depth, and severity, and is an important consideration when planning future patient care.

Skin is made up of two distinct layers: the epidermis and dermis, histologically depicted in Figure 2.1. The epidermal cells originate in the basal layer and gradually migrate to the surface. As they approach the surface, the cells undergo a process of keratinization in which a fibrous protein, keratin, is produced, the cellular structure is lost and the cells become flattened, leaving a thin layer of keratin fiber on the surface. The keratin layer forms an important protective barrier on the skin, preventing bacterial invasion as well as the loss of essential body fluids. Keratin which is lost is rapidly replaced by the underlying epidermal cells. Epidermal cells are found not only in the basal layer of the epidermis, but they also line the hair follicles and sweat glands which are located in the deep dermis (Fig. 2.1). These epidermal cells in the deep dermis are the source of epithelium for the healing of deep second degree burns.

The dermis is made up of a vascular connective tissue which supports the epidermis and provides nutrients to the epidermal layer and the skin appendages—sweat glands, hair follicles, and sebaceous glands. The dermis is composed of dense interlacing collagen fibers with interspersed elastic fibers, giving the skin strength and elasticity. Together the two layers of the skin are supported on subcutaneous fat. The depth of subcutaneous fat is dependent on body habitus. The thickest subcutaneous fat is found over the buttocks and thighs with only a thin layer over the nose, ears, and digits.

Skin thickness (including both dermis and epidermis) varies with age and location. The thinnest skin is located on the prepuce and eyelids (.013 inches or .33 mm). Intermediate thickness skin is found on the anterior thorax and arm (.050 inches or 1.28 mm). The thickest skin, .085 inches or 2.16 mm, is located in the intrascapular area (1). Thinner skin generally is

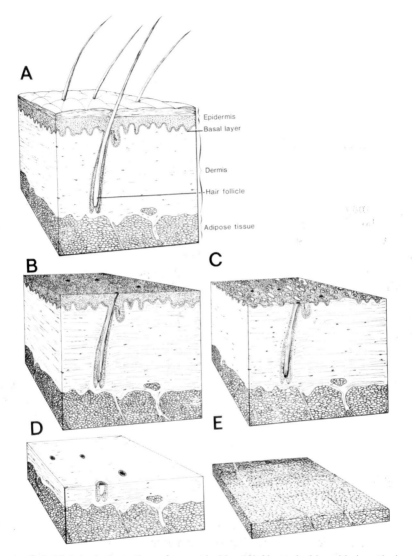

Figure 2.1. Histological section of normal skin. (*A*) Normal skin with keratin layer, epidermis, and dermis intact. (*B*) First degree burn; keratin and superficial epidermis destroyed. (*C*) Superficial second degree burn; most of basal layer remains. (*D*) Deep second degree burn, only the basal layer lining the skin appendages remains. (*E*) Third degree ("full-thickness") burn; total destruction of all epidermal elements, including those at the base of skin appendages. NOTE: Burn injury does not cleave away the destroyed skin. Therefore, in the clinical situation, necrotic skin elements would remain. (Reproduced with permission from Fisher SV: Rehabilitation Management of Burns. In Basmajian JB, Kirby RL: *Medical Rehabilitation.* Baltimore, Williams & Wilkins, 1984.)

found in areas which are relatively protected such as the medial thigh and medial portion of the upper arm, whereas thicker skin is found over the back and posterior neck. Skin appendages penetrate to varying depths with the deepest penetration being found in the scalp and in the male beard.

Classification by Etiology

Burns can be classified by etiology with thermal injuries being the most frequent. Thermal injuries include burns caused by contact with hot liquids (spills or immersion scalds), hot solid objects, or flames. Thermal injuries make up approximately 95% of all burns treated. Chemical and electrical injuries comprise about 5% of burns admitted to a regional burn center. Radiation injuries, the fourth category of burns, are extremely rare.

Classification by Depth of Burn

Burn injuries are customarily classified into first, second, and third degree burns. First degree burns involve only the outer layers of the epidermis leaving the deep layers of epidermis intact. These burns never blister and usually are caused by ultraviolet exposure such as sunlight or a tanning lamp, or a very short exposure to flame (flash burn). First degree burns are painful, particularly during the initial 48 hours after injury. Normal skin functions are retained and infectious complications do not occur. First degree burns heal uneventfully in three to six days as the epidermis flakes off leaving no permanent alteration of the skin. First degree burns are not included when burn surface area is calculated.

Second degree burns may be classified as either superficial or deep second degree. Prognostically, superficial second degree burns are much less severe, involving only the epidermis but sparing the basal layer. The burns usually form blisters and the superficial layers of skin may be readily wiped away. Once the vesicles are removed, these burns are erythematous, wet, weeping, and painful. Superficial second degree burns typically follow a brief contact with hot liquids or flames. They heal spontaneously within three weeks, and exhibit minimal permanent changes such as hypopigmentation or hyperpigmentation.

Deep second degree burns involve all of the epidermis and extend deep into the dermis, but spare the base of the skin appendages (hair follicles, sweat glands, and sebaceous glands). This wound is frequenty waxy white in appearance, and the skin is soft, dry, and relatively insensitive. The remaining epidermal elements at the base of the skin appendages are very fragile. Before the introduction of effective topical antimicrobials, deep second degree burns frequently were converted to third degree burns by bacterial proliferation and infection. Deep second degree burns are caused by longer exposure to intense heat such as immersion scalds or contact with flames. They require more than three weeks to heal and nearly always result in significant scarring.

Third degree ("full-thickness") burns are characterized by total destruction of both the epidermis and dermis. Third degree burns of any significant size (i.e., greater than 3 or 4 cm in diameter) always require split-thickness skin grafting because no epidermal cells remain. Third degree burns are caused by longer exposure to flames, prolonged immersion scalds, chemical contacts, and electrical flash or conduction injuries. Third degree burns involving tendon, muscle, or bone are most common on digits, hands, feet, and over bony prominences such as the iliac crest, patella, anterior tibia, and cranium as these areas have only a thin covering of subcutaneous tissue. Electrical injuries may expose bone in almost any area due to the extreme destruction associated with high voltage conduction.

Third degree burns have a characteristic appearance, usually being tan or fawn in color. The skin may be thinned ("parchment-like") with thrombosed vessels visible in the subcutaneous tissue. The skin is cold, hard, and insensitive. It is frequently leathery as the elasticity of the dermis has been destroyed. This loss of elasticity also causes abnormal wrinkling or folding of the skin, particularly over bony prominences or joints. Full-thickness burns, unlike superficial burns, have the unmistakable odor of burned flesh.

Determination of burn depth is difficult for the experienced observer and nearly impossible for the occasional observer. First degree burns, frequently seen about the margins of deeper burns, are the most easily identified. Differentiation between second and third degree burns becomes more difficult. Appearance (Table 2.1) remains the most reliable indicator. Historically, several methods have been utilized in attempts to judge depth more accurately, including evaluation of both capillary refill (with or without intravenous dyes) and sensation. Capillary refill may be visible in superficial second degree burns shortly after injury, but not on the second or third post-injury day as edema increases. Theoretically, intravenous dyes such as Patent Blue V and fluorescein will flow only into viable tissue which has patent capillaries. However, there is always associated stasis and frequently thrombosis, which decreases flow into the intradermal burns. Passive diffusion by capillary leak into full-thickness burns may produce false-positive results. Also, severe anaphylactic reactions have been described with these dyes. Therefore, these dyes are not only inaccurate, they may have deleterious side-effects.

Sensation may be used as an indicator of depth because superficial burns usually have intact sensation. However, Bull and Lennard-Jones (2) studied experimentally induced burns on their own bodies and found that at least 10 pin pricks per square inch were necessary to evaluate sensation reliably. Obviously, the clinician and the patient would not be willing to cooperate for such extensive sensory testing.

Generally, it is impossible to make an accurate determination of burn depth in the first few hours or days. Burn depth is more reliably determined 21 days after injury by the rate and completeness of healing.

Table 2.1.
Burn Classification by Depth, Clinical Findings, Cause and Healing Characteristics

Burn Depth	Skin Elements Involved	Clinical Findings	Cause	Healing
First degree	Superficial epidermis	Erythema Edema Painful	Ultraviolet exposure Sunburn Short flash	3–7 days No scar
Second degree Superficial	Epidermis	Blistered Weeping Red Painful	Scald Short exposure to flame	<21 days Minimal scar (pigment changes)
Deep	Epidermis and dermis	Pale or cherry red ± pain Skin pliable	Immersion scald Flame	>21 days May develop severe hypertrophic scarring
Third degree	Total destruction of skin May involve deeper tissues—subcutaneous fat, muscle, tendons, bone	Tan Leathery Nonpliable Wrinkled Parchment-like Thrombosed vessels	Flame Electrical Chemical	Require grafting

Body Surface Area Burn

The skin is a very large organ. At birth, the average child has .25 square meters of skin which expands to 1.2–1.9 square meters as an adult. The total volume of skin (surface area times thickness) is nearly 4 liters in the average adult. Surface area in square meters may be calculated by the formula: body weight (in kg) × height (in cm) × 71.84 (a constant) (5). The *patient's* palm print is approximately 1% of his or her total body surface area and may be conveniently used when estimating the size of small burns.

The Rule of Nines (Fig. 2.2) devised by Pulaski and Tennison is a simple and rapid but relatively inaccurate method of determining the size of burn injury. The body is represented by nines or multiples of nines and the perineum makes up the final 1%. This method is particularly unreliable in children less than 15 years of age as it underestimates the burn area of the head and neck and overestimates burn area of the legs.

A much more accurate estimation of the total body surface area burn was developed by Lund and Browder (3) in 1944 at Boston City Hospital (Fig. 2.3). Nonburned area should be calculated independently as a check when determining the area of large surface area burns, i.e., greater than 50% total body surface area.

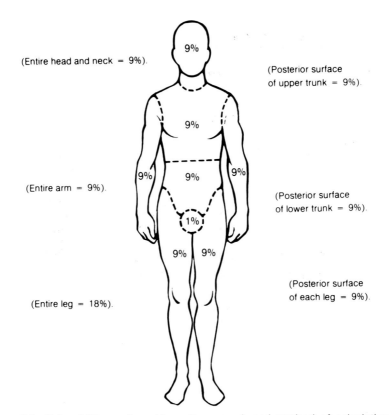

(Entire head and neck = 9%).

9%

(Posterior surface of upper trunk = 9%).

9%

(Entire arm = 9%).

9% 9% 9%

(Posterior surface of lower trunk = 9%).

1%

(Posterior surface of each leg = 9%).

9% 9%

(Entire leg = 18%).

Figure 2.2. Rule of Nines: A rapid, easily remembered method of calculation, but relatively inaccurate.

Burn Triage

Appropriate treatment decisions can be made after calculation of the severity of the burn by following the American Burn Association (4) treatment guidelines. Patients with minor burns may be treated as outpatients, i.e., burns of less than 15% second degree in adults or 10% second degree in children and third degree burns of less than 2%. Moderately severe *uncomplicated* burns may be treated in a community hospital by an experienced surgeon or physician. This would include second degree burns of 15–25% total body surface area (10–20% in children). Major burn injuries are treated appropriately at a burn center. Burns which should be referred to a burn center include larger second degree burns (greater than 25% in adults or 20% in children), all third degree burns greater than 10%, burns of difficult areas such as the hands, face, eyes, ears, feet, and perineum, burns with associated injuries including inhalation or electrical injuries, fractures, or other trauma, and all poor risk patients.

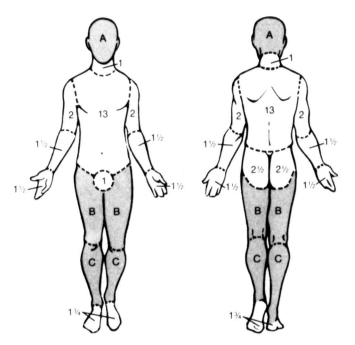

Relative percentages of areas affected by growth

Age in years	Half of head (A)	Half of one thigh (B)	Half of one leg (C)
Infant	9½	2¾	2½
1	8½	3¼	2½
5	6½	4	2¾
10	5½	4¼	3
15	4½	4½	3¼
Adult	3½	4¾	3½

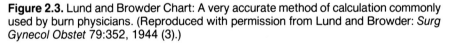

Total percent burned _____ 2° + _____ 3° = _____

Figure 2.3. Lund and Browder Chart: A very accurate method of calculation commonly used by burn physicians. (Reproduced with permission from Lund and Browder: *Surg Gynecol Obstet* 79:352, 1944 (3).)

REFERENCES

1. Artz CP, Moncrief JA, Pruitt BA: *Burns—A Team Approach.* Philadelphia, W.B. Saunders, 1979.
2. Bull JP, Lennard-Jones JE: The impairment of sensation in burns and its clinical application as a test of the depth of skin loss. *Clin Sci* 8:155, 1949.
3. Lund CC, Browder NC: The estimation of areas of burns. *Surg Gynecol Obstet* 79:352, 1944.
4. Specific Optimal Criteria for Hospital Resources for Care of Patients with Burn Injury. American Burn Association, April 1976.
5. Stark RB: *Plastic Surgery.* New York, Harper and Row, 1962.

3

Pathophysiology

ALAN R. DIMICK

Pathophysiology of Burns

Thermal destruction of the skin initiates a significant chain of events unparalleled either in magnitude or duration in other types of trauma. There are physiological changes in the local wound as well as severe multiple systemic responses in almost all organ systems initially, and also throughout the protracted coruse of burn illness. Optimal medical care for the burn patient requires understanding the many mechanisms of thermal trauma causing tissue injury.

MECHANISMS OF HEAT INJURY AND DEPTH OF BURN

The mechanisms involved in the severity of tissue destruction by heat are relatively simple. However, the amount of tissue destroyed is dependent on both local and systemic reactions to the heat damage. The amount of immediate injury to the tissues exposed to heat is dependent on the duration and intensity of the thermal exposure as well as the specific characteristics of the area. The longer the contact of flaming materials to the skin, the more severe the tissue destruction. Scald due to immersion produces greater damage than do scalds due to hot liquids which have brief contact with the skin. Also of importance is the conductivity of the tissue which varies with its density, water content, and vascularity. Both epidermal and dermal components of skin vary in thickness and somewhat in composition over different parts of the body. In adults, the well developed rete pegs increase the thickness of skin. In children, rete pegs have not developed in most areas of the body, and in the elderly they have become thin and atrophic, thus, increasing the damage because there are fewer protective layers of epithelium. The water content of the tissues, local natural oils or secretions, the amount and distribution of local pigmentation, and the presence of cornified keratin in the skin are the most significant factors in determining specific tissue conductivity. In addition, alterations of the local circulation have a profound effect on heat transfer and distribution not only in the

16

local area but in the body in general. The circulation determines the speed with which heat transfer takes palce. Heat dissipation is maximal in areas of the best blood supply.

The total amount of cell death and extracellular destruction is dependent on local chemical responses to the initial insult, and to systemic factors set in motion by the systemic response to burn injury. The release of histamine in the local area of the burn occurs immediately following thermal injury causing intense vasoconstriction. Within a few hours vasodilation occurs, probably as a result of kinins released locally. The vasodilatation unmasks the increased capillary permeability that permits whole plasma to be extravasated into the burn wound. The protein composition of edema fluid in a third degree burn is exactly the same as plasma. Damaged, but not necrotic, tissue cells imbibe large quantities of isotonic solutions through damaged cell walls. Within 24 hours post burn both platelets and leukocytes exhibit abnormal aggregation, sticking firmly to vessel walls producing thrombosis. This results in progressive vascular obstruction, which may produce an area of ischemia three to seven times greater in depth than the initial cellular damage caused by the heat. Transfer of oxygen and nutrients to damaged cells is impaired by the edema, increasing the likelihood of additional cellular damage. This thrombotic tendency in the burn wound is present for a minimum of five days. Other factors may decrease the arterial pressure or aggravate the hypercoagulable state, and may further contribute to cell destruction and greater depth of injury.

For these reasons even experienced observers cannot be certain of the depth of burn for three to five days post burn. Classification of the depth of burn, first, second and third degree, will be addressed in another chapter. Only a few general comments will be made here since they are pertinent to the discussion. First degree burns are characterized by simple erythema of the skin with destruction of only the superficial layers of epidermis. This is typically seen as a moderate to severe sunburn, and has little clinical significance. Second degree burns have more tissue destruction, located principally in the epidermis, but may also involve the more superficial areas of the dermis. However, if epithelial elements in the hair follicles and sweat glands still remain, regeneration can occur from these epithelial islands. If regeneration of the epithelium occurs and results in a new epithelial covering for the area, by definition the burn will be second degree in depth. Since restoration can occur from remaining epithelial elements, second degree burns are described as partial-thickness burns. The nerve endings in the partial-thickness second degree burns have been damaged but not destroyed. Therefore, they are hypersensitive and interpret all stimuli far out of proportion to their actual magnitude. This is the reason patients with partial-thickness burns complain so bitterly about pain in their burns. As the second degree burns heal, the nerve endings heal and their pain becomes significantly less. Blister formation is a hallmark of second degree burns.

Third degree burns by definition are characterized by total, irreversible destruction of all the skin including the dermal appendages. Therefore, spontaneous regeneration of epithelium is not possible and this is a full-thickness burn. Since all layers of the skin are coagulated and destroyed in third degree burns, the nerve endings are also destroyed and, therefore, are not present to perceive pain. Therefore, the burn that has the most destruction does not have nerve endings with which to perceive pain. This is a point that is often forgotten by the physician and his colleagues, and frequently the physician overreacts to this devastating injury by administering large doses of narcotics to alleviate pain when actually there is little if any pain in the areas of full-thickness third degree burn. This subject will be discussed further in a subsequent chapter so we will not proceed further at this point.

Because skin varies in thickness in different parts of the body, application of the same intensity of heat for given periods of time results in different burn depth. Thus, in the very old in whom dermal papillae and appendages are atrophic, and in the young in whom they have yet to develop fully, deeper burns result from heat of the same intensity that produces a moderate second degree burn in the average adult. The skin is thickest on the back and on the palm of the hands, but is thinnest on the inner arm. Dermal appendages (primarily hair follicles and sweat glands) penetrate to varying depths in different areas with those in the scalp and the male beard being notable deep. Burned parts involving the thickest areas of skin regenerate faster.

LOCAL RESULTS OF THERMAL INJURY

Both second and third degree burns result in loss or impairment of the functional integrity of the body's largest organ. The most important of those clinically apparent functions include loss of the ability to regulate evaporative water loss, impairment of the body's first line of defense against infection, and the loss of massive amounts of body fluids through open wounds.

The excessive loss of water by evaporation has several important consequences, not the least of which is the severe heat loss. This heat loss results in a tremendous calorie drain on the patient. Thus, it is necessary to supply large amounts of additional calories to replace those used for water evaporation.

Skin performs a major protective function in our body's resistance against infection. Skin protects us against the continual assault of bacteria present in our environment. The loss of the barrier of skin allows bacteria to enter the body. Because of thrombosis in blood vessels in third degree burn, it is avascular. Without an effective blood supply the host resistance of the patient is severely impaired by being unable to deliver humoral factors to fight infection. Thus, a third degree burn characteristically shows extensive vascular thrombosis and almost complete lack of inflammatory reaction. In contrast by the third day, the second degree burn shows patent blood vessels and an active inflammatory response. If bacterial infection goes unchallenged, a progressive thrombosis ensues in the area of second degree burn, and there is subsequent devitalization of tissue. This necrosis resulting from the proliferation of bacteria in the original partial-thickness burn causes a conversion to full-thickness skin destruction—"infectious conversion."

Bacterial contamination of the burn wound occurs almost immediately after thermal injury. Proliferation of the bacteria usually occurs primarily in sweat glands and hair follicles, but also may be contaminated from adjacent normal skin. The type of bacteria first colonizing the wound is dependent on the treatment and the environment to which the patient is exposed. Generally, burns that are not treated with topical antibacterial agents develop streptococcal or staphylococcal colonization. Hospitalized patients usually become colonized with gram-negative bacteria which frequently exist in the hospital environment.

The term "burn wound sepsis" has been defined as the presence of bacteria in the concentration of 100,000 or more per gram of tissue. However, invasive sepsis has been demonstrated in either lower or higher concentrations. This definition is important because once colonization of the burn has been established, there is usually rapid invasion culminating in systemic sepsis.

It should be noted that blood cultures are seldom positive in burn patients. The bacteria present in burn wound sepsis usually invade the body by way of the lymphatics, and are cultured from the blood only much later. Therefore, death may occur from burn wound sepsis without blood stream invasion. Because of this the presence of a positive blood culture suggests strongly a secondary source of infection, such as pneumonia or septic thrombophlebitis.

SYSTEMIC EFFECTS OF BURN INJURY

A major burn initiates many pathophysiological changes, which affect the function of almost every organ system in the body. The most immediate life-threatening response to burn injury is the syndrome of burn shock. The most significant component of burn shock is the loss of large volumes of plasma and extracellular fluid. One component of burn shock is the loss of body fluids into the burn wound. Also, heat damage to the tissues causes a change in the molecular configuration of collagen which then chemically binds both sodium and water. Acute hypovolemia results from the losses into the extravascular compartment.

Another component of burn shock has been identified. This occurs 48–72 hours after injury, and is thought to be due to the increase in concentration of fibrinogen polymers in the edema fluid. These polymers are of molecular weights ranging between 700,000 and 1 million, and physically are gels. It is probable that these polymers produce mechanical obstruction of the lymphatics and venules draining the burn area.

The clinical significance of this second phase of burn edema relates primarily to the severe swelling and stiffness noted in the first few days of burn injury. Obviously, this severe edema inhibits active and/or passive motion of the involved areas, and delays rehabilitation of these injured parts. In this situation, the primary therapeutic measure that should be utilized is appropriate positioning and/or splinting of the involved area which would tend to facilitate the resolution of the edema fluid while maintaining appropriate positioning of the involved body parts. Careful positioning of the patient minimizes edema formation. Burns of the hands or feet and circumferential burns of an extremity should be treated by elevation. Such extremities should be constantly assessed for decreased blood flow due to pressure produced by excessive edema formation.

Although pulmonary complications of thermal injury are a major hazard to survival, changes in pulmonary function show nothing characteristic of thermal injury as opposed to any other type of trauma. Increased ventilation is universally present and is generally proportional to the magnitude of the injury. Hyperventilation is usually seen during the first five days following injury, but unless other complications supervene it gradually declines to normal. Oxygen consumption shows a marked increase, but is apparently independent of ventilatory performance in the absence of any significant impairment in respiratory gas exchange. There have been no significant changes in pulmonary function studies of burn patients without pulmonary inhalation injury. Airway resistance may be elevated in some cases of inhalation, but is usually normal. There is no striking variation in blood gas changes in patients without inhalation injury.

Although the lungs play a major role in the clinical response to major thermal injury, the effect of a peripheral burn on pulmonary function appears to be of little significance. The high incidence of pulmonary dysfunction observed in some reported series of burn patients is usually related to direct damage produced by the inhalation of noxious gases resulting in atelectasis or upper airway obstruction. Later, the lungs participate significantly in the systemic response to invasive sepsis, and the incidence of "late" pneumonia is high.

Blood viscosity increases rather rapidly following thermal injury and is proportional to the increase in hematocrit. The polymerization of some of the larger protein molecules such as fibrinogen adds to this, and viscosity remains elevated for a considerable interval after the hematocrit has returned to normal. Viscosity of the blood is influenced by the effectiveness of fluid resuscitation therapy. Platelet adhesiveness is greatly influenced by the burn injury, with an initial rapid drop in platelet count and platelet survival time in the first five days post burn. This is usually followed by a slow rise in platelets with counts remaining elevated for several weeks.

Gastrointestinal changes following thermal injury are common, and are manifest by the gastric aspirate having coffee-ground material in it. The pathogenesis of the gastric lesion is not clear but is probably related to the severity of burn shock. Acute gastric dilation frequently accompanies severe stress of any nature, and total gastrointestinal ileus commonly occurs during the first three days post burn. These initial changes do not appear to be related directly to the late appearance of Curling's ulcer, which may be manifest by significant bleeding or perforation, and occurs most often in the duodenum and less frequently in the stomach. The precise mechanism is unknown, but there appears to be no relation to gastric hypersecretion or pre-existing ulcer disease. Curling's ulcers are frequently associated with episodes of generalized sepsis, and often herald a septic episode for the patient.

Immunological competence is severely depressed for many reasons in the burn patient. Initially, leukocyte adhesiveness produces leukopenia of varying degrees. Complement and other antibodies have varying degrees of depression, which are frequently related to septic episodes. Immunoglobulins are usually depressed for two to three weeks following injury, and also appear to make the patient more at risk for infection. These immunological factors are still being defined, and currently are undergoing active investigation of many researchers.

MECHANISM OF CHEMICAL INJURY

Chemical agents produce direct tissue damage by a variety of reactions. Chemical injuries have a relatively low incidence, and therefore, the experience of individual physicians is limited. Since many chemical agents continue to act until neutralized or removed, emergency therapy should be instituted as rapidly as possible. Copious lavage with water dilutes, neutralizes, or removes a wide variety of chemicals effectively. There are specific exceptions to the use of water, and the reader is referred to the suggested readings for several good articles which review this subject.

Except for the emergency therapy to minimize the severity of chemical injury, the principles of treatment for chemical burns are the same as for thermal burns. Long-term sequelae are also the same as those seen in thermal burns.

In general, there is a notable difference in the results of burns due to acid and burns due to alkali. In general, acid burns tend to be superficial in depth whereas alkali burns tend to burrow deeper into the tissues and cause more significant destruction. Therefore, it is imperative to remove as much of the alkali as soon as possible from the tissues to prevent this significantly greater tissue destruction.

MECHANISM OF COLD INJURY

Cold injury may be manifest in several forms. Local injury to distal parts exposed to low environmental temperatures is the most common. Highly volatile liquid stored at low temperatures may produce a rapid freezing of tissues.

Frostbite results when tissues are exposed to intense cold. The severity of injury varies with the intensity of cold and duration of exposure. The depth of injury is classified into four clinical types: first degree injury— edema and redness of the affected part without necrosis; second degree injury—formation of blisters with subsequent epidermal healing; third degree injury—necrosis of the skin resulting in full-thickness skin loss; and fourth degree injury—gangrene of the affected area.

Diagnosis seldom can be made on initial examination before rewarming is accomplished. The rewarmed tissues become reddened, hot, and edematous, and the signs of the depth of injury become apparent. Fortunately, the degree of gangrene is often much less than initially feared, because the skin may be gangrenous while the underlying tissues are viable. For this reason, amputation should be delayed until the extent of gangrene is definitively known, unless infection supervenes.

After healing of the injured area, there is frequently a permanent increase in vasoconstrictor tone, resulting in hyperhidrosis and an abnormal sensitivity to cold. Pain and paresthesia are common, probably the residual of ischemic neuritis.

The most important aspect of treatment is the rapid rewarming of the injured tissue. The frozen tissue should be placed in warm water between 40° and 44°C. Complete rewarming usually takes about 20 minutes. Higher temperatures are injurious to the tissues. Blankets and other forms of rewarming are inadequate. Following rewarming, the injured area should be elevated to minimize edema, and should be protected from bacterial contamination preferably with the use of a topical chemotherapeutic agent such as Mafenid or silver sulfadiazine. Blisters should be debrided, and necrotic tissue is debrided as it separates. Hydrotherapy and physiotherapy are employed to maintain mobility of the part. Amputation is delayed until the extent of gangrene is accurately determined, which usually is at least one or more weeks following the injury. Sympathectomy and heparinization currently are not recommended for therapy of frostbite.

Rapid freeze injuries may occur from the sudden escape of gases stored under very high pressure in liquid form. Contact produces instant freezing of varying depth. The injured skin is intensely blue to purplish color. Extremely massive edema occurs rapidly within one to four hours, and pulses are frequently absent. The tissues have been destroyed immediately by ice crystal formation. Muscle may appear viable on initial examination, but within 7 to 10 days may become obviously necrotic. Excision of necrotic areas and/or amputation are preferably withheld until demarcation is complete, unless infection supervenes.

The sequelae of cold injuries has many of the same characteristics of healed burn injury; i.e., pruritis, hypertrophic scarring, and contractures. In addition, neuritis and/or neuromas due to nerve damage are frequent.

Severe total body hypothermia with the core body temperature being below 90°F is a severe injury with uniformly poor survival. Therefore, it is elected not to discuss this particular cold injury because the reader will seldom be faced with this type patient.

HEALING AND REGENERATION OF PARTIAL-THICKNESS BURNS

Regeneration of epithelial elements in partial-thickness injury to resurface the area comes from the epithelial cells lining every hair follicle and sweat gland. Therefore, it is important to keep partial-thickness burns as clean as possible to diminish the number of bacteria in the wound. If bacteria are allowed to proliferate in the wound and cause invasive infection, this will result in vascular thrombosis and a loss of blood supply to the area, causing an infectious conversion of the partial-thickness second degree burn to a full-thickness third degree burn. For these reasons topical antibacterial agents are utilized to diminish the total number of bacteria in the burn wound thereby preventing invasive infection. Several topical agents are currently in use in many burn units. However, the prime reason for each of these agents being used is to keep the number of bacteria in the burn wound as low as possible. They do not sterilize the burn wound but keep the concentration of bacteria in the wound as low as possible.

Healing of the partial-thickness burns usually takes 14 days, but if the burn is sufficiently deep these burns may take 21 days for complete healing. As the epithelium grows from around every hair follicle and sweat gland to resurface the area of partial-thickness second degree burn, the normal pigmentation gradually and progressively returns. In the Black race, one can see the regeneration of epithelial cells containing melanin pigment as they slowly but progressively grow out from every hair follicle and sweat gland to resurface the area of the partial-thickness second degree burn completely.

As the epithelium regenerates and resurfaces the area of partial-thickness second degree burns, the new skin progressively becomes more involved in temperature regulation. As this regenerated epithelium differentiates and forms the keratin layer of the skin once again, the epithelium becomes involved in the temperature regulatory process again by maintaining and conserving the core body temperature.

As all burn areas, skin grafts, and donor sites heal with progressive growth and covering by epithelium, the patient becomes more comfortable. However, this is only the beginning. Although epithelial coverage has been gained, several factors still continue in the healing process. One of these is the continuing regeneration of peripheral nerves in the area of burn injury. As nerves regenerate, they may cause the patient extreme discomfort due to varying uncomfortable sensations. There may also be pruritic discomfort in the area of healing burns, skin grafts, and donor sites, which may persist for four to six months until the nerve endings in these areas have completely regenerated.

Currently there is not a good medication which can completely alleviate this pruritis. Because the B-complex vitamins are so important to nerve metabolism, some physicians instruct patients to take vitamins containing the B-complex to facilitate this nerve tissue regeneraton. However, one must keep in mind that nerves take much longer to regenerate than does epithelium, and therefore, these symptoms of pruritis may exist long after the epithelial cover for the wound has been accomplished.

Patients frequently have abnormal or odd sensations in their burn wounds, which are probably due to the regeneration of the nerve endings into the burned areas. As the nerve endings grow through the areas of burn tissue they frequently come up against an obstruction which may cause an area of hypersensitivity, causing unusual or odd sensations in the wound. Small neuromas may occur in scattered areas throughout the burned area, and this may be the problem causing hypersensitivity in this area. Densensitization may be required for these patients.

Several long-term disabilities occur as a result of skin grafting required for third degree burns. When the skin is transplanted to the area of third degree burn, no hair follicles or sweat glands are included. Therefore, these grafted areas do not have the specialized skin appendages. Without these, the grafted area has none of the normal body oils, which results in excessively dry skin. Therefore, the patient must apply some type of lotion or cream to the area. Instructions should include the caution not to put too much lotion or cream on the area because this results in excessive moisture and masseration of the tissues. If the patient can see the lotion or cream on the surface, he/she has applied too much.

A problem for patients with extensive skin grafting is created because of the absence of sweat glands in grafted skin. The grafted areas cannot sweat, and therefore, are unable to dissipate the core body temperature if it is too high. Patients with extensive areas of skin grafting are usually cautioned about this problem, and warned to avoid environments with high heat and/or humidity, since they may have trouble dissipating their core body temperature.

As results of burn care improve, patients with more extensive burns survive. However, we need to keep in mind the manifestations of healing wounds involving large surfaces. Recently, patients with decreased exercise tolerance and high resting pulse rates have been noted. Although this has not been noted in the literature, there is a high index of suspicion that there are many small arteriovenous fistulae in the extensive healing scars of these patients, resulting in a high-output heart failure. As the scars mature, these fistulae become obliterated and the patient's exercise tolerance and resting pulse return to normal. This may explain why patients who have recovered from their burn injury have poor exercise tolerance with elevated resting pulse rates.

HYPERTROPHIC SCARRING

Although this subject will be covered in another chapter, several comments should be made regarding the pathophysiology of the healing burn wound. Although the growth of epithelium with subsequent coverage of the burn wound is the primary objective, one must keep in mind that dermal scarring occurs in the burn wound on a continuing basis for several months after injury. Therefore, the burn team needs to continue to evaluate the burn scars for at least six months to one year to determine if the dermal scarring is becoming hypertrophic. If this does occur, continuous compression garments will be required to keep the scars as soft, pliable, and flexible as possible.

Most burns have a satisfactory flat appearance upon healing. However, the true prognosis can not be known until a minimal of six months has elapsed, as the healed burn wound does not become elevated and hard until two or three months after healing. The process of healing in burn wounds is conducive to the formation of hypertrophic scars and contractures, as it is characterized by a marked increase in vascularity, fibroblasts, myofibroblasts, and collagen deposition.

The vascularity of healed burn wounds influences the formation of hypertrophic scars. Healed burn wounds that lose their redness within two to three months usually do not become hypertrophic. If this is the case, the scars will not require pressure dressings. On the other hand, a scar that remains highly vascularized for two months after healing, and becomes progressively firmer will become hypertrophic. Such hypertrophic scars will lose their red color (vascularity) only when they mature and become soft and flat. This may not occur from six months to two years after injury. The application of pressure dressings providing a capillary pressure of at least 25 mm Hg will significantly decrease the amount of scarring.

CONTRACTURES

The burn wound will shorten until it meets an opposing force. For example, the force exerted by myofibroblasts in the wound can be severe enough to dislocate joints. The position of comfort for most patients is that of flexion of the joints, and they will assume this position if allowed to do so. This permits new collagen fibers in the wound to fuse together resulting in contracture formation. Eventually the scar will mature, becoming a solid mass of fused collagen. The resulting mass of collagen will have a Swiss-cheese appearance due to the continuing reabsorption of the collagen. But the contracture will remain because of fusion of some of the collagen fibers into the shortened position.

Scar contractures and hypertrophic scar formation following thermal injury can be decreased with proper patient positioning, by the use of splints to maintain good position of all joints, and by maintaining proper joint alignment. Patient positioning begins immediately after injury and continues throughout the treatment process. Following healing of the wounds, splints and pressure dressings may be necessary on a long-term basis. The dynamic nature of collagen in the wound has been well-demonstrated by many investigators. This build-up and breakdown of collagen is very similar to the same process that occurs in bone. The realignment along the lines of stress which occurs in the healing burn wound is very similar to the stress lines seen in healing bone.

As detailed in other chapters of this book, significant advances in the treatment of burns have been made in many areas. However, the development of scar tissue hypertrophy is frequently overlooked as attention is directed primarily at survival. Certainly survival must be the primary immediate goal, but this does not preclude the need to decrease scar formation and the resulting deformities. Too often, severe deformity is accepted because the burns were thought to be too extensive. The patient's survival is obviously a major goal, but the associated grotesque appearance and crippling contractures are frequently overlooked in the process of treatment. Physicians caring for burn patients should always ask what kind of life each patient can expect. If this questioning is done, survival will no longer be the sole end point of care, and therapy will be directed toward the goal of maximum rehabilitation.

ADDITIONAL READINGS

1. Anon: Medical progress—Burns. N Engl J Med 288:444, 1973.
2. Artz CP, Moncrief JA: The Treatment of Burns. Philadelphia, W.B. Saunders, 1969.
3. Baxter CR: Crystalloid resuscitation of burn shock. In Polk HC Jr, Stone HH (Eds): Contemporary Burn Management. Boston, Little, Brown, 1971.
4. Baxter CR, Cook WA, Shires GT: Serum myocardial depressant factor of burn shock. Surg Forum 17:1, 1966.
5. Baxter CR, Shires GT: Physiological response to crystalloid resuscitation of severe burns. Ann NY Acad Sci 150:874, 1968.
6. Burke JF, Quinby WC, Bondoc CC, et al: Immunosuppression and temporary skin transplantation in the treatment of massive third degree burns. Ann Surg 182:183, 1975.
7. Cook WA, Baxter CR, Ferrell JM: Pulmonary circulation after dermal burns. Vasc Surg 2:1, 1968.
8. Davis L, Scarff JE, Rogers N et al: High altitude frostbite: Preliminary report. Surg Gynecol Obstet 77:561, 1973.
9. Fox CL: Silver sulfadiazine: A new topical therapy for pseudomonas in burns. Arch Surg 96:184, 1968.
10. Harrison HN, Bales H, Jacoby F: The behavior of mafenide acetate as a basis for its clinical use. Arch Surg 103:449, 1971.

11. Heck EL, Browne L, Curreri PW, et al: Evaluation of leukocyte function in burned individuals by *in vitro* cellular oxygen consumption. *J Trauma* 15:486, 1975.
12. Jelenko C: Chemicals that "burn." *J Trauma* 14:65, 1974.
13. Lange K, Boyd LJ: The functional pathology of frostbite and the prevention of gangrene in experimental animals and humans. *Science* 102:151, 1945.
14. Lindberg RB, Moncrief JA, Switzer WE, et al: The successful control of burn wound sepsis. *J Trauma* 5:601, 1965.
15. Loebl EC, Baxter CR, Curreri PW: The mechanisms of erythrocyte destruction in the early postburn period. *Ann Surg* 178:681, 1973.
16. Meryman HT: Tissue freezing and local cold injury. *Physiol Rev* 37:233, 1957.
17. Monafo WW: *The Treatment of Burns: Principles and Practice.* St. Louis, W.A. Green, 1971.
18. Moncrief JA: Burns of specific areas. *J Trauma* 5:278, 1965.
19. Moncrief JA, Switzer WE, Teplitz C: Curling's ulcer. *J Trauma* 4:481, 1964.
20. Order SE, Mason AD Jr, Switzer WE et al: Arterial vascular occlusion and devitalization of burn wounds. *Ann Surg* 161:502, 1965.
21. Pruitt BA Jr, Erickson DR, Morris A: Progressive pulmonary insufficiency and other pulmonary complications of thermal injury. *J Trauma* 15:369, 1975.
22. Rayfield D, Vaught M, Curreri PW et al: Extravascular fibrinogen degradation in experimental burn wounds—A source of circulating fibrin split products. *Surgery* 77:86, 1975.
23. Schumaker HB, White BH, Wrenn EL, et al: Studies in experimental frostbite—The effect of heparin in preventing gangrene. *Surgery* 22:900, 1947.
24. Wilterdink ME, Curreri PW, Baxter CR: Characterization of elevated fibrin split products following thermal injury. *Ann Surg* 181:157, 1975.

4

Surgical Management

CHARLES E. HARTFORD

Criteria for Hospital Admission

The initial problem in the management of a patient with thermal injury is to determine whether it is advantageous to admit that patient to a hospital or whether he or she can safely be treated as an outpatient. In the following circumstances, patients with burns are usually considered for admission:

(1) most infants;
(2) when child abuse is suspected;
(3) young children with burns in excess of 10% of the body surface area;
(4) older children and adults with burns in excess of 15% of the body surface area;
(5) most aged patients;
(6) those with chemical injury beyond obviously superficial or limited extent;
(7) those with high voltage electrical injury;
(8) those with burns to parts of the body which render the patient incapacitated, e.g., of the face with swelling of the eyelids resulting in obstruction of vision, of both hands, of the perineum or of both feet;
(9) when respiratory tract complications (smoke inhalation syndrome, upper airway obstruction from edema, or carbon monoxide poisoning) are a possibility, i.e., when a patient is injured by flame in a closed space;
(10) when intercurrent injury, illness, or pre-existing medical condition might enhance morbidity or mortality.

Priorities in Management of Patients Admitted to the Hospital

A rapid estimate of the surface area involved by burn and overall condition of the patient is first made to determine the need for immediate lifesaving measures, such as the need for endotracheal intubation, ventilatory support, control of bleeding, etc., and whether intravenous fluid therapy is needed to prevent or treat burn shock.

If fluid therapy is necessary, an intravenous line is secured and fluid delivery begun. Next, the urinary bladder is catheterized to help monitor fluid therapy and a nasogastric tube inserted to decompress the stomach to prevent the possibility of vomiting and aspiration. Laboratory studies, roentgenograms, an electrocardiogram, and consultation with physicians of other disciplines are obtained as clinically appropriate.

The successful treatment of a patient at high risk from burns begins with a good data base. The medical history and physical examination should be as complete and as thorough as possible. The extent of burn is carefully drawn on an appropriate burn diagram sheet (Fig. 4.1) and a calculation made of the percentage of body surface area involved by the burn (Figs. 2.2 and 2.3) (26). Only after these tasks are accomplished and the immediate

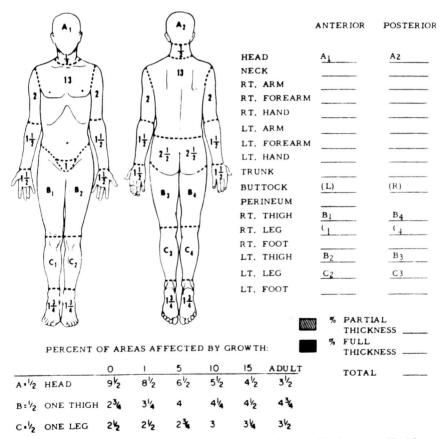

Figure 4.1. A method for calculating the surface area involved by burn modified from Lund and Browder (26). This technique takes into account that as an individual grows from infancy to adulthood, the relative size of the head decreases while that of the lower extremities increase.

life-threatening conditions other than the burn wound are cared for or excluded is attention turned to the care of the wound.

Often, pain is an early and prominent complaint. If medication for control of pain is to be given, there are two important considerations. First, restlessness from lack of oxygen must not be interpreted as pain. Second, to ensure effective absorption, the drug must be given intravenously.

The intravenous administration of narcotics in small incremental doses until the desired effect is obtained is an effective method of achieving pain control. Because of the obligatory sequestration of body fluids away from the circulation, drugs given subcutaneously have delayed and erratic absorption during the first several days following a large burn injury.

Burn Shock and Fluid Resuscitation

Burn injury causes translocation of body fluids, the net result of which is intravascular hypovolemia. If the burn is large enough and the patient is not properly treated, circulatory failure occurs; this is known as burn shock. The shift in body fluid occurs as a consequence of a lesion in the microcirculation in which capillaries become abnormally permeable (12). This results in the obligatory sequestration of an ultrafiltrate of plasma into the extravascular space. Edema, at times massive, in both the injured and uninjured tissues occurs (Fig. 4.2). The loss of fluid from the intravascular

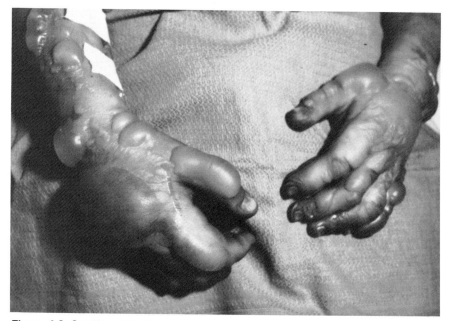

Figure 4.2. Swelling with blisters occurs from translocation of body fluids induced by burns.

space progressively diminishes plasma volume, blood volume, and cardiac output and leads to hemoconcentration, poor tissue perfusion, lactic acidemia, and metabolic acidosis. If treatment is inadequate or the patient does not respond to the resuscitative effort, acute renal failure and death ensue. Prevention of or resuscitation from burn shock is usually the most important item in the early management of the seriously burned patient.

The rate of obligatory sequestration of fluid, maximal soon after injury, decreases progressively until about 18–30 hours after injury when, with proper treatment, there is spontaneous restoration of microcirculatory integrity. The timely administration of fluids to patients with large surface burns prevents death from burn shock. These fluids must contain sodium (35) but whether colloids are needed or even desirable is controversial. Until the capillary leak stops, intravenous fluid therapy is necessary to maintain the circulation and perfusion of tissues. At the time microcirculatory integrity is restored, the edema is maximal. There is then gradual resorption of edema concurrent with an increase in intravascular volume, cardiac output, and urine production. During this phase, congestive heart failure and pulmonary edema may occur, especially among the elderly.

Several formulas have been advanced for calculating fluid requirements for burned patients. These formulas are only guides and the response of each patient to treatment must be assessed repeatedly and adjustments made in fluid therapy on an individual basis.

The Brooke formula, published in 1953 (45), is a modification of the Evans formula which was described in 1952 (17). According to the Brooke formula, the volume of fluid recommended for each of the first two 24-hour postburn periods is calculated from the body weight and the percentage of surface area of burn. A percentage of this fluid is given as crystalloid and a percentage as colloid.

BROOKE FORMULA

First 24 Hours:

Crystalloid: 1.5 ml/kg. body weight/% burn as lactated Ringer's solution.
Colloid: 0.5 ml/kg body weight/% burn as plasma, Plasmanate, or dextran.
Maintenance: 2000 ml as 5% dextrose in water.
Half the calculated volume is given during the first eight hours, the other half during the next 16 hours.

Second 24 Hours:

Half of the first 24 hours calculated colloid and crystalloid.
Maintenance: 2000 ml as 5% dextrose in water.

To avoid fluid overload, the authors of these two formulas recommended that the initial estimate should not exceed the estimated volume for a 50% surface area burn. However, in actual practice, the calculation predicts with reasonable accuracy the fluid requirements for a burn of up to 50% of the body surface; above that the volumes increase almost linearly as the extent of the burn increases (44).

Many patients are successfully resuscitated with balanced salt solution alone. This method is based on the premise that sodium is the essential substance for successful resuscitation (35) and that any colloid given during the first 18–24 hours after injury does not augment the plasma volume (3). However, after the leaky capillaries seal, colloid will augment the plasma volume by the amount of colloid given. The use of balanced crystalloid solution was first employed by Moyer and co-workers (35) and has been modified by Baxter (3). The latter recommends 4 ml of lactated Ringer's solution per kg body weight per % body surface area burn, with half of the calculated volume to be given in the first eight hours and the remainder over the next 16 hours. After all of the calculated fluid has been given, the patient is evaluated for adequacy of resuscitation; if signs are less than optimal, the patient is cautiously given colloid (plasma) to expand the patient is cautiously given colloid (plasma) to expand the plasma volume.

By adding albumin to lactated Ringer's solution (e.g., 25 g of albumin to each L of crystalloid) (43) or increasing the concentration of sodium (e.g., hypertonic lactated saline containing 200–250 mEq/L of sodium) (29), the volume of fluid needed for successful resuscitation can be reduced substantially below that required from the use of lactated Ringer's solution alone. However, as yet there is no evidence that this reduction in fluid requirement has or will translate into a reduction in mortality.

Most previously healthy young adults with burns on less than two-thirds of the body surface area are successfully resuscitated by a variety of regimens. However, the following circumstances may make treatment difficult: deep burns in excess of two-thirds of the body surface, extremes of age, smoke inhalation injury, premorbid impairment of cardiovascular, respiratory, and renal function, and delay in treatment. It is also evident that those physicians who attend their patients with frequent, careful, and knowledgeable assessment, making the necessary adjustments in therapy, will have the best results.

With respect to fluid therapy, as soon as the patient is admitted, the extent of injury and the patient's overall condition are rapidly assessed. Infants and young children with burns larger than 10% of the body surface area and older children and adults with burns larger than 15% of the body surface should receive intravenous fluids to prevent burn shock.

Immediately, a large bore cannula is placed in a vein. If no practical unburned site is available, the cannula is inserted through burned tissue. Venous blood is drawn for laboratory studies and crossmatching of blood. Arterial blood is obtained for measurement of pH and blood gasses. Because urine output is a highly regarded sign in the clinical assessment of adequacy of fluid resuscitation, the urinary bladder is catheterized and each hour the urine volume is measured. Since many patients develop an ileus, a nasogastric tube is inserted ╈ decompress the stomach to prevent vomiting and aspiration.

Currently, the fluid for resuscitation recommended by most authorities is lactated Ringer's solution, but, as noted above, by increasing either the osmolality or tonicity of the fluid, the amount of fluid needed can be reduced. Fluid is administered intravenously and rapidly until urine flow is established and then the rate of delivery is adjusted to keep the patient comfortably alive, out of shock, lucid, and making urine at a rate of at least 30–50 ml per hour, with corresponding lesser amounts of urine for children. The amount of fluid required to maintain the circulation and the desired urine flow decreases gradually during the first day or two after injury. Hourly assessments are made of the urinary output, pH, and specific gravity; blood pressure; pulse rate and rhythm; respiratory status; and level of consciousness. From these observations and re-examination of the patient, the physician adjusts the rate of fluid administration and determines whether additional kinds of therapy or laboratory tests are needed.

Between 18–30 hours after injury the patient should, in most instances, be satisfactorily resuscitated. Burn shock persisting beyond this time is usually not the result of the burn and other causes should be sought, e.g., heart, respiratory, or renal failure. When the need for the intravenous cannula and urinary bladder catheter has been met, these should be removed to prevent infection. When the patient regains gastrointestinal function, enteral alimentation is instituted.

Elevated Tissue Pressure

The accumulation of edema in extremities with circumferential burns of either partial- or full-thickness depth may cause a rise in tissue pressure. The burn prevents expansion of the underlying tissues often with progressive obstruction of lymphatic and venous outflow from the extremity and, if allowed to progress, eventual arterial inflow. There is evidence that at even modest but sustained elevations of tissue pressure of 40 mm Hg, permanent injury to nerve and muscle will occur (47). This may contribute to residual muscular weakness after recovery from burn injury.

While ischemia is easily detected clinically by finding cool, pale, painful, immobile digits with poor capillary refill or absence of pulse by physical examination or altered flow characteristics on examination with a Doppler flowmeter, the detection of modest elevations of tissue pressure cannot be done accurately by physical diagnosis. Therefore, tissue pressure should be measured. Several methods, including the needle technique described by Whitesides et al. (51), and the wick catheter technique (38) employing a transducer, have been used clinically. The wick catheter can be left inlying to obtain continuous or intermittent readings of tissue pressure. The Whitesides technique measures the tissue pressure directly with sufficient accuracy using relatively inexpensive material readily available in any hospital (Fig. 4.3). In most instances in which there is a pathological elevation of tissue pressure, the elevation has already occurred by the time the pressure is first measured and therefore the occasional need to reinsert the needle to remeasure the pressure is not a practical disadvantage.

Escharotomy, incision through the burn, is used to relieve the pressure and to restore circulation (Fig. 4.4). It is done when the tissue pressure exceeds 40 mm Hg. The incisions are made along the medial and lateral aspects of the limb taking care not to cross flexion creases. The proximal incision should extend to the limit of the burn. As the tissues are released, the subcutaneous fat bulges through the incision, tissue tension is relieved, and effective circulation is restored. When possible, escharotomy should be done in the operating room under general anesthesia using aseptic technique and cautery. It is fallacious to believe that this is a painless procedure. It is essential that bleeding be meticulously controlled. Among those with large surface burns when multiple extremity escharotomy is needed, the clotting mechanism should be assessed preoperatively and preparation made to correct these factors if the levels are dangerously low or the patient begins

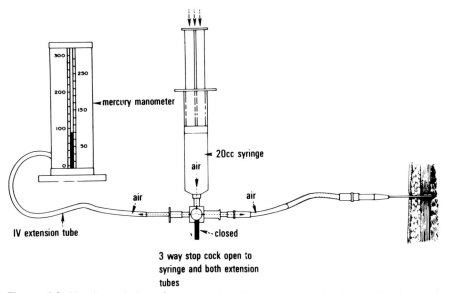

Figure 4.3. Needle technique for measuring tissue pressure is shown. A column of sterile saline is drawn through needle to create meniscus between needle and three way stop cock. Needle is then inserted into tissue compartment and three way stop cock opened to manometer, syringe and tubing to tissue compartment simultaneously. Plunger of syringe is slowly compressed. When meniscus moves, the tissue pressure is read off the mercury manometer. Reprinted with permission: Whitesides et al. (51) copyright 1975, American Medical Association.

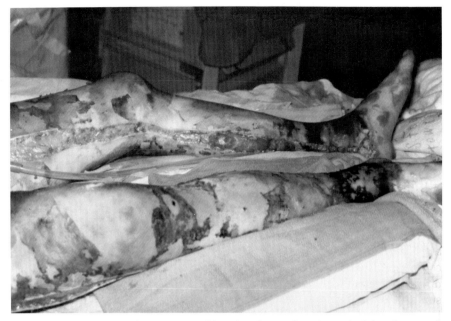

Figure 4.4. Deep burns of lower extremities showing escharotomy. Incision deepened to fasciotomy in leg revealing necrotic muscle. Note wide spreading of burned skin which effects a reduction in tissue pressure allowing restoration of circulation.

to ooze blood uncontrollably from multiple escharotomy sites during or after the procedure.

Among patients with deep burns (Fig. 4.4) or high voltage electrical injury involving muscle, fasciotomy may be necessary to relieve elevated pressure in fascial compartments unrelieved by simple escharotomy.

Care of the Burn Wound

COOLING THE BURN

As long as the temperature in tissues exceeds 45°C, thermal damage occurs (33). It makes sense to try to reduce the temperature in heated tissues as rapidly as possible. However, spontaneous cooling occurs rapidly and, in most instances, the temperature of the injured tissue has spontaneously cooled below 45°C before exogeneous cooling can be initiated. Additionally, cooling large surfaces may reduce the patient's core temperature to dangerously low levels initiating shivering and predisposing to arrhythmias. Therefore, the patient should not be packed in ice, and cool compresses, if used, should be applied to no more than 10% of the body surface area at one time. During cooling the body temperature should be carefully monitored. The time needed to cool burn tissue to below 45°C is brief.

Among patients with small-area partial-thickness of depth burns, cool compresses may be used effectively to relieve pain.

BLISTERS

Intact blisters provide a superb biological dressing for a burn and should be left intact (Fig. 4.2). Removal of the blister usually converts a painless wound into one which is painful and exposes the raw surfaces to bacterial colonization and potential infection.

OUTPATIENT CARE OF BURNS

The wound is first cleansed of dirt and loose devitalized debris. A topical antibacterial agent, currently silver sulfadiazine, 1% cream, is usually applied on the thesis that infectious complications will be reduced. There are no data to support this contention and it may be equally effective to cover the wound with either a nonadherent petrolatum gauze which permits drainage or only a plain dry dressing. Whatever is placed next to the wound surface is then covered with 20 thicknesses of sterile coarse mesh gauze held in place with a loosely wrapped elastic gauze bandage. The dressing provides some measure of protection and isolation of the wound and serves to absorb exudate and drainage. To help reduce the extent of the swelling, the patient is instructed to keep the injured part elevated above the level of the heart. No antibiotics are given.

The wound should be reinspected by a physician the next day. Then the patient or a responsible person is instructed in wound care, i.e., to remove the dressing once daily, gently cleanse the wound with soap and water, and reapply the dressing with or without the topical antibacterial agent. Additionally, instruction is given in appropriate modalities of physical and occupational therapy. Thereafter, the patient is re-examined at weekly intervals at which time loose devitalized debris is trimmed away and, if needed, treatment altered. Other arrangements are made if the above recommended scheme for wound care is inadequate or if the patient fails to maintain progress in his or her unsupervised physical or occupational therapy efforts. The patient is instructed to notify the physician of pain, redness in the tissues around the wound, persistent edema, or fever.

INPATIENT CARE OF BURN WOUNDS

After fluid resuscitation has been started and a detailed history and physical examination completed, attention is directed to care of the burn. Wounds are gently cleansed of debris, loose devitalized tissues trimmed away, and a topical antibacterial agent is applied.

Topical Antibacterial Agents

There are several agents available which when applied topically to wounds are thought to modify favorably the bacterial growth on wounds without doing appreciable damage to viable tissue and are thought to have a salutary effect on survival. Although none of these agents is capable of perpetually sustaining sterilization of all wounds, they are capable of temporarily delaying colonization and reducing bacterial counts on or in wounds. In many instances, organisms not affected by the topical agent are selected out or find their way to the wound. These agents are 0.5% silver nitrate soaks (34), mafenide (32), silver sulfadiazine (4), silver sulfadiazine with cerium nitrate (30), and povidone-iodine (19). Data is unavailable which proves superiority of one agent over the others for survival of patients (20). Silver sulfadiazine is currently in widest use, probably because of its low incidence of side-effects. The use of topical antibacterial agents is only one among many adjuncts used for successful treatment of a patient with a burn and these agents are not substitutes for meticulous care of the wound based on well-established surgical principles.

Should Burn Wounds be Dressed?

While dressings are needed to employ 0.5% silver nitrate soaks successfully and mafenide is most advantageously used without dressings, other topical agents may be used with or without dressings.

The lipid complex in the stratum corneum provides the skin's water integrity (23). When heat deranges the epidermis and destroys the lipid complex, there is an obligatory loss of water through the wound. Patients with large wounds are, therefore, in a permanent state of uncontrolled sweating until their wounds are healed. The loss of water by evaporation is energy consuming; for each liter evaporated, 580 kcal of heat are lost. While the patient with a large surface burn has an increase in thermal load because of postburn hypermetabolism (52), and the evaporative water loss through the wound provides a convenient route for the removal of this heat, excessive loss of heat sufficient to cause shivering or a fall in core temperature below normal levels must be prevented. Therefore, patients with biologically significant burn injury, i.e., those with burns over 20% body surface area and burned infants and elderly patients should, in some way, have thermal support to achieve comfort, to minimize metabolic expenditure, and to prevent hypothermia.

When wounds are treated by the open technique, i.e., without dressings, external warmth must be provided. The temperature of the air that surrounds the patient with a large surface burn must be above 30°C (6, 53). If the entire room is warmed to this level, conditions are too uncomfortable and fatiguing for individuals attending the patient. To obviate this problem, individual or banks of heat lamps and reflectors, or heat shields can be employed, or the patient can be nursed in the unit surrounded by a plastic envelope in which ambient conditions can be optimally regulated for the patient without altering desirable working ambient conditions outside.

Dressings, even when wetted, can be constructed in such a way as to maintain body heat (40). In a dressing composed of 20 thicknesses of coarse mesh gauze held in place with an elastic gauze bandage and maintained with a dry top layer, the temperature in the dressing just above the wound surface will be 35.4°C in spite of lower ambient room temperatures which are well within the comfort range for attendants. It is imperative that the top layer be dry. If the outer layer is wet, heat will be conducted rapidly through the dressing away from the patient and the patient will soon become cool. Patients with dressed wounds are more comfortable than those with exposed wounds. Furthermore, dressings serve to absorb wound exudate and drainage.

Surgical Care of the Burn

As soon as the patient's condition is stabilized, the wounds are assessed for the purpose of developing a plan for wound closure. This assessment is considerably hampered by no currently available reliable noninvasive method of accurately determining depth of injury.

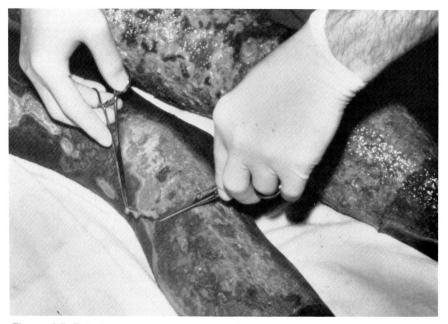

Figure 4.5. Epluchage or piecemeal removal of necrotic tissue which has separated spontaneously.

Necrotic tissue produced by the burn must be removed. This not only reduces the possibility of bacterial wound invasion and systemic infection but also is a necessary step in preparing the wound for closure by skin graft. There are two commonly employed methods of removing eschar: (1) epluchage or piecemeal removal of necrotic tissue which has spontaneously separated (Fig. 4.5); and (2) excision either (a) directly to fascia (8) (Fig. 4.6), or (b) tangentially, i.e., shaving sequential levels until viable tissue is exposed (22) (Fig. 4.7).

In using epluchage the wounds are inspected daily and the necrotic tissue which has separated is gently cut away (Fig. 4.5). This should not produce pain or bleeding. It usually takes three to five weeks for the eschar to separate completely. Separation of eschar is delayed among the elderly, hastened by bacterial autolysis, and occurs rapidly with infection. In recent years with better bacterial control in burn wounds, spontaneous eschar separation has, among some patients, been considerably delayed. Therefore, operative débridement is often used to prepare the wound for skin grafting.

The use of hydrotherapy, once a hallmark of burn care, especially with epluchage, is decreasing. It is this author's contention that there is no evidence that it helps improve outcome. However, with proper safeguards for intravenous lines or tracheostomy tube if present and if immersion is not prolonged, a bath may be used when needed for reasons of hygiene.

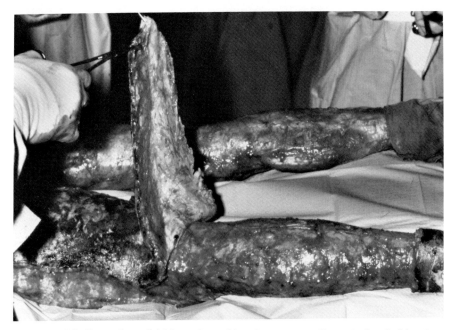

Figure 4.6. Resection of thick eschar with subcutaneous tissue to level of fascia.

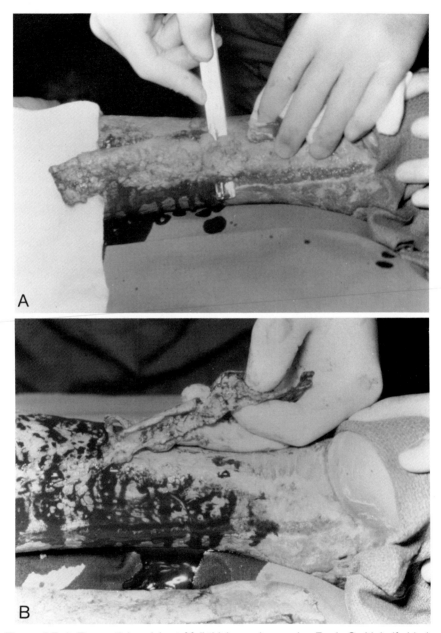

Figure 4.7. A. Tangential excision of full-thickness burn using Ferris-Smith knife blade. A variety of knives and devices can be used for this kind of excision. B. Viable tissue (fat) exposed. C. Bleeding controlled and wound being covered with nonviable sterile pigskin. D. Pigskin coverage of wound completed. The grafts may then be covered with nylon net as shown here. This net is a convenient way to ensure that grafts are not inadvertently dislodged and yet permit access for visual inspection of the grafts to detect complications that might occur. The net can be used with or without other dressing.

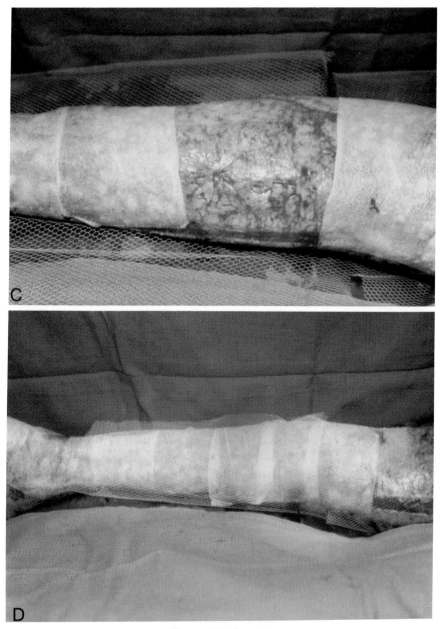

Figure 4.7. C and D.

In general, wounds that will heal spontaneously within three to four weeks after injury are allowed to do so. When wounds will not heal spontaneously within this time, when practical, the residual necrotic debris and granulation tissue may be debrided or tangentially excised and the wound then closed with autogenous split thickness skin grafts. The debrided area may first be covered with a biological dressing (Fig. 4.7) and the skin graft applied during a second anesthetic several days later. This delay in autografting ensures precise control of bleeding and avoids disastrous loss of skin grafts when, as occasionally happens, exposed fat becomes devitalized by infection. This sequence of tangential excision followed by skin grafting is repeated until all wounds are healed. The areas of full-thickness burns are closed first. Unless spontaneous healing is imminent, wounds of deep partial-thickness depth should also be closed with skin grafts, provided, of course, that donor skin grafts are available. It is the author's contention that, in most instances, this approach will result in a better quality of skin covering with a lower incidence of hypertrophic scarring than if deep partial-thickness wounds are allowed to heal spontaneously.

With increasing frequency, some burn surgeons, disappointed with epluchage and realizing that eschar must be removed, have turned to excision down to fascia (8) (Fig. 4.6). This is done as soon as possible after admission and especially among those patients at excessive risk of dying because of large areas of deep partial-thickness and full-thickness burns. One tries to do the excision before excessive bacterial colonization of the burn eschar has occurred. Excision to fascia is used because blood loss is less than that when tangential excision is employed. Experience has shown that it is safe to excise only up to about 20% of the body surface at one operation. Therefore, when there is a large burn, several procedures are required. The excised wound is immediately covered with as much autograft as can be obtained or with a biological dressing. If a biological dressing is used, a donor-related or viable cadaver allograft is preferred. More recently, synthetic coverings have also been employed. When autogenous donor skin becomes available, the biological or synthetic dressing is removed and the wound closed with an autogenous skin graft. More recent advances in anesthetic management and general supportive care have allowed burn surgeons to extend their capability in the field of excision. However, the blood loss may be prodigious and total replacement of the blood volume may be necessary unless hypotensive anesthesia, cutting cautery or one of the newer instruments of excision, e.g., a carbon dioxide laser (18), are employed. Excision, as advantageous as it may seem must not be undertaken lightly nor by one who only sometimes treats burns. That excision has a salutary effect on survival among young children is fairly well accepted (10, 27), but the data on adults are not so convincing, especially among the elderly (13). Furthermore, the cosmetic and functional result of grafted split-thickness skin on muscle or fascia, particularly over joints, may be less than desired.

Although the removal of eschar by enzymatic digestion is appealing and the proteolytic enzyme sutilains ointment has been used clinically with apparent effectiveness (14), their use has not been widely accepted. To be effective, the eschar must be moist. Because the enzyme is not lipolytic, fat which has been devitalized by heat will remain undigested. The most disquieting problem with the use of enzymatic ointment are reports of an increase in the incidence of infection (21, 24). Wound sepsis is said to be reduced when the enzyme is mixed with the topical antibacterial agent, silver sulfadiazine (39).

Biological Dressings

Biological dressings consist of viable or once viable tissues used to temporarily cover wounds in place of conventional dressings or leaving the wound exposed (49). There are several benefits derived by closing wounds with these materials: the loss of protein, fluid, electrolyte, and other substances are much reduced thereby improving the patient's nutritional and overall condition; the wound becomes pain free; bacterial growth is inhibited when the biological dressing is placed on viable uninfected wounds; the healing of partial-thickness burns is enhanced; and adherence of the biological dressing ensures that wound conditions are favorable for autografting. Frequently used materials are partial-thickness skin grafts from relatives of the patient (9) or deceased humans (48), human fetal membranes (46) (homografts or allografts), and partial-thickness skin grafts from pigs (7) (heterografts or xenografts).

Viable homografts are usually used in the following manner. After removal of eschar, usually by one of the techniques of excision, the wounds, for which autograft is not readily available, are closed with viable split-thickness skin homografts from either a donor closely related to the patient or from a cadaver. These grafts "take", i.e., they become vascularized. However, eventually, usually in one to three weeks, rejection of the homograft occurs. Rejection may be delayed among patients with sepsis. Immunosuppressants have been used to delay rejection of homografts (39). These methods help provide wound closure until autograft donor sites can heal and be recropped to replace the homograft. Eventually all full-thickness wounds covered by homograft must be covered with autografts. The viability of homografts can be prolonged by freezing (5).

All biological dressings, viable and nonviable, can be used for short-term, several-day, wound coverage (49) (Fig. 4.7). After removal of eschar and other debris, homograft or xenograft is placed on clean uninfected wounds. If adherence does not occur, a new biological dressing is applied. When there is adherence, the biological dressing can be replaced by autogenous skin grafts or changed every several days until it becomes feasible to substitute autografts. Changing viable homografts and xenografts every several days prevents rejection and allows the patient to derive all the benefits of a closed wound. Although true vascularization, i.e., anastomosis of blood vessels between wound and nonviable biological graft materials does not occur, blood vessels from the wound do grow into the interstices of the graft material so that when the biological dressing is removed, fine, easily controlled capillary bleeding occurs.

The technique of changing the biological dressing every several days is most advantageously employed to cover and protect wounds for several days after they are surgically prepared for autografting (Fig. 4.7). Transfer of autografts is delayed until a second operation is performed several days later. This delay ensures precise control of bleeding and avoids loss of skin grafts if freshly exposed fat becomes devitalized by infection.

Biological dressings may also be effectively employed to protect wounds which have been covered by widely meshed or widely placed pieces of skin graft. Used in this way, the wounds between the autografts are closed as well. The biological dressing may be removed in two days before vascular ingrowth makes removal of the biological dressing difficult and to prevent the possibility of impeding the spread of epithelium from the new autografts. However, viable cadaver homograft may be left on the wound until it is rejected or until it desiccates and flakes off after the epithelium has spread resurfacing the underlying wound (Fig. 4.8).

Biological dressings may be used in the management of burns of partial-thickness depth, particularly scald burns (28). If, after blistered skin is removed and there is no eschar, these wounds are protected with the biological dressing, they are much less painful and are said to heal more rapidly.

The demand for homograft skin is great and at times the supply is limited. An effective alternate for short-term use is porcine xenograft (Fig. 4.7). This material in the nonviable form is available commercially and is in wide use. Fetal membranes, thought to be superior to nonviable pig skin, is also readily available, but not commercially.

The coverage of wounds containing infected or devitalized tissue with biological materials makes no sense.

Synthetic Wound Coverings

Although satisfactory substitutes for either temporary or permanent use have been found for joints, the heart, the kidney, and blood vessels, no suitable synthetic replacement exists for the skin. However, there are several materials available which can be advantageously used in the management of large wounds.

The first, a membrane dressing, is composed of a thin transparent elastic adhesive coated polyurethane film (Opsite) permeable to water vapor,

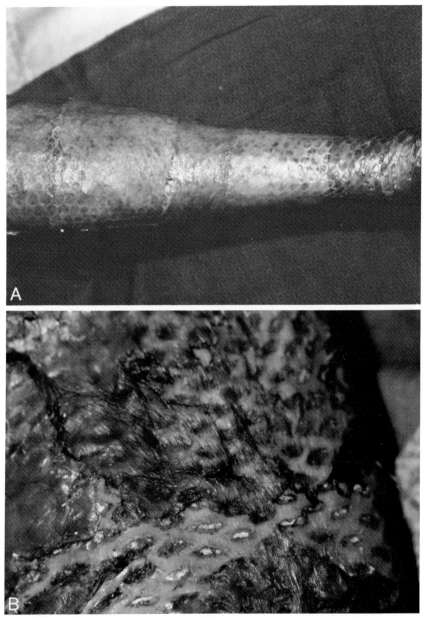

Figure 4.8. A. Wound of forearm excised to level of fascia then grafted with split thickness meshed autogenous skin covered with viable cadaver homograft to completely close the wound. B. Same patient as in A two weeks later showing desiccated and sloughing cadaver skin as autograft expands beneath.

oxygen, and carbon dioxide, but not to liquid, water, or bacteria. This membrane, used to cover skin donor sites (15) and clean uninfected partial-thickness wounds, creates an environment which virtually eliminates pain and decreases healing time.

Another synthetic dressing is a composite of an ultrathin poly-dimethyl-siloxane rubberlike membrane to which is bonded a mixture of hydrophilic collagen peptides obtained from dermal collagen (50). This flexible knitted nylon fabric (Biobrane) of fine denier has been used to cover clean partial-thickness burns, temporarily close excised full-thickness burns, and to dress meshed autograft and donor sites.

Touted as a synthetic skin, a highly porous polymer of collagen fibers obtained from cowhide covalently bonded to chondroitin-6-sulfate, a major polysaccharide of cartilage obtained from sharks, covered with a sheet of medical grade silicone rubber that serves as a barrier to infection and fluid loss has been developed (11) and is undergoing clinical trial. This material is used to cover excised wounds. Mesodermal cells, including blood vessels, grow into the polymer, biodegrading it over a 20-day period and creating a neodermis. The wound is ultimately resurfaced by removing the sheet of silicone rubber and replacing it with ultrathin autografts.

Wound Closure and Skin Grafting

A patient with a burn is not successfully treated until all wounds are healed. Unless of small size, all full-thickness wounds require skin grafts. Wounds of partial-thickness depth which do not heal spontaneously in a reasonable time, may, if donor skin is available, be closed with a skin graft. In general, by one month after injury, a decision should have been reached as to whether a particular wound will be allowed to heal spontaneously or whether it will be closed by skin graft. Furthermore, it is the burn surgeon's responsibility to make certain the patient's wounds heal and stay healed. If the latter principle is adhered to, the incidence of epidermoid carcinoma arising in burn scars should be nil.

Skin autografting refers to the transfer of skin from one part of the body to another on the same individual. In the treatment of patients with unhealed burn wounds for which skin grafts are needed, split-thickness skin grafts are used almost exclusively. This implies that the grafts are cut through a partial-thickness of depth of skin leaving epidermal regenerative cells which cause re-epithelization of the donor site. Full-thickness skin grafts and flaps are used in some late burn reconstructive procedures.

Skin grafts must lie quietly and be undisturbed to take. Fibrin causes initial adherence. The cells of the graft are nourished by tissue fluid until inosculation (anastomosis) of blood vessels between the wound and the graft establishes a nutritive blood flow in the graft. Inosculation occurs in about two days. Because thin skin grafts have less tissue to be nourished while the graft is being vascularized, thin grafts have a better chance of surviving than do thick skin grafts. However, thicker grafts, if they do survive, produce a better cosmetic result. The thickness of split-thickness skin grafts used in human burn work vary from .006 inch to, at most, .015 inch. For split-thickness skin grafts on full-thickness wounds to be durable, the graft must contain dermis.

There are three kinds of instruments used to cut split-thickness skin grafts: (1) drum dermatomes which are accurate and versatile but slow and tedious to use when large amounts of skin are needed; (2) knives with or without depth guards which require considerable skill to use well; and (3) currently in widest use for resurfacing burns, electric or air driven dermatomes which have a reciprocating blade and which are capable of cutting long even strips of skin quickly.

Skin grafts may be cut from virtually any area of the body. However, the face and hands are not used. The foot as a skin donor source is generally impractical. The scalp is a superior donor site. It has an excellent blood supply with deep closely placed hair follicles which are able to effect re-epithelization in four or five days. Regrowth of scalp hair hides the donor site. Donor sites of the torso and extremities heal more slowly. Nonhealing and infection of donor sites are unusual. However, past middle age, the healing of skin donor sites below the level of the knees may be extremely slow and occasionally the wound may be converted to full-thickness injury by infection. Although donor sites may be recropped several times, there is a limit to the number of harvestings and one must be careful not to leave a wound of full-thickness depth at the donor site.

Donor sites may be dressed in a number of ways, or left open. If they are left exposed, after control of bleeding, a crust forms under which healing occurs. Dry fine mesh gauze or a gauze impregnated with scarlet red or one of several other substances may also be used. Donor sites treated in this way may also be allowed to dry. If suppuration or maceration occurs, the crust or dressing should be removed and a topical antibacterial agent employed to help control bacterial growth. Among patients with large burns or when the donor site is adjacent to an unhealed burn wound, the donor site is often treated as the burn. With the use of membrane dressings, pain can be virtually eliminated from donor sites and healing time is shortened. However, to employ membrane dressings effectively, the donor site must be surrounded by intact skin so that the pressure-sensitive adhesive of the membrane can adhere completely around the wound.

Failure of a skin graft to take is unnecessary and disastrous. Not only does the grafted wound remain open, but the partial-thickness wound made at the donor site adds to the area of open wounds. Skin grafts fail because of: (1) movement of grafts; (2) foreign material and other substances under the graft, e.g., blood serum, necrotic tissue, sutures, etc., which separate the graft from the wound preventing vascularization of the graft; and (3) infection, e.g., invasive infection of the wound or the dissolution of the graft from streptolysin elaborated from *Group A beta hemolytic streptococci.* A skin graft should never be placed on a wound on which the skin graft is not expected to take. The wound bed for successful grafting must have viable uninfected tissue free of foreign material. To accomplish this, all necrotic burn tissue, debris, and granulation tissue needs to be removed. The best place to complete preparation of a wound for grafting is in the operating room with the patient anesthetized. The bleeding must be perfectly controlled. Pressure, thrombin, and time are the most effective methods. Coagulation cautery and sutures, while necessary, should be used sparingly. If bleeding cannot be precisely controlled or the wound and other conditions are not optimal, the transfer of skin grafts should be delayed. In this instance, the wound is covered temporarily with a biological dressing to protect the wound and to serve as a test graft.

In skin grafting, it is preferable to cover the wound completely from edge to edge (Fig. 4.9). However, with a large wound and with limited donor skin, it is often advantageous to use one of the techniques of skin expansion. The simplest method is to cut the grafts into small pieces and distribute them evenly over the wound. This is known as the postage stamp graft method (Fig. 4.10). The cosmetic result of this technique is poor. Mesh grafting, made practical by the development of the Tanner-Vanderput skin meshing device, is now widely practiced. In this method, sheets of split-thickness skin are placed on grooved carriers and passed through a device with a series of sharp edges on a roller which cuts slits in the sheet of graft. The graft is pulled apart as lace and placed on the wound. Practical expansions are 1.5:1 and 3:1. Expansion of 6:1 is used but this and wider expansions are flimsy, difficult to work with, and have poorer cosmetic outcomes. Often meshed skin, particularly wider meshes and widely placed stamp grafts are covered with biological dressings to completely close the wound between grafts until the autografts can take and expand (Figs. 4.8 and 4.10).

Securing thin, split-thickness skin grafts by suture or staple, while frequently done, is unnecessary. These grafts need only to be laid on properly prepared wounds and left undisturbed for about four days for them to take. An excellent and rapid way to secure grafts so they are not inadvertently dislodged is to cover the grafts with a nylon net fixed with collodion or tacked in place with sutures (Fig. 4.7D). If a dressing is employed, which we usually prefer to do, the dressing can be changed down to the level of the nylon net without fear of disturbing the skin grafts. In this way, the new grafts can be inspected as frequently as necessary.

There are a wide variety of techniques, tricks, and devices with and without dressings employed by surgeons to secure grafts and immobilize parts to allow grafts to take. Joints must be held immobile until the take of the skin graft is assured. This is usually accomplished by splinting. Because there are alternate techniques of immobilization and positioning the body

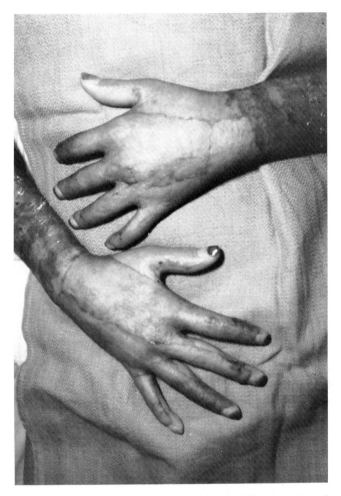

Figure 4.9. Burn wounds of dorsum of hands tangentially excised and completely closed with sheets of split-thickness skin grafts. This is the preferred method of closing burn wounds requiring skin grafts and when sufficient donor skin is available.

parts satisfactorily to allow skin grafts to take, the use of skeletal traction for this purpose is unnecessary and may lead to annoying infections. The use of wires through joints, as has been recommended for immobilization of fingers for skin grafting, is to be condemned because disastrous septic arthritis will occasionally occur.

The aftercare of grafts should be the responsibility of the surgeon until the take of the graft is secure. This takes about four days. Grafts should be inspected daily for complications; e.g., seromas which should be drained;

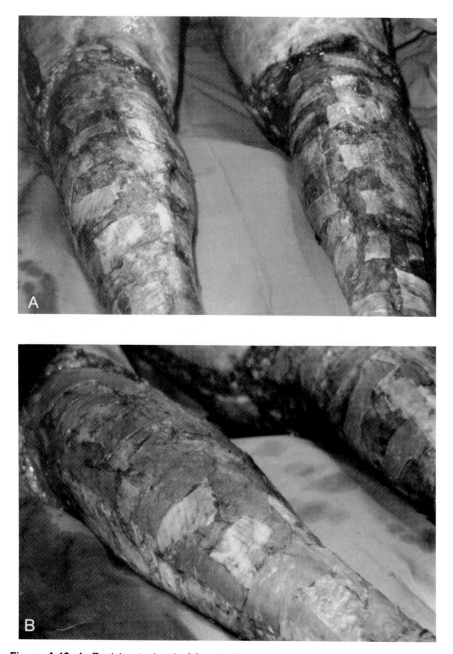

Figure 4.10. A. Excision to level of fascia. Postage stamp skin grafts donated from scalp applied. B. Same patient as in A. Postage stamp autografts are intermingled with cadaver homograft skin in attempt to completely close the excised wound.

hematomas which should be evacuated; and slippage of graft which should be corrected or the exposed area covered with a new piece of skin graft, if any skin graft was left over and preserved from the operation. If nylon net was used to protect the skin grafts it is removed on the fourth postgraft day. If a biological dressing, other than viable homograft, is placed over the exposed parts of a wound between grafts, it is usually removed in two days. If the biological dressing is left in contact with the wound bed longer than two days, adherence will be too great to allow easy removal. In this case, it should be allowed to remain undisturbed and it will slough, usually by desiccation and flaking off, when epithelialization is completed underneath the biological dressing.

The following is a laundry list of effective methods usually employed by the author to obtain immobilization to allow grafts to take. The face and neck are always grafted with sheets of skin and are not dressed. Movement is prevented by positioning, sand bags, and sedation. When the dorsum of the hand is grafted, the hand is sewn into a custom-made splint for immobilization and sheet grafts are used. When grafts are applied to other sites of the upper or lower extremity or to the torso, the grafts are covered first with nylon net and then a dressing composed of 20 thicknesses of coarse mesh gauze held in place with an elastic gauze bandage. Joints are held immobile with custom made splints prepared preoperatively. The skin grafted axilla is held open by positioning the shoulder in 90 degrees of abduction. The back, the posterior aspect of the head and neck, and buttocks are skin grafted last. To ensure take of the grafts on these areas the patient is placed on his abdomen. For skin grafting the back, we have occasionally quilted a dressing over the graft. In this method, sutures are passed at intervals through the dressing into the tissues to secure it to the fascia. The patient may then be nursed on the back. The survival of grafts when this technique is employed has been quite good.

In most instances there is enough tensile strength between the graft and the wound to permit active range of motion on the fourth and certainly by the sixth day after skin grafting. Gentle passive range of motion can be added on the sixth or seventh day.

The hydrostatic pressure from the column of venous blood when the patient is in the upright position may cause hemorrhage under skin grafts newly placed on the lower extremity. Therefore, the safest approach among patients with grafts at these sites is to keep the patient in bed with his grafted lower extremity nondependent for 10 days. The more distal the graft and the older the patient, the longer the patient should be protected up to 10 days. When ambulation is allowed, the grafted lower extremity should be wrapped carefully with an elastic bandage.

In the overwhelming majority of instances, wounds of the hands, face, and neck take precedence for skin grafts. However, when life is at stake

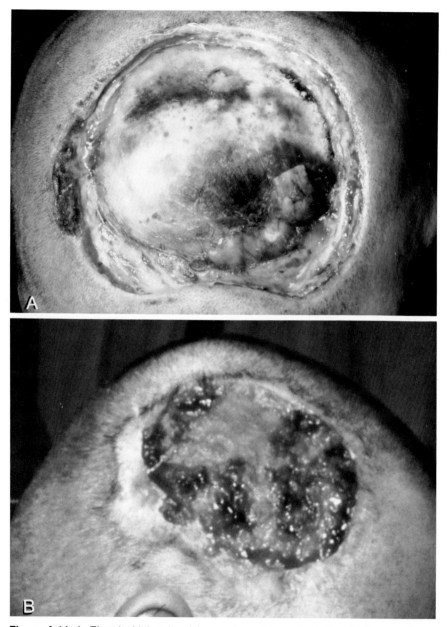

Figure 4.11. A. Electrical injury involving scalp and outer table to calvarium. B. Same patient as in A. Outer table of calvarium was removed permitting granulation tissue to form from diploe. C. Same patient as in A and B. Split-thickness skin graft applied to granulation tissue. Often, there remain small pieces of necrotic bone which need to be debrided to complete wound closure. If a more pleasing cosmetic result is desired, a flap, preferably bearing hair, can be moved into the defect.

and there is limited donor skin, consideration must be given to covering larger areas to try to reduce the size of the wound to attempt to first preserve the patient's life. The next priority for skin grafts after the hands, face, and neck is the skin over joints.

In the management of patients with large burns, one seldom has the luxury of choosing skin for optimal color match. However, when practical and among patients with smaller burns who need skin grafts on cosmetically sensitive areas such as the face, neck, and hands, consideration should be given to this matter.

When necrosis of soft tissue extends to bone, regardless of site and provided an amputation is not needed, the nonviable tissue surrounding the bone is removed and the bone left alone until the soft-tissue wounds are healed. If left undisturbed, eventually, in months, the devitalized portion of bone would slough leaving a wound covered with granulation tissue. However, to hasten wound closure, the bone may be decorticated exposing viable bone. Granulation tissue will start to form and the wound can then be covered with a split-thickness skin graft (Fig. 4.11). All devitalized bone must be removed before the wound can heal completely. If a flap would provide a more desirable cover, it may be transferred later. However, even in acute burn work, it is occasionally desirable to cover a defect such as an exposed joint with a flap rather than use a split-thickness skin graft. For a flap to close a wound successfully, all necrotic tissue must first be removed.

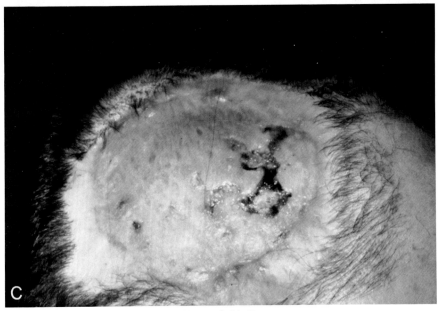

Figure 4.11. C.

Viable tendon will accept a thin split-thickness skin graft. Peritendineum has an excellent vascular supply and will reliably accept a skin graft, and the graft will not be bound to the tendon. If, however, exposure of the tendon does occur, it may be dressed as any other wound. Usually, the superficial portion of an otherwise viable tendon will slough but granulation tissue will eventually grow up through the tendon. When this occurs, the granulation tissue is shaved off with a *very* sharp knife, bleeding controlled with thrombin and pressure—no cautery!—and a split-thickness skin graft applied.

Complications That May Affect Rehabilitation

SMOKE INHALATION SYNDROME

When smoke is inhaled, the irritating noxious gases may cause a clinical illness known as smoke inhalation syndrome. This syndrome occurs frequently among those burned in closed spaces. There may be a symptom-free interval, but clinical manifestations usually occur within 72 hours of the accident. Early signs include tachypnea, dyspnea, and wheezing caused by bronchospasm or debris in the lower airway. There is a high incidence of burns of the face with singed nasal vibrissae, superficial burns of the cornea, and burns of the oral mucosa. This condition is identified by finding soot in the sputum; soot, erythema, and ulcerations in the lower airway on fiberoptic bronchoscopy (36); abnormalities on xenon[133] ventilation-perfusion scan of the lungs (37); and changes of respiratory acidosis and hypoxia on arterial blood gas analysis. Initially, the chest roentgenogram may be normal, but in the full blown syndrome, noncardiogenic pulmonary edema occurs.

Treatment in the early stages and of milder cases consists of humidified air with increased levels of inspired oxygen, chest physical therapy, and postural drainage.

If the exposure to smoke is severe, progressive pulmonary insufficiency may occur. If indicated, positive pressure ventilation is instituted. While some patients require ventilatory support for only a brief period, others may not be successfully weaned from the ventilator for several weeks or longer.

The principle complication of smoke inhalation is superimposed bacterial pneumonia (1). When the injury is severe enough to require ventilatory support, especially when there is an accompanying large surface burn, the mortality is high.

If ventilatory support is required, the difficulty of delivering physical and occupational therapeutic efforts is enhanced. First, the patient is also likely to be clinically ill, at least for a time, from infection. Second, an endotracheal tube adds discomfort to a patient who is already uncomfortable. Third, a patient who is immobile from the injury to the skin is further restricted by the equipment necessary to support respiration. Furthermore, the patient is more distracted and less willing to participate in physical activities. Lastly, even after successful treatment, the patient may have exercise intolerance because of residual impairment of pulmonary function. Also, as a result of prolonged intubation either with a tracheostomy or endotracheal tube, the patient may have temporarily impaired phonation and swallowing.

INFECTION

Infection remains the most frequent cause of morbidity and death among burned patients (2). Over one-half of the deaths are from septicemia and pneumonia. The risk of infection varies with the extent and depth of the burn, and the age of the patient and is greatly enhanced in the presence of smoke inhalation syndrome. When the burn is small, the risk of septicemia is small, but when the burn exceeds 30% of the body surface area, the risk is great and increases exponentially thereafter. Infants and the aged are at much greater risk for septicemia than are older children and young adults. The most common sources of systemic infection among patients with burns are: the wound (31); the lungs from the infectious sequelae of smoke inhalation syndrome (1); veins from septic thrombophlebitis caused by prolonged venous canalization (42); and pressure sores from either prolonged immobilization in one position or from ill-fitting or improperly positioned splints.

Serious infection occurs much earlier in the postburn period and in a more insidious fashion than may be generally appreciated. It is crucial to recognize the early subtle manifestations of septicemia because if one waits for overt signs to become manifested before starting appropriate therapy, the patient will be in danger of developing shock and losing his life from infection. The important manifestations which should make one suspicious of septicemia are: body temperature greater than 39°C, or hypothermia; leukocyte count greater than 20,000 cells/mm^3 or leukopenia; change in sensorium, ileus; gastroduodenal bleeding or perforation; persistent thrombocytopenia; unexplained oliguria; impaired utilization of glucose; unexplained anemia; gain in body weight in conjunction with the decrease in caloric intake; and an unexplained decrease in pulmonary function. The presence of two of these clinical manifestations provides enough suspicion of septicemia to justify obtaining the necessary cultures and to begin appropriate therapy. Systemic antibiotic therapy is instituted on the clinical suspicion of septicemia and the most likely microorganism or organisms responsible for the clinical state of the patient. Treatment is then modified based on the patients clinical response to treatment and on specific bacteriological culture data and antibiotic sensitivity tests.

Because of the unique relationship between the patient and physical and occupational therapists, therapists are able to make observations which are of great value in helping to detect changes which are suggestive of systemic infection. For instance, because the therapist works with the patient each day, he or she is able to detect subtle and early changes in the patient's sensorium and any alteration in the state of consciousness, intellectual capacity, or confusion. Any such changes should be reported to the physician. Also, deterioration in exercise tolerance may indicate pulmonary insufficiency from infection.

Scars and Contractures

The principal late complications of burns are hypertrophic scars and contractures.

Hypertrophic scars, scars which are red, raised, and indurated, occur frequently among convalescent burn patients and in wounds which are deeper than superficial partial-thickness. They occur when wounds heal spontaneously as well as in those which have been skin grafted (Fig. 4.12). The longer a wound remains open, the more likely is the possibility of a hypertrophic scar. For this reason, it may be advisable to close deep partial-thickness wounds by skin graft as soon as practical rather than to allow spontaneous healing to occur; provided donor skin is available.

While all the factors which lead to the formation of hypertrophic scars are not completely known, the disorder results in fused, tightly packed, heaped up collagen. Hypertrophic scars are dynamic lesions. Most burn wounds are flat when they heal. However, in several weeks those areas which are destined to become hypertrophic begin to raise. They reach their zenith in several months. However, with time, some of the collagen is resorbed and that which remains tends to realign into a more orderly and linear pattern. Gradually the scar loses its redness, becomes softer, more pliable, and usually flattens. This process is known as maturation of the scar. In some cases all the hypertrophic qualities do not disappear and the scar remains raised. It is known that a scar can be flattened with pressure (25). Also, maturation is thought to be aided and hastened by applying pressure, usually in the form of an elastic rubber bandage or a custom made elastic garment. It takes about 18 months or longer for the majority of changes that occur with maturation of scars to occur. Only then can one make a definitive estimate of permanency and esthetic quality of scars.

In addition to natural maturation and the application of pressure, atrophy of hypertrophic scars can be caused by injection of steroids into the scar. Injecting an indurated scar is both difficult and painful and there is always the danger of depositing the drug into the subcutaneous tissue causing unsightly atrophy of the fat. In spite of these problems, excellent results can be obtained. Hypertrophic scars have been treated surgically by excision and either closing the defect primarily or by skin graft, or by shaving off

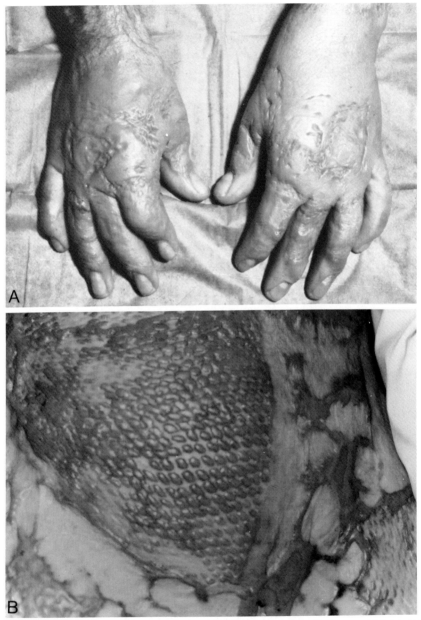

Figure 4.12. A. Hypertrophic scars from partial-thickness of depth burns which healed spontaneously. Severe limitation of range of motion of the hand was corrected by excision of entire hypertrophic scar and the defect closed with thick split thickness skin grafts. B. Hypertrophic scars between skin grafts on the anterior abdominal wall. These wounds were caused by electricity with tissue loss to the level of transversalis fascia. Therefore, hypertrophic scar must have come from dermis exposed at edge of grafts.

the scar and skin grafting the wound. Before one uses steroids or does a surgical procedure to alter hypertrophic scars, particularly extensive ones, consideration should be given to natural resolution that might yet occur.

Contraction is a property of all healing wounds (Fig. 4.13). As a result, contractures, which limit range of motion, develop. Prevention is the key. This includes the use of proper techniques of positioning and splinting in the anticontracture position (e.g., the elbow extended) and conscientious active and passive physical therapy until the proclivity to form contractures is past.

A contracture may involve any joint. In recent years, techniques have been developed which aid in preventing most contractures. For instance, contractures of the antecubital and popliteal fossae rarely occur. The incidence of contractures of the neck, ankles, feet and hands has decreased yet still can be a significant problem. Definitive prevention of contractures of the axilla continues to be difficult. Contractures of the face are particularly dangerous because contraction of periorbital tissues may cause ectropion of the eyelids exposing the cornea to drying with all its horrible infectious sequelae and contraction or perioral tissues may result in microstomia of such extent that eating, oral hygiene, and dental manipulations are difficult and delivery of general anesthetics excessively dangerous.

If a contracture forms, splinting, exercise, skeletal traction, serial casting, or other nonsurgical techniques may be used to try to reverse the process.

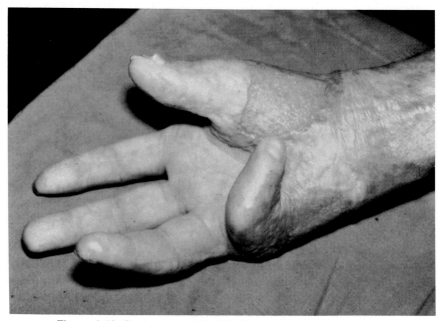

Figure 4.13. Contracture of the little finger and palm from burns.

While these methods may be successful, especially for contractures of minor extent, surgical treatment for the contracture is often needed when the contracture is uncontrolled and well advanced. It is generally considered undesirable to relieve contractures early, that is, during the phase of active scar formation and as long as the scar is erythematous. However, uncontrolled contractures at important sites, such as of the eyelids, the neck, or the hands, may be so disabling that surgical release will be required before scars mature. For instance, if a contracture of the dorsum of the hand is causing progressive subluxation of the metacarpophalangeal joints, release and skin grafting should be done to preserve the integrity of the joint and a better splinting position for the hand.

It is most desirable to delay reconstructive procedures until maturation of the scar is well advanced. The principal surgical procedures used to preserve functional integrity and improve cosmesis are: excision of scars with primary wound closure or skin grafting; release of contracture with skin grafting; rotational, tube, free, or myocutaneous flaps; and Z-plasty. The two most frequently used procedures are release of contractures with skin grafting and Z-plasty. In releasing contractures surgically the incision is made perpendicular through the contracture, or the entire scar responsible for the contracture is excised. Often the underlying fascia has contracted as well and it may be necessary to incise it to release the contracture completely. The defect, which is often amazingly large, is usually closed with a relatively thick split-thickness skin graft. The joint is held in the antecontracture position. When scars have matured and are supple, a Z-plasty procedure will often suffice, especially to relieve band contractures.

An extremely difficult period for the surviving burn patient, especially among those with large and deep burns, is that period shortly after wound closure has been completed. For several months hypertrophic scars develop, wound contraction is continuing, and itching and sweating to an annoying extent are all occurring. Gradually these changes abate as the wounds mature. Among the severely and extensively burned, it takes about two years to complete maturation of scars and the necessary reconstructive procedures.

Heterotopic Bone Formation

The heterotopic formation of bone around joints may cause a disabling complication which occurs in about 2–3% of convalescent hospitalized burn patients (16). If the calcification bridges a joint, the joint is rendered immobile (Fig. 4.14).

While ectopic calcification among the burned occurs most frequently at the elbow (Fig. 4.15), it also develops at the shoulder, radioulnar joint, wrist, knee, hip, and in the hand (41). Although its cause is unknown, heterotopic bone formation occurs most frequently in adults and usually among those recovering from deep large surface burns. With respect to the elbow, the

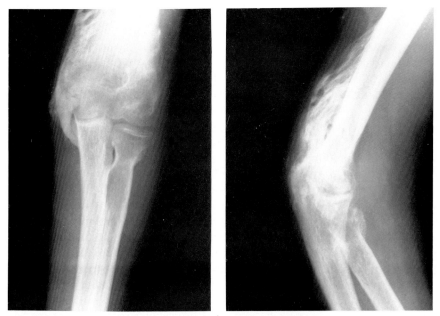

Figure 4.14. Roentgenograms showing heterotopic bone bridging elbow joint following burns. Calcification is usually located posterior and medially.

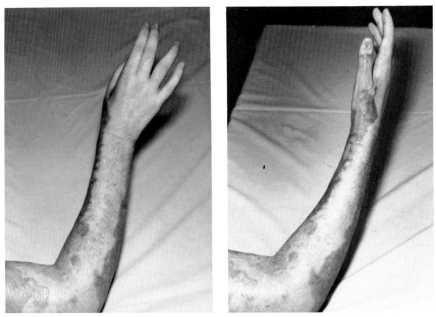

Figure 4.15. Case of heterotopic bone bridging elbow joint completely preventing flexion-extension of the elbow. However, patient can pronate-supinate forearm indicating that radio-ulnar joint is not involved.

upper extremity is usually, but not always burned, requires skin grafts and a period of immobilization to ensure the take of those grafts. Subsequently, during the latter stages of the hospital stay, the physical therapist notices progressive decrease in active and passive range of motion with increasing pain and resistance to physical therapy efforts beyond any limitation imposed by tight skin. At this point, a roentgenogram may or may not yet show calcification. The calcification at the elbow is located posteriorly and medially with a bony bridge between the olecranon of the ulna and the medial epicondyle and intercondylar portion and posterior shaft of the humerus (Fig. 4.14). When the radioulnar joint is involved, the patient is unable to supinate-pronate the forearm.

Even without roentgenographic confirmation, when the clinical manifestations of heterotopic bone formation are present, the joint involved should be kept in the best functional position when not being exercised, i.e., the elbow should be in 90 degrees of flexion. Further treatment consists of continuing physical therapy efforts at remobilization of the joint. With respect to the elbow, the heterotopic bone disappears spontaneously in about one-half of the cases. However, by six months it is unlikely that the calcification will resorb spontaneously and surgical excision should be considered. Preoperatively, a vigorous program of isometric exercises will help with active motion in the early postoperative period. Postoperatively, supervised active and passive exercises are essential and are begun on about the fourth postoperative day. Postburn heterotopic ossification usually does not reform after it has been surgically removed, but if it does, the ossification is usually not to the original extent.

REFERENCES

1. Achauer BM, Allyn PA, Furnas DW, et al: Pulmonary complications of burns: The major threat to the burn patient. *Ann Surg* 177:311, 1973.
2. Alexander JW: The body's response to infection. In Artz CP, Moncrief JA, Pruitt BA Jr: *Burns: A Team Approach.* Philadelphia, W.B. Saunders, 1979, p. 107.
3. Baxter CR: Crystalloid resuscitation of burn shock. In Polk HC Jr, Stone HH: *Contemporary Burn Management.* Boston, Little, Brown, 1971, p. 7.
4. Baxter CR: Topical use of 1.0% silver sulfadiazine. In Polk HC Jr, Stone HH: *Contemporary Burn Management.* Boston, Little, Brown, 1971, p. 217.
5. Berggren RB, Lehr HB: Clinical use of viable frozen human skin. *JAMA* 194:149, 1965.
6. Birke G, Liljedahl SO: Studies on burns. XV. Treatment with warm dry air, clinical results compared with those of earlier treatment series. *Acta Chir Scand (Suppl)* 422:1, 1971.
7. Bromberg BE, Song IC, Mohn MP: The use of pig skin as a temporary biological dressing. *Plast Reconstr Surg* 36:80, 1965.
8. Burke JF, Bondoc CC, Quinby WC: Primary burn excision and immediate grafting: A method shortening illness. *J Trauma* 14:389, 1974.
9. Burke JF, Quinby WC, Bondoc OC, et al: Immunosuppression and temporary skin transplantation in the treatment of massive third degree burns. *Ann Surg* 182:183, 1975.
10. Burke JF, Quinby WC Jr, Bondoc CC: Primary excision and prompt grafting as routine therapy for the treatment of thermal burns in children. *Surg Clin North Am* 56:477, 1976.
11. Burke JF, Yannas IV, Quinby WC Jr, et al: Successful use of a physiologically acceptable artificial skin in the treatment of extensive burn injury. *Ann Surg* 194:413, 1981.

12. Cotran RS, Remensnyder JP: The structural basis of increased vascular permeability after graded thermal injury—light and electron microscopic studies. *Ann NY Acad Sci* 150:495, 1968.

13. Curreri PW, Luterman A, Braun DW Jr, et al: Burn injury: Analysis of survival and hospitalization time for 937 patients. *Ann Surg* 192:472, 1980.

14. Dimick AR: Experience with the use of proteolytic enzyme (Travase) in burn patients. *J Trauma* 17:948, 1977.

15. Dinner MI, Peters CR, Sherer J: Use of a semipermeable polyurethane membrane as a dressing for split-skin graft donor sites. *Plast Reconstr Surg* 64:112, 1979.

16. Evans EB: Orthopaedic measures in the treatment of severe burns. *J Bone Joint Surg* 48A:643, 1966.

17. Evans EI, Purnell OJ, Robinett PW, et al: Fluid and electrolyte requirements in severe burns. *Ann Surg* 135:804, 1952.

18. Fidler JP, Law E, Rockwell RJ Jr, et al: Carbon dioxide laser excision of acute burns with immediate autografting. *J Surg Res* 17:1, 1974.

19. Georgiade NG, Harris WA: Open and closed treatment of burns with povidone-iodine. *Plast Reconstr Surg* 52:640, 1973.

20. Hartford CE: The bequests of Moncrief and Moyer: An appraisal of topical therapy of burns. *J Trauma* 21:827, 1981.

21. Hummel RP, Kautz PD, MacMillan BG, et al: The continuing problem of sepsis following enzymatic debridement of burns. *J Trauma* 14:572, 1974.

22. Janzekovic Z: A new concept in the early excision and immediate grafting of burns. *J Trauma* 10:1103, 1970.

23. Jelenko C III, Smulyan WI, Wheeler ML: VI: Studies in burns. The role of lipids in the transmissivity of membranes. *Ann Surg* 167:521, 1968.

24. Krizek TJ, Robson MC, Groskin MG: Experimental burn wound sepsis—evaluation of enzymatic debridement. *J Surg Res* 17:219, 1974.

25. Larson DL, Abston S, Evans EB, et al: Techniques for decreasing scar formation and contractures in the burned patient. *J Trauma* 11:807, 1971.

26. Lund CC, Browder NC: The estimation of areas of burns. *Surg Gynecol Obstet* 79:352, 1944.

27. MacMillan BG: Early excision. *J Trauma* 7:75, 1967.

28. Miller TA, Switzer WE, Foley FD, et al: Early homografting of second degree burns. *Plast Reconstr Surg* 40:117, 1967.

29. Monafo WW: Hypertonic sodium solutions for the treatment of burn shock. In Polk HC Jr, Stone HH: *Contemporary Burn Management.* Boston, Little, Brown, 1971, p. 33.

30. Monafo WW, Robinson HN, Yoshioka T, et al: Lethal burns: A progress report. *Arch Surg* 113:397, 1978.

31. Moncrief JA, Teplitz C: Changing concepts in burn sepsis. *J Trauma* 4:233, 1964.

32. Moncrief JA, Lindberg RB, Switzer WE, et al: Use of topical antibacterial therapy in the treatment of the burn wound. *Arch Surg* 92:558, 1966.

33. Moritz AR, Henriques FC Jr: Studies of thermal injury: II. The relative importance of time and surface temperature in the causation of cutaneous burns. *Am J Pathol* 23:695, 1947.

34. Moyer CA, Brentano L, Gravens DL, et al: Treatment of large human burns with 0.5% silver nitrate solution. *Arch Surg* 90:812, 1965.

35. Moyer CA, Margraf HW, Monafo WW Jr: Burn shock and extravascular sodium deficiency—Treatment with Ringer's solution with lactate. *Arch Surg* 90:799, 1965.

36. Moylan JA, Adib K, Birnbaum M: Fiberoptic bronchoscopy following thermal injury. *Surg Gynecol Obstet* 140:541, 1975.

37. Moylan JA Jr, Wilmore DW, Morton DE, et al: Early diagnosis of inhalation injury using [133]xenon lung scan. *Ann Surg* 176:477, 1972.

38. Mubarak SJ, Owen CA, Hargens AR, et al: Acute compartment syndromes: Diagnosis and treatment with the aid of the wick catheter. *J Bone Joint Surg* 60-A:1091, 1978.
39. Pennisi VR, Abril F, Capozzi A: The combined efficiency of Travase and silver sulfadiazine in the acute burn. *Burns* 2:169, 1976.
40. Polk HC Jr: Aqueous silver nitrate (0.5%) for topical wound care. In Polk HC Jr, Stone HH: *Contemporary Burn Management*. Boston, Little, Brown, 1971, p. 177.
41. Pruitt BA Jr: Complications of thermal injury. *Clin Plast Surg* 1:667, 1974.
42. Pruitt BA Jr, Stein JM, Foley FD, et al: Intravenous therapy in burn patients: Suppurative thrombophlebitis and other life-threatening complications. *Arch Surg* 100:399, 1970.
43. Recinos PR, Hartford CE, Ziffren SE: Fluid resuscitation of burn patients comparing a crystalloid with a colloid containing solution: A prospective study. *J Iowa Med Soc* 65:426, 1975.
44. Reckler JM, Mason AD Jr: A critical evaluation of fluid resuscitation in the burned patient. *Ann Surg* 174:115, 1971.
45. Reiss E, Stirman JA, Artz CP, et al: Fluid and electrolyte balance in burns. *JAMA* 152:1309, 1953.
46. Robson MC, Krizek TJ, Koss N, et al: Amniotic membranes as a temporary wound dressing. *Surg Gynecol Obstet* 136:904, 1973.
47. Rorabeck CH, Clarke KM: The pathophysiology of the anterior tibial compartment syndrome: An experimental investigation. *J Trauma* 18:299, 1978.
48. Shuck JM: The use of homografts in burn therapy. *Surg Clin North Am* 50:1325, 1970.
49. Shuck JM: Biologic dressings. In Artz CP, Moncrief JA, Pruitt BA Jr: *Burns: A Team Approach*. Philadelphia, W.B. Saunders, 1979, p. 211.
50. Tavis MJ, Thornton JW, Bartlett RH, et al: A new composite skin prosthesis. *Burns* 7:123, 1980.
51. Whitesides TE Jr, Haney TC, Harada H, et al: A simple method for tissue pressure determination. *Arch Surg* 110:1311, 1975.
52. Wilmore DW: Nutrition and metabolism following thermal injury. *Clin Plast Surg* 1:603, 1974.
53. Wilmore DW, Aulick LH: Metabolic changes in burned patients. *Surg Clin North Am* 58:1173, 1978.

5

Splinting and Positioning*

GERRY F. PULLIUM

Care of the burned injured patient traditionally has been directed at treatment of burn shock and prevention of sepsis. Advances in these areas have significantly reduced mortality and increased emphasis can now be placed on other aspects of early post-burn care. Burn shock and infection control continue to be primary concerns in the acute management, but function and cosmesis should also be addressed in this early post-burn period. An example of this increased emphasis has been the development of therapeutic positioning techniques for the acute period. Credit for the advancement of early splinting techniques properly belongs to Barbara Willis Galstaun, O.T.R., formerly of the Shriner's Burn Institute in Galveston, Texas. She pioneered this concept in the acute phase of burn care and most of the splinting techniques used today are based on her original work.

Functional loss and deformity are outcomes of burn injury which can be avoided with the prompt institution immediately after injury, of rehabilitation techniques. The positioning program is directed at preserving function, preventing contractures, and compensating for functional loss secondary to neurological deficit.

Positioning

Most burn patients develop contractures to some degree, therefore, an anticontracture positioning program is essential to offset the severity. Since scar contracture can cause permanent deformity and functional disability, immediate institution of proper positioning is imperative. Specific injury site and total body positioning are combined to control edema, maintain functional range of motion, and facilitate good wound care. Good positioning

---

* Illustrations by Mary Reid, O.T.R.—formerly an occupational therapist at Parkland Memorial Hospital.

is effective both when the patient is confined to bed and when the patient is active. Patients who can sit or walk accomplish their positioning programs in various planned activities.

One of the many values of an early positioning program is that of reducing edema in the extremities, thus allowing return to functional movement. Edema which may become organized can lead to freezing of the joints. Elevating the extremities allows reduction of edema, utilizing the pull of gravity.

Positioning also helps maintain range of motion throughout the acute burn period. When movement becomes painful, patients often assume positions of comfort which equate directly to positions of contracture. Often patients are hospitalized and bedridden for extended periods. In many instances, the severely burned patients are unable to feed themselves or attend to personal or grooming needs. Proper positioning can preserve a potential for functional return and counteract contracture by maintaining proper length of connective tissue and skin.

Positioning must be individualized to the patient needs, but in some cases, ideal positions must be compromised to achieve patient tolerance. A series of positions should be designed for each involved joint, whereby the patient alternates position every two to four hours, as static positioning is not well tolerated.

When skin grafts or biological dressings are required, specific positioning contributes to good wound coverage. When possible, the position chosen should incorporate the best aspects of positioning for wound care and for a good functional recovery.

Pain tolerances and positioning needs vary greatly among patients. Children usually have more difficulty understanding the long-range benefits of positioning procedures, and require constant patience and supervision. Often, splinting is the most appropriate and effective control for proper positioning, especially during unsupervised periods and during sleep, when deformity positions are often assumed. Conversely, adults may voluntarily maintain proper positioning when its purpose, method, and long-range benefits are thoroughly understood, except during sleep. When patients are unable or unwilling to cooperate in positioning regimens, 24-hour splinting is indicated to maintain anticontracture positioning. When the patient is able to be active during the day, night splinting may be indicated to maintain range of motion gained during the day.

Complications may impose limitations on the anticontracture positioning program. These include associated injuries sustained at the time of the burn injury, airway trauma, fractures, and other wounds. Pre-existing conditions may also complicate care, such as arthritis and neuromuscular deficits. The positioning regimen can also be compromised by the use of catheters and endotracheal tubes which restrict movement.

Since grafting and surgery are priority procedures, they often necessitate temporary curtailment of ideal positioning of involved body segments. Critical to the grafting success is postgraft positioning which may not coincide with the established positioning program. The proper graft positioning takes priority when a compromise cannot be attained.

Splinting

Splinting is an extension of therapeutic positioning in the acute burn period. Splinting is indicated when the patient cannot voluntarily maintain proper positioning, when voluntary positioning is ineffective, or when the patient must be immobilized, as after grafting procedures. Depending upon individual needs and functional range of motion, splinting can be instituted at any time in the acute burn period. Hands especially require immediate splinting to aid in edema resolution and to maintain functional joint position.

Peripheral neuropathies with loss of function may result from injury or dysfunction of the nervous system. Electrical trauma or pre-existing disease may cause neuromuscular deficit, and when voluntary movement is impaired, the area must be continuously splinted to avoid contracture formation.

Splints are also indicated for 24-hour wear with burn wound edema in the hands, exposed tendons, peripheral neuropathies and with uncooperative or unresponsive patients. Immediately following burn trauma, edema begins to form in the injured tissues and continues to accumulate for the next 24–72 hours. Therefore, 24-hour splints are applied to support the hand, and the extremity is elevated. Exposed tendons quickly become dry and denatured, and if stressed, may snap or rupture. They must be covered immediately with moist wraps or biological dressings to prevent drying, and positioned to prevent tension. The 24-hour splint maintains slack on the exposed tendon until wound closure occurs.

Optimal rehabilitative care requires frequent and thorough patient assessment. Splints must be checked at least once daily; 24-hour splints are checked at least three times per day. Assessment of the splint is made at each stage of removal and application to ensure proper fit and effectiveness in preventing deformity. Prior to removing the splint, the body part is observed for proper alignment of the splint; malfitting or improperly applied splints can result in pressure necrosis of burned and unburned areas. Range of motion is assessed when the splint is removed, as is the wound. Pain, numbness, tingling, inflammation, and wound masceration indicate that immediate adjustment is necessary to prevent further damage.

Acute Site by Site Positioning and Splinting

THE HAND

Edema—failure to decompress the hands in the first 48–72 hours can result in organized edema components creating a fixed deformity.

Full-thickness dorsal burns—failure to position the extensor mechanism on a slack may result in rupture of the mechanism, i.e., Boutonniere deformity.

Full- or partial-thickness volar burns—failure to provide a counter stretch to the granulating tissue may result in a palmar contracture.

Positioning Techniques

(1) The hand is positioned with a Kling roll supporting the transverse palmar arch, and the thumb is placed in abduction around the roll. The hand is then wrapped to secure this position. The extremity is elevated using an intravenous (I.V.) pole with Flexinet or stockinette for suspension.

(2) Alternate positioning methods for elevation include commercial positioning stands or stacked pillows.

Dorsal Surface Burns

Dorsal surface burns are the most commonly seen hand involvement. The extremity should be elevated and a volar positioning splint applied within 12–24 hours of admission. Excluding dressing changes, splints are worn until edema subsides. Splints are then worn for night positioning to preserve range of motion gained from daily exercise. Splinting is discontinued when the patient can actively achieve flexion to the midpalmar crease. Splint immobilization past this point may cause decreased strength and coordination, secondary to muscle imbalance.

Exposed Tendons on the Dorsal Surface

These occur during the acute period usually after eschar separation or tangential excision. The exposed tendon must be covered immediately with moist gauze or biological dressing to prevent drying and denaturation of the tendon. Continuous splinting is used to maintain the tendon in a slack position until permanent closure is obtained. Finger gutter splints (Fig. 5.1) are used if damage is limited to the extensor hood. If more extensive damage is apparent, a volar positioning splint is used. Immobilization of the hand for six weeks with involved fingers in extension will allow scar tissue to

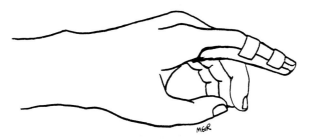

Figure 5.1. A finger gutter splint is shown.

form across the extensor surface. This will provide a substitute for the destroyed or damaged extensor mechanism.

Volar Surface Burns

Volar surface hand burns are more common in children, and usually result from touching a hot surface. The extremity is elevated and a dorsal positioning splint is applied. Dorsal positioning splints should be worn at night until healing is achieved.

Circumferential Full- and Partial-Thickness

The full- and partial-thickness circumferential burns that usually occur in large total body surface area burns are markedly edematous. During the first 72 hours, elevation of the upper extremities to aid in edema resolution is the most important consideration. The application of a volar positioning splint should be delayed until (1) Doppler ultrasonic flowmeter or palpation indicates that pulses are intact distally, (2) escharotomies are considered, and (3) fluid resuscitation is complete. Once applied, the volar positioning splint is worn continuously in the acute phase.

Volar Positioning Splint (Fig. 5.2)

This splint is designed to:
(1) preserve anatomical alignment.

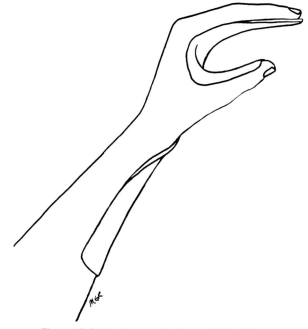

Figure 5.2. A volar positioning splint is shown.

(2) oppose patterns of contracture.

(3) aid in the resolution of edema.

Its design varies from one burn center to another but the fundamental positioning components are the same: (1) wrist extension, (2) metacarpophalangeal flexion, (3) proximal and distal interphalangeal extension, and (4) thumb in short abduction.

Construction. In the acute burn period, splints require frequent assessment and adjustment to ensure proper fit. For this reason, Orthoplast, a pliable, light-weight, low-heat thermoplastic material with good memory, is desirable. To construct the splint:

(1) A drawing of the patient's hand is made, identifying anatomical land marks.

(2) Using this pattern, the splint is cut from heated Orthoplast.

(3) While the material is warm and pliable, the splint is molded on the therapist's hand, or that of a suitable model, allowing for the difference in size.

(4) The splint is then fitted to the patient with any alterations made to ensure correct fit.

Correct Fit.

(1) The palmar arch is supported.

(2) Metacarpophalangeal joints are placed in flexion.

(3) The wrist is extended and ample depth is provided for the hypothenar eminence.

(4) The medial and lateral borders of the finger platform are precise in width.

(5) Splint modification is made to accommodate arterial or intravenous catheters.

(6) The proximal forearm and hypothenar edges are sufficiently flared to decrease edge effect.

Application.

(1) A topical agent is applied to the wound.

(2) Each finger is wrapped individually with gauze squares.

(3) A layer of fine mesh is placed in the splint to prevent masceration of burned and nonburned tissue.

(4) The splint is then placed on the patient and secured with a bandage wrap, using equal tension.

(5) Nail beds are left exposed to monitor circulation.

(6) Bulky dressings should be avoided as they interfere with the fit of the splint and compromise alignment.

Adjustment. As edema subsides in the acute period, splints require daily assessment and frequent alteration. Inspections are made at each dressing change and splint removal with routine alteration of the splint completed:

(1) The medial and lateral borders of the finger platform are trimmed.

(2) The palmar arch is increased.

(3) Bandaging techniques are assessed.

(4) Range of motion is assessed.

Pain, numbness, or masceration of good tissue indicate a malfitting or improperly applied splint. Immediate adjustment is mandatory to prevent further damage.

Dorsal Positioning Splint (Fig. 5.3)

This splint is designed to provide a stretch on contractile healing tissue.

Construction. To decrease the possibility of irritation and breakdown over bony prominences, this splint is molded directly on the patient. The splinting material should contour precisely and cool and harden rapidly. Polyflex and Kay Splint are good examples of the correct materials to use.

Correct Fit.

(1) The wrist is placed at 30 degrees of extension.

(2) Metacarpal and interphalangeal joints are placed in full extension.

Application. As with the volar positioning splint, bulky dressings should be avoided to ensure proper fit. It is secured with a Kling bandage wrap.

Adjustment. Red irritated areas over bony prominences usually indicate improper application. Volar surface burns are especially susceptible to

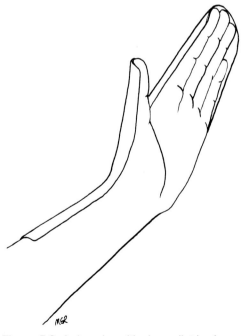

Figure 5.3. A dorsal positioning splint is shown.

contracture and should be monitored closely as healing occurs. Splint intervention methods for this problem will be discussed later in this chapter.

THE ELBOW

The optimal position is full extension and supination. Burns to the cubital fossa and circumferential burns to the extremity tend to produce flexion contractures. Prolonged elbow flexion can produce ulnar nerve neuropathy. Prolonged, forced elbow extension may contribute to the development of calcification in the elbow joint, producing extension contractures.

Positioning Techniques

Positioning equipment is utilized in the early acute stage for elevation to reduce edema and for anticontracture positioning throughout the patient's hospital stay:
   (1) A commercially available stand is bolted to the bed frame; it is adjustable in height and angle.
   (2) Over-bed tables can be utilized for voluntary positioning.
   (3) The patient should be provided with an alternate positioning schedule to ensure compliance with the program.
Positioning splints are indicated:
   (1) when the patient is unable to comply voluntarily with the positioning progam; this is often true of young children.
   (2) immobilization of the elbow is necessary following excisional therapy.
   (3) when the combined motions of elbow extension and forearm supination cannot be achieved actively in daily exercise periods.

Three-Point Extension Splint (Fig. 5.4)

This splint is described widely in the literature and utilized in the acute period as a night splint.
Construction.
(1) Two cuffs of splinting material are molded to conform to the anterior

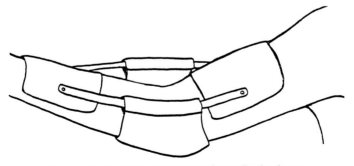

Figure 5.4. A three-point extension splint is shown.

surface of the upper arm and middle of the forearm in the neutral position.

(2) The two cuffs are bridged with two parallel aluminum bars riveted in place at the midpoint of each cuff.

(3) An adjustable strap secures the splint and leverage point at the posterior elbow.

Correct Fit.

(1) The splint is applied over dressings.

(2) The cuffs should distribute pressure over the maximum area.

(3) Strapping material should have some "give" to disperse pressure around the bony prominences of the elbow.

Application. The splint is applied over light dressings.

Posterior Elbow Extension Splint (Fig. 5.5)

This splint is used for immobilization following autografting or homografting to the anterior surface of the elbow.

Construction. The splint is molded on the patient prior to surgery.

Application. It is applied following surgery over bandages approximating the surgical dressing. The arm is positioned in the splint with full elbow extension and the forearm in the neutral position.

Anterior/Volar Conforming Splint (Fig. 5.6)

This splint is used in the subacute period when the patient cannot extend the elbow and supinate the forearm simultaneously. It is best tolerated by the patient if worn intermittently, four hours of wear followed by two hours of rest. Prolonged continous wear produces pain in the elbow joint and may contribute to an elbow extension contracture in circumferential burns.

Construction. It is molded directly on the extremity. To ensure total contact and distribute pressure evenly a malleable, fast-setting splint material, such as Polyflex, is recommended.

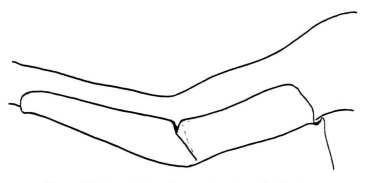

Figure 5.5. A posterior elbow extension splint is shown.

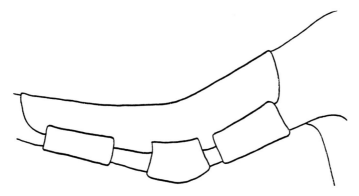

Figure 5.6. An anterior/volar conforming splint is shown.

Application. The splint is applied over a minimal layer of dressing. The elbow is positioned in extension, the forearm supinated, and the wrist slightly extended. The splint is secured with an ace bandage, wrapping distally to proximally, using equal tension.

THE SHOULDER AND AXILLA

The optimal position is 90 degrees of abduction and external rotation. Burns involving the axilla result in shoulder adduction contractures. Burns sparing the axilla, but involving the anterior chest and upper arm or lateral posterior trunk, may produce axillary banding in the normal skin with subsequent shoulder contracture. Prolonged prone positioning may result in brachial plexus injury. Abduction of the shoulder past 90 degrees for even brief periods in older patients may produce severe joint pain.

Positioning Techniques

(1) Commercial positioning stands may be utilized; they are adjustable to varying degrees of shoulder abduction. Strapping is included on the arm trough to restrain the unresponsive patient.

(2) Over-bed tables padded with bed pillows are useful for positioning when the patient is sitting in a chair.

(3) Simple shoulder boards, constructed in the hospital carpentry shop, are useful for voluntary positioning.

(4) A foam wedge (Fig. 5.7) may be used, the arm held in place with Velcro strapping inserted through slits in the foam. It remains fairly secure during ambulation. The wedge is available commercially or may be cut from a six-inch block of firm density foam.

Patients should be encouraged to include external rotation of the shoulder in the positioning schedule.

Positioning splints are indicated to:

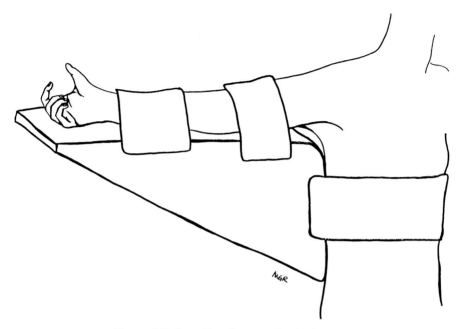

Figure 5.7. An axillary foam wedge is shown.

(1) facilitate axillary healing.
(2) immobilize and position the shoulder at 90 degrees of abduction after surgical excision and skin grafting to the axilla.
(3) maintain range of motion and axillary contour in children during the subacute period.

Weight-bearing Axillary Splint (See Fig. 5.25)

This splint is designed to immobilize the axilla in 90 degrees of abduction.
Construction.
(1) The splint is molded directly on the body while the patient is in a seated position.
(2) An arm trough is molded of fast setting material, such as Polyflex. It should be of sufficient length to displace pressure equally, but may or may not include the elbow, forearm, or wrist, depending upon the positioning goals.
(3) The trunk portion is molded of Polyflex as well, to extend around the trunk from the midline anteriorly to the midline posteriorly. Modification is made for the female breast.
(4) The trunk piece is held in place with an elastic wrap until the splinting material cools.
(5) The two sections are strapped in place. The trunk portion should be

secured with two broad straps around the trunk to prevent slippage and one strap across the opposite shoulder to decrease downward displacement.

(6) With the two sections in place, an aluminum support bar is cut and bent to the proper angle. Position for attachment of the bar is marked on the two sections. The sections are then removed and the bar riveted in place.

Correct Fit.

(1) The fit of this splint varies in sitting, lying, and standing positions. Strap adjustments, tightening and loosening, are made as the patient changes position.

(2) Padding may be added to the strapping and trunk piece to prevent irritation or pressure necrosis.

(3) The proximal portions of the arm trough and trunk piece should not interfere with areas to be skin grafted; the splint may require modification accordingly.

Conforming Axillary Splint (Fig. 5.8)

This splint is applied in the subacute period subsequent to decreased range of motion and the threat of axillary banding. It is most often used with young children. The splint may be worn continuously or for night positioning until the patient can actively achieve range of motion.

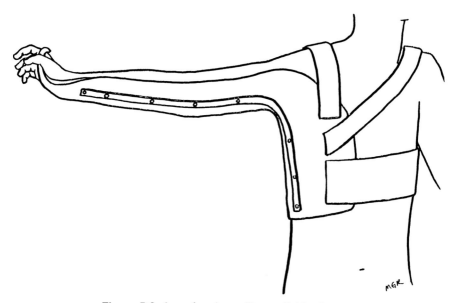

Figure 5.8. A conforming axillary splint is shown.

Construction.
(1) The splint is molded directly on the patient using precise contouring material. A perforated material is recommended as it allows some ventilation.
(2) The arm is positioned in 90 degrees or more of abduction; variable forward flexion may be included if the posterior axillary fold is the major involvement.
(3) Elbow and wrist extension should be incorporated in the splint if those joints are also involved.

THE TRUNK

The optimal position is straight body alignment, shoulder abduction, and neck extension. Improper body alignment discourages proper chest expansion. Improper positioning, sitting or lying, may contribute to rotation or curvature of the spine. Failure to stress proper body alignment throughout the acute and subacute periods may result in contractures and produce protraction of the shoulders and flexion of the neck.

Positioning Techniques

(1) A small towel roll is placed along the thoracic spine to promote scapular adduction and thoracic spine extension and provide stretch for the anterior chest.
(2) A double mattress is the most effective way to position the neck and anterior chest and it provides maximum stretch to the burned area. Care should be taken to avoid hyperextension of the neck in elderly patients who may have cervical spine abnormalities. Patients exhibiting respiratory complications should not be positioned with a double mattress.
(3) When sitting, a straight back chair should be used to provide support to the trunk.

THE HIP

The optimal position is full extension, no external rotation, and 20 degrees of abduction. Failure to position properly may lead to hip flexion, external rotation or adduction and knee flexion contractures. Failure to stress good body alignment throughout the acute and subacute periods may contribute to the development of scoliosis in children.

Positioning Technique

A triangular foam wedge (Fig. 5.9), purchased commercially or fabricated, is placed between the legs to provide hip abduction.

Hip Abduction Extension Splint (Fig. 5.10)

This splint is used primarily in children and indicated for:
(1) facilitating wound care.

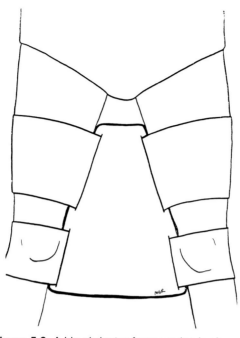

Figure 5.9. A hip abductor foam wedge is shown.

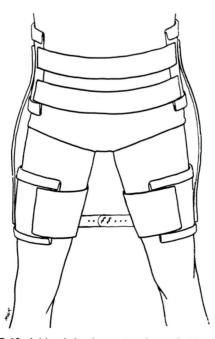

Figure 5.10. A hip abduction extension splint is shown.

(2) immobilizing following excisional therapy.

(3) preventing hip flexion contracture.

Construction.

(1) A body piece is molded around the posterior and lateral trunk and secured with a wide front closure.

(2) Two shells are molded to fit the lateral sides of the legs and secured.

(3) Two aluminum bars are measured and marked to join the body and leg shells at 15 degrees of abduction.

(4) The components of the splint are removed and rivets set. An additional bar is placed between the leg shells for reinforcement.

Correct Fit.

(1) The splint body and leg shells should be as broad as possible to distribute pressure evenly.

(2) The reinforcement bar can be made adjustable to vary the degree of abduction.

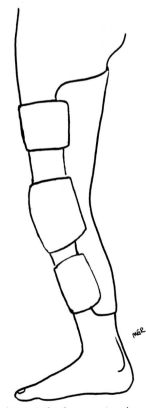

Figure 5.11. A posterior knee extension splint is shown.

THE KNEE

The optimal position is 0 degrees of extension. Failure to position in extension may produce knee flexion or hip flexion contracture. Continuous frog-lying position causes pressure or stretch on the peroneal nerve and may produce peroneal nerve palsy or "drop foot" with subsequent shortening of the Achilles tendon.

Positioning Techniques

(1) Trochanter rolls, used with voluntary positioning, are of some assistance in maintaining hip and leg alignment.

(2) To reduce edema, the foot of the bed is raised and two pillows supporting the lower leg but excluding the knee, encourage knee extension.

Posterior Knee and Three-Point Extension Splints (Figs. 5.11 and 5.12)

The criteria for use is essentially identical with that of the elbow, as are design and construction. Splint intervention is usually routine with young children but delayed in adults until specific problems threaten or voluntary positioning cannot be achieved.

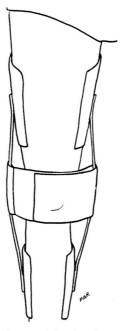

Figure 5.12. A three-point extension splint is shown.

THE ANKLE AND FOOT

The optimal position is 90 degrees dorsiflexion and 0 degrees inversion. Burns to the posterior leg and ankle and plantar foot tend to result in plantar flexion contractures with inversion of the foot. Burns to the anterior leg or ankle and dorsum of the foot may result in ankle dorsiflexion contracture with hyperextension of the toes. Failure to alternate positioning of circumferential burns to the feet and ankles usually results in contracture deformity.

Positioning Techniques

(1) Commercial splints consisting of a rigid plastic shell and contoured foam liner provide static ankle dorsiflexion. Soft straps secure the splint and some splints are equipped with a bar to prevent external hip rotation.

(2) When prone, the patient's feet and ankles should be positioned over the end of the mattress where they will drop in a near neutral position.

(3) When supine, pillows are placed under the posterior leg to prevent pressure necrosis to the heel.

Foot and ankle splints are indicated for:

(1) shortening of the Achilles tendon due to improper positioning.

(2) peroneal nerve palsy.

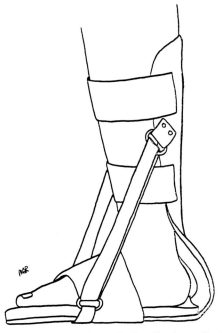

Figure 5.13. A posterior dynamic dorsiflexion splint is shown.

(3) intervention to prevent hyperextension and subluxation of the toes in the subacute period.

Posterior Dynamic Dorsiflexion Splint (Figs. 5.13 and 5.14)

This splint is utilized for:

(1) positioning the ankle at 90 degrees; elasticity allows dorsiflexion. Although it is not likely to cause pressure necrosis on the plantar surface of the foot, necessary precautions need to be observed.
(2) constant elastic tension which reduces plantar flexion contracture.
(3) positioning the entire lower extremity in combination with a posterior or three-point knee extension splint.

Construction.

(1) It may be molded directly on the patient or on a model with similar foot size.
(2) Padding is placed on the heel before molding to displace heel pressure in the finished splint.

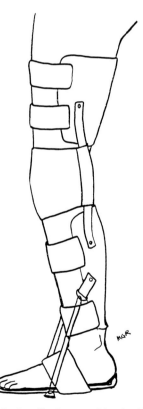

Figure 5.14. A posterior dynamic dorsiflexion combined with three-point knee extension splint is shown.

(3) With the ankle and foot positioned at neutral, heated splint material is drapped over the posterior leg and foot.

(4) The splint material is contoured to the leg and foot and the medial lateral borders at the ankle are rolled. This serves to clear the maleoli and acts as a reinforcement for the heel offset.

(5) If a model is used, the rough splint is then fitted on the patient to make any necessary fitting adjustments.

(6) The splint is trimmed.

(7) Wide strapping is applied across the leg, ankle, and foot. Strapping material should be soft and flexible to distribute pressure evenly over the bony prominences of the tibia and maleoli, and dorsum of the foot.

(8) "D" rings are attached to the leg and foot portions of the splint.

(9) Elastic or rubber tubing is threaded through the corresponding "D" rings which act as the dynamic component for dorsiflexion.

Correct Fit.

(1) The foot strap should be secured firmly or the leg portion will migrate downward and cause pressure on the heel.

(2) Elastic tension should be equal to prevent forefoot supination or pronation.

(3) Elastic tension should not exceed the amount required to put moderate stretch on the Achilles contracture. Excessive tension produces migration of the splint.

Sole Plate with Elastic Straps (Fig. 5.15)

This may be used in conjunction with a knee extension splint to position the knee, ankle, or foot.

Construction.

(1) Heated splinting material is molded directly on the patient with special care taken to contour the heel, instep, and metatarsal heads.

(2) When the material has cooled, the foot is outlined and excess material is trimmed.

(3) Strapping is applied over the instep and "D" rings added to the distal portion of the knee splint.

(4) Adhesive backed foam padding is used to line the splint and decrease any likelihood of skin breakdown.

Correct Fit.

(1) The same considerations apply as with the posterior dynamic dorsiflexion splint.

(2) A pillow should be placed under the posterior leg to clear the heel and keep it from touching the bed.

The sole plate may be used as a counter-resistive support if the patient tends toward metatarsal subluxation. The sole plate may be secured with

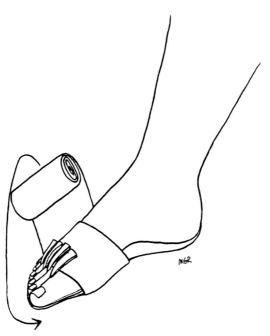

Figure 5.15. A method of securing sole plate and web spacers is shown.

an Ace bandage or straps (Fig. 5.15). Web spacers may be added to encourage toe separation and force skin excursion on the dorsum of the foot.

Total Contact Sandal (Fig. 5.16)

Ambulation provides a major tool to counteract the debilitating effects of immobilization. Mild to moderate burns to the foot do not preclude the early institution of gait. Dressings with extra padding aid in reducing the discomfort of weight bearing. Full-thickness burns, or tissue deficits, such as those produced by electrical injury, do require special attention. Total contact sandals distribute the weight of the body over the entire plantar surface of the foot. If a tissue defect is present, displacement of the material into the defect decreases the possibility of graft loss.

Construction.
(1) The patient is seated in a chair and the foot is placed on a piece of four to six inches of soft density foam.
(2) A piece of soft density Plastazote, four inches by 12 inches, by one-half inch is cut and placed in an oven.
(3) The material is heated for three minutes at 300° Farenheit, removed from the oven, and placed on the foam cushion.
(4) The patient's foot is immediately placed on the Plastazote and pressed downwards at two points, at the knee and the top of the

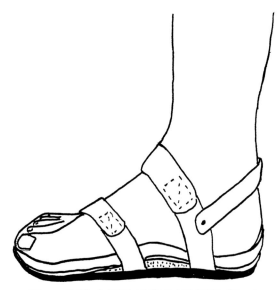

Figure 5.16. A total contact sandal is shown.

foot. The pressure may be released after approximately 10 seconds, but the foot should be held in place for three minutes, allowing the Plastazote to set.

(5) The outline of the foot is traced, the Plastazote removed, and the excess trimmed.

(6) The molded Plastazote insole is placed on the foot and strap placement marked.

(7) Straps are then glued to the bottom of the insole.

(8) A mixture of six tablespoons of cork dust and one tablespoon of liquid latex is applied to the bottom surface of the insole for leveling. This is allowed to dry overnight.

(9) The bottom of the insole is buffed until level.

(10) An undersole of one-quarter inch microcellular rubber is then glued to the molded insole.

(11) The sandal is ready for wear when the patient is medically cleared for ambulation. Ace wraps are used to provide vascular support to the feet and legs.

Convalescent Phase

With closure of the burn wound, the burn victim enters the convalescent phase of care. During this period, the transition from hospitalization to home care is made and the long process of re-establishing a suitable life style is begun. Throughout this phase, the burn wound remains a focal point in patient care. Initially, wound management is directed at two inter-related concerns, skin care and scar control. A third aspect of care during the convalescent phase involves the prevention and/or correction of functional deficits.

Contractile bands of scar tissue crossing joints, hypertrophic scar and neurological deficits are frequent causes of functional disability in the convalescent period. Exercise techniques and early institution of gradient pressure are important in limiting the risk of functional deficits as scarring develops. However, many problems require specialized splinting to correct or avert deficits. Specialized splinting employed when problems first become apparent can prevent contracture by decreasing band formation. It can also be used to reduce existing contracture and, therefore, preclude or minimize the need for extensive reconstructive surgery. When splinting is indicated, the following factors must be considered:

(1) Skin readiness—The newly healed skin must be assessed to determine whether or not it can tolerate shear force and pressure, and if so, for what periods of time.

(2) Location—The contracture or band formation must be evaluated to determine if it would respond better to constant static pressure or dynamic tension and stretch.

(3) Priorities—If there are conflicting deformities requiring equal attention, a priority must be established in the treatment plan.

(4) Patient acceptance—The patient must fully understand the purpose of the device and be able to live with the restriction and cosmetic appearance.

(5) Muscle imbalance—The exercise program must effectively compensate for prolonged immobilization.

CONFORMING SPLINTS

Conforming splints are utilized primarily on flexor surfaces. Patients who are developing contractures or banding over the volar aspect of the hand, wrist, elbow, posterior knee, or dorsum of the ankle and foot are fitted with conforming splints to oppose contracture formation. Frequently, these splints are worn at night only, and the patient is encouraged to use the part actively during the day.

Splinting material is heated and then molded directly on the patient for maximum contact with the scar or band formation. The hard, nonyielding pressure exerted by conforming splints produces a softening and flattening effect on the scar band, which then allows increased skin excursion.

In the event of existing deformity, conforming splints may be used for nonsurgical correction of contracture. The splints are designed to apply maximum tension and constant pressure to the contracture. As the contracture resolves, the splint is remolded progressively until proper alignment of the part is achieved. These splints are worn for 24-hour periods with biweekly serial adjustments. The splints should be removed four to six times daily for exercise, skin care, and splint cleaning.

DYNAMIC SPLINTS

Dynamic splinting is the most effective method of correcting contractures involving the extensor surfaces of the wrist, hand, and posterior elbow. The superficiality of the extensor tendons to the burned surface may result in scar adhesions forming around or attaching to the tendon. Dynamic splints, which apply elastic tension in opposition to the contracture, but allow controlled resistive motion, force excursion of the tendon through the scar formation.

PROBLEM-ORIENTED SPLINTING

Specialized splints are utilized for problems encountered in the convalescent period. All are subject to modification or innovation as dictated by individual need. Only the more commonly seen problems are addressed and the appropriate splint described.

Wrist/Palm Contracture (Fig. 5.17)

Splint   Palmar conforming splint
Purpose   Prevent flexion contracture of wrist and fingers

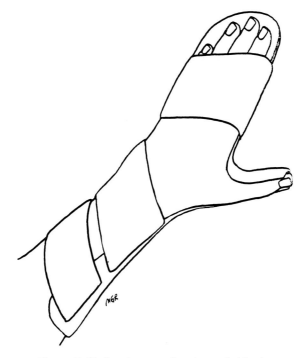

Figure 5.17. A palmar conforming splint is shown.

Optimal position	Wrist in maximum extension
	Fingers in maximum extension
Wear	At night for maintenance
	Continuous as tolerated for serial management

Hand/Wrist Radial Contracture (Fig. 5.18)

Splint	Radial wrist conformer with thumb and index finger
	Thumb web space (Fig. 5.19)
Purpose	Decrease existing contracture
	Increase thumb web space
Optimal position	Maximum ulnar deviation with contour to thumb
	web space
Wear	At night

First and Fifth Finger Palmar Contracture (Fig. 5.20)

| Splint | First and fifth palmar conformer |
| Purpose | Prevent cupped hand deformity |

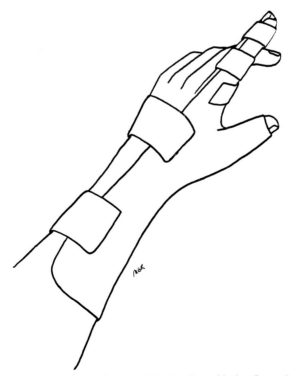

Figure 5.18. A radial wrist conformer with thumb and index finger is shown.

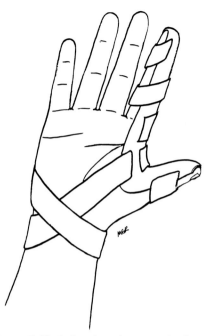

Figure 5.19. A thumb web spacer is shown.

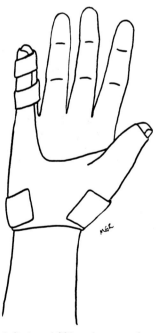

Figure 5.20. A first and fifth palmar conformer is shown.

	Decrease existing contracture
Optimal position	Finger in maximum extension
	Thumb in maximum abduction and extension
Wear	At night for maintenance
	Continuous as tolerated for serial management

Dorsal Hand Burn/Extension of Metacarpophalangeal (MCP) Joint (Figs. 5.21 and 5.22)

Splint	Cock-up with MCP cuffs
	Cock-up with flexion wrap
	Nail hooks may be added to include flexion of proximal interphalangeal (PIP) and distal interphalangeal (DIP) joints
Purpose	Increase flexion of MCP joints
Optimal position	Wrist at 0
	Elastic tension to tolerance for flexion
Wear	Continuous as tolerated

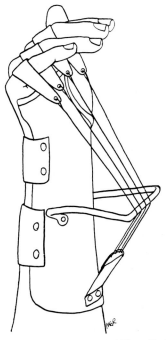

Figure 5.21. A cock-up with MP cuffs is shown.

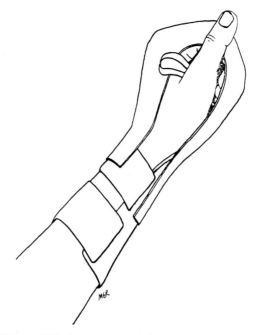

Figure 5.22. A cock-up with flexion wrap is shown.

Extension Contracture of PIP/DIP Joints (Fig. 5.23)

Splint	Wrist cock-up with nail hooks
Purpose	Increase joint range of motion
Optimal position	Wrist at 0
	MCP joints blocked at 10 degrees flexion
Wear	Continuous as tolerated

Individual finger flexion contracture

Splint	Finger guard (See Fig. 5.1)
	Fifth finger extension splint (Fig. 5.24)
Purpose	Prevent finger flexion contracture and banding
	Decrease existing contracture
Optimal position	Finger in maximum extension
Wear	Continuous as tolerated for serial management
	At night for maintenance

Elbow/Axillary Contracture (Fig. 5.25)

Splint	Segmental axillary/elbow splint
Purpose	Serial management of elbow and axillary contracture
	Increase external rotation of the shoulder

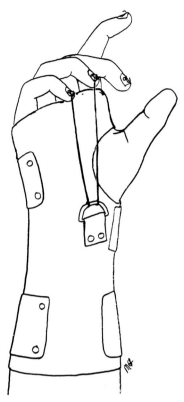

Figure 5.23. A wrist cock-up with nail hooks is shown.

Optimal position	Shoulder at 90 to 100 degrees abduction
	Elbow in maximum extension
Wear	Continuous as tolerated for serial management

Elbow Extension Contracture (Fig. 5.26)

Splint	Dynamic elbow flexion splint
Purpose	Increase elbow flexion
Optimal position	Maximum flexion
	30 to 40 degrees flexion required for splint application
Wear	Continuous as tolerated

Elbow Flexion Contracture (See Fig. 5.6)

Splint	Elbow extension conformer splints
Purpose	Pressure to control contracture
	Maintain elbow extension

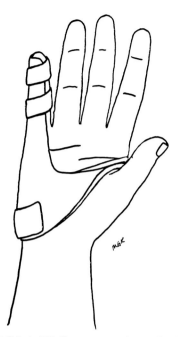

Figure 5.24. A fifth finger extension splint is shown.

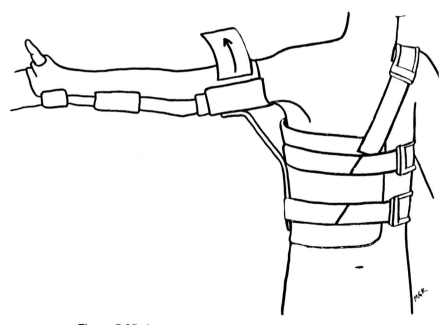

Figure 5.25. A segmental axillary/elbow splint is shown.

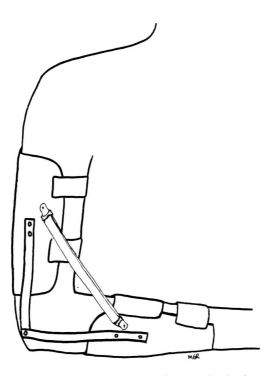

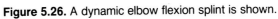

Figure 5.26. A dynamic elbow flexion splint is shown.

	Serially decrease existing contracture
Optimal position	Maximum extension
	Contact with scar band
Wear	Continuous as tolerated for serial management
	At night for maintenance

Knee Flexion Contracture/Skin Banding (See Fig. 5.11)

Splint	Posterior knee conformer
Purpose	Control band formation
	Serially decrease contracture
Optimal position	Knee at 0 degrees extension
	Contact with scar band
Wear	At night

Anterior Foot/Ankle Burn/Subluxation of Metatarsals (Fig. 5.27)

Splint	Anterior conformer with metatarsal bar
Purpose	Prevent dorsiflexion contracture

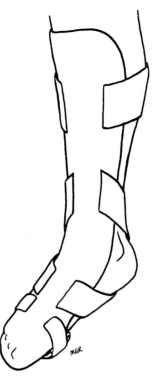

Figure 5.27. An anterior conformer with metatarsal bar is shown.

	Prevent hyperextension of toes
	Serially correct subluxation of metatarsal joint
Optimal position	Maximum plantar flexion
	Conforming pressure to ankle and dorsum of foot
Wear	At night

Loss of function and deformity are avoidable outcomes of burn injury in most instances, provided there is intervention in the early acute period and follow-up throughout the convalescent periods with aggressive and individualized positioning and splinting programs. These can preserve function and prevent or minimize scar contracture deformity. As with any aspect of the rehabilitation plan, all personnel, the patient, and his family cooperate in ensuring compliance with the positioning and splinting program for successful functional and cosmetic outcome.

ADDITIONAL READINGS

1. Bruster J, Pullium G: Segmental axillary splinting. Abstract. *Am Burn Assoc*, p. 97, March, 1980.
2. Drury FA, Burke JE, Nelson MK, et al: Construction of Sandals for Prevention of Injuries

to Insensitive Feet. Social Rehabilitation Service, Department of HEW, Washington, DC, 1969.

3. Fess E, Gettle K, Strickland J: *Hand Splinting Principles and Methods*. St. Louis, C. V. Mosby, 1981.

4. Head MD, Pullium G, Nothdurft D, et al: Thermal injury: Therapeutic exercise in the acute period. A slide tape presentation developed by the Texas Regional Burn Care System, Dallas, 1979.

5. Head MD, Pullium G, Nothdurft D, et al: Thermal injury: Positioning in the acute period. A slide tape presentation developed by the Texas Regional Burn Care System, Dallas, 1978.

6. Helm PA, Kevorkian CG, Lushbaugh M, et al: Burn injury: Rehabilitation management in 1982. *Arch Phys Med Rehab* 63:6–16, 1982.

7. Larson DL, Abston S, Evans EB, et al: Techniques for decreasing scar formation and contracture in the burn patient. *J Trauma* 11:807–823, 1971.

8. Lushbaugh M, Nothdurft D, Pullium G, et al: Thermal injury: Convalescent phase rehabilitation. A slide tape presentation developed by the Texas Regional Burn Care System, Dallas, 1979.

9. Malick MH: *Manual on Dynamic Hand Splinting with Thermoplastic Materials*. Pittsburgh, Harmarville Rehabilitation Center, 1974.

10. Malick MH: *Manual on Static Hand Splinting—New Materials and Techniques*. Pittsburgh, Harmarville Rehabilitation Center, 1974.

11. Nothdurft D, Pullium G, Bruster J: Management of feet and ankle burns. *J Int Soc Burn Inj* 5:221, 1970.

12. Pullium G, Nothdurft D, Head MD, et al: Thermal injury: Principles of splinting in the acute period. A slide tape presentation developed by the Texas Regional Burn Care System, Dallas, 1978.

13. Redford JB (Ed): *Orthotics Etcetera*. Baltimore, Williams & Wilkins, 1980.

14. Weeks PM, Wray RC: *Management of Acute Hand Injuries: Biological Approach*, Ed 3. St. Louis, C.V. Mosby, 1978.

15. Willis G: Follow-up: Use of Orthoplast splints in treatment of acutely burned child. *Am J Occup Ther* 24:187–191, 1970.

16. Willis G: Use of Orthoplast isoprene splints in treatment of acutely burned child: Preliminary report. *Am J Occup Ther* 23:57–61, 1969.

17. Wynn-Parry CB: Restoration of hand function: Rehabilitation of the injured hand. *Trans Med Soc Lond* 90:101–104, 1974.

6

Exercise and Treatment Modalities

DONNA NOTHDURFT
PATRICIA S. SMITH
JEAN E. LeMASTER

Introduction

Physical treatment, including exercise and the use of specific therapeutic modalities, is a key element in a burn patient's reach toward functional recovery. It is imperative that these physical treatment programs be carefully integrated into the total rehabilitation effort. Although individuals with expertise in the area of physical medicine hold primary responsibility for implementation of these programs, optimal physical restoration will largely depend upon the combined and concentrated efforts of all team members, the patient, and his family.

The goal of the patient's treatment program is restoration of optimal function as quickly as possible. This is accomplished by a coordinated program to assist and augment the surgical care. Treatment protocols have been developed by observing the deformities resulting from inadequately treated burns and then "working backward" to devise programs to prevent these expected deformities which often lead to functional impairment (9).

It is the focus of this chapter to provide guidelines for the use of exercise and modalities in the physical treatment of burn injuries in order to maximize the patient's functional ability in the home and community. Therapeutic exercise is addressed initially as it is a major thrust of treatment throughout all phases of burn rehabilitation. The use of therapeutic modalities, primarily associated with the post-acute phase of rehabilitation, is discussed in detail later in the chapter.

Planning an Exercise Program

Many factors influence the therapist's ability to provide adequate exercise for the victim of burn injury. The severe pain of the burn wound is a major factor. Surgical procedures, wound complications, and patient and family adjustment to the injury affect therapy. The therapist's skill in timing the initiation of exercise, choosing the type of exercise, and the timely transferring of care to the patient and family are important to the level of function attained and the duration of the rehabilitation program.

The consequences of patient immobilization imposed by the burn injury are additional factors which must be considered when designing an exercise program. These consequences often include decreased cardiovascular fitness, disuse osteoporosis, increased risk of thromboemboli, pulmonary complications, decubiti, and muscle atrophy (21). Positions of comfort are the patient's natural reaction to the pain imposed by the burn injury. The patient tends to avoid movement, or at best, movement is rigid and slow. Planned exercise programs, therefore, are needed to prevent undesirable burn wound healing sequelae.

Exercise prescription is an ongoing process which is altered according to the patient's medical status and changing needs. Reviewing past medical history provides the therapist with a general idea of potential complications, procedures which need emphasis, the amount of time required per treatment session, and probable degree of participation by the patient. The exercise program is then tailored to meet the individual patient needs.

The treatment regimens used in burn care are not in themselves unusual or difficult. Providing these regimens in the constantly changing physiological and psychological milieu of the burn patient is the challenging task. The therapist must establish clear and reasonable goals, yet must be flexible in choosing the means to achieve them. It is best to prepare for the unexpected and keep the treatment program open for review. Even the patient with a small localized area burn can become a difficult management problem when wound complications, or the patient's reaction to the injury, are unusual. A few standard exercise regimens and principles can be followed, but the therapist's imagination is needed to elicit patient motivation in the presence of the painful burn injury. Adding humor, variety, and quiet conversation times keeps the treatment sessions more agreeable to both the patient and therapist.

EXERCISE DURING THE EMERGENT PERIOD

During the emergent period, exercise goals are (1) resolution of edema, (2) maintenance of joint mobility, and (3) prevention of respiratory complications. The patient's medical status is assessed daily, prior to the initiation of any physical treatment. During the resuscitation period, emphasis of treatment is placed on positioning and splinting. However, if the patient is alert, he may be able to engage in some movement activities such as bed mobility and positioning of extremities for dressing applications. As soon as adequate signs of burn shock resuscitation have been observed, generally within the first 24–72 hours after injury, exercise is initiated for most patients.

Guidelines in the literature are vague as to the optimal intensity, duration, and type of exercise which a severely ill person can tolerate without detrimental effects. Careful observation of vital signs is imperative upon initiation of an exercise program. Poor tolerance of exercise may be indicated by dyspnea, rapid respiration, diaphoresis, immediate increase of over 20 mm Hg systolic blood pressure and tachycardia. Many of these stress responses are also triggered by other conditions such as poor nutritional status, hypermetabolism, fluid and electrolyte imbalance, anxiety, infection, age, and environmental status. When these responses become apparent upon initiation of exercise, positioning and splinting remain the primary focus of treatment.

During the emergent period, resolution of edema is imperative. The presence of edema compromises circulation as well as joint mobility. In the presence of deep burns and circumferential injury, thick inelastic eschar often necessitates escharotomy in order to release pressure allowing outward expansion of underlying tissues. Escharotomies do not preclude exercise, however. Gentle passive and active assistive range of motion is encouraged two to four times daily for maintenance of joint mobility (Fig. 6.1).

In the absence of escharotomy, frequent intermittent periods of slow, gentle active or active assistive motion are preferred. The pumping action of muscular contraction facilitates reduction of edema. Caution is taken in cases where deep burns are circumferential as vigorous active motion may further constrict the already compromised circulatory status. Rapid passive stretching techniques are also avoided as they might cause bacteria from an infected area to enter the blood stream (12).

In conjunction with exercise, elevation of edematous parts is crucial as long as swelling persists. Edema fluid has a high protein component which can congeal, thereby preventing joint mobility when it surrounds joint capsules, ligaments, and other fibrous structures. If not quickly resolved, edema often leads to fibrous ankylosis of joints. Light compressive dressings in conjunction with splinting during periods of elevation also aids in edema resolution.

During the emergent period, special attention to certain medical conditions is required. For example, inhalation injury can cause mild to severe bronchial and alveolar changes which interfere with respiratory function. Inhalation injury, edema formation, and constricting eschar of the neck can obstruct the trachea necessitating intubation and mechanical ventilation. Physical therapists or respiratory therapists, in conjunction with the nursing staff, provide pulmonary hygiene through postural drainage, with percussion, vibration, and suctioning. When the patient requires ventilation, the frequency of treatment is usually every four hours. Another respiratory concern includes possible mechanical restriction of deep breathing due to pain or constricting circumferential eschar of the chest. The physical therapist assists this type of patient in deep breathing and coughing exercises three to four times a day. For some patients, an incentive spirometry device is used five to ten times an hour to help prevent atelectasis as well

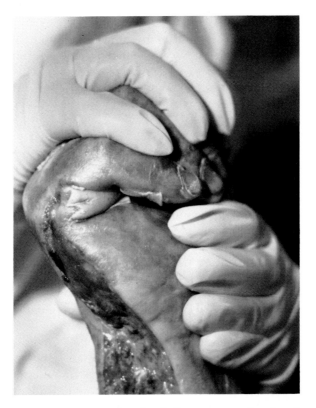

Figure 6.1. Active assisted range of motion in the presence of escharotomy is shown.

as to exercise respiratory muscles. In all respiratory treatment, the frequency and focus of treatment depends on lung field auscultation, the patient's response to treatment, and the patient's activity level.

Caution is taken in implementing exercise programs for patients with cardiac involvement. Even passive range of motion, positioning, and splinting may increase stress levels for these patients. Stress reactions are often characterized by premature ventricular contractions observed on the cardiac monitor and rapid changes in pulse. For these reasons, the patient with cardiac involvement is carefully monitored.

In the presence of tracheostomy, cutdowns, and conditions requiring intravenous and arterial catheterization, exercise may be contraindicated. Exercises which would compromise or dislodge lines and airways are withheld and emphasis is placed on positioning.

Medical treatments and procedures remain the priority in the emergent phase. However, physical measures to resolve edema, maintain joint range of motion, and prevent respiratory complications can often be executed without interfering with necessary lifesaving measures in this phase.

ACUTE REHABILITATIVE EXERCISE

As the patient makes the transition from the emergent phase to the acute phase of burn rehabilitation, the physical treatment program must also change to meet the patient's needs. The acute phase generally refers to the time period after emergent care through wound coverage, when the foundations of scarring are just beginning to form. Functional impairment is a major threat during this period.

Therapeutic exercise comprises one of the most important factors in preventing functional loss. Goals of exercise during this phase of burn rehabilitation include:

(1) stretching of healing skin;
(2) maintaining full joint range of motion;
(3) preserving motor skill coordination;
(4) promoting functional independence;
(5) maintaining strength and endurance to minimize muscular atrophy.

Three primary techniques are used to accomplish these goals of exercise during acute rehabilitation: (1) range of motion exercises, (2) participation in activities of daily living (ADL), and (3) ambulation. The use of these techniques follows a natural progression into later stages of rehabilitation. Integration of exercise techniques throughout the rehabilitative effort greatly minimizes the long-term consequences of burn injury.

Many factors influence the degree to which the exercise regimens can be accomplished in the acute phase. When burn wound edema is resolved, range of motion exercise is directed at maintaining full joint mobility. Gently stretching the wound surface, preventing adherence or shortening of tendons and preventing tightening of capsular structures aid in minimizing potential contractures. Patients can be assisted with their exercise programs two to four times daily by the therapist (Fig. 6.2). Patients with severe injury only tolerate very brief exercise sessions, and if so, sessions should be more frequent.

In addition to sessions with the therapist, specific exercises are also taught to the patient to be performed at prescribed intervals in the therapist's absence. Unless carefully instructed, the patient may elect to engage in those exercises he can most easily perform, often favoring muscles that contribute to contracture formation. Unnecessary and undesirable exercises can needlessly exhaust the patient.

Energy expenditure and nutritional requirements are major considerations when planning an exercise program. The nutritional requirements of burn patients are considerably increased. Weight loss and muscle atrophy are difficult to prevent during acute rehabilitation when the patient is in a catabolic state. Recognized physical therapy measures commonly used for rehabilitation and strengthening are too excessive for the severely burned. Expenditures of energy, therefore, should be limited to maintaining range

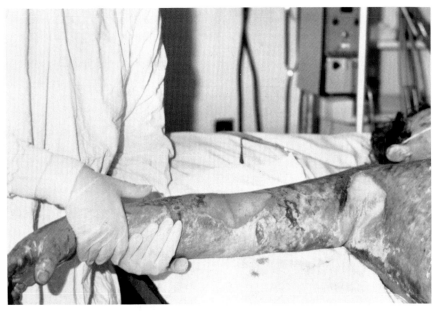

Figure 6.2. Patient is assisted with exercise at bedside early in the acute phase of rehabilitation.

of motion of involved joints, simple ADL, and functional ambulation early in the acute phase of rehabilitation (1). Because the nutritional status of a patient takes medical precedence, unless the aim of treatment is providing increased mobility for independent feeding, exercise therapy never interferes with mealtime.

Exercise is best tolerated after the wound has been cleansed and a topical cream or biological dressing has been applied. The topical agents generally promote pliability of the wound surface, thereby decreasing pain associated with stretching. Dressings applied over topical agents affect range of motion if they have been applied in such a way as to restrict or resist motion, or if they bridge joints. Whenever possible, dressings over joints should be loose and applied with minimal bulk.

Occasionally, range of motion exercises are performed during hydrotherapy. Advantages to brief periods of exercise during hydrotherapy include (1) reduced pain and the relaxation effects of warm water, (2) reduced energy expenditure and ease of exercise due to buoyancy of limbs, and (3) increased wound observation.

Traditionally, exercise is accomplished at the patient's bedside during the acute phase of rehabilitation. Active exercise by the patient and active assistive exercise by the patient and therapist are encouraged during this phase of burn care. Exercises are performed with each isolated joint through

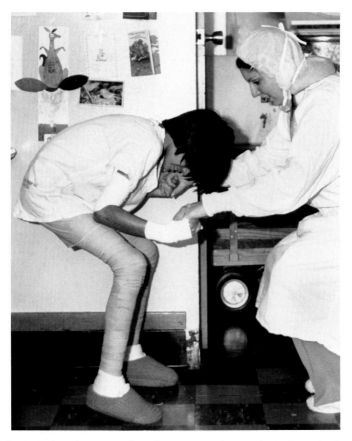

Figure 6.3. Limitations in range of motion are noted as patient attempts the multiple joint motion of deep knee bends.

appropriate planes of motion attempting completion of motion through the entire range permitted by the joint. Overall patterns of motion for groups of joints are then encouraged emphasizing gentle sustained stretch for each burned area. Even though the patient may have normal range in each isolated joint, he may be limited when a coordinated overall pattern of motion is attempted (Fig. 6.3). This limitation is due to the scar tissue involving multiple joints. However, multiple vigorous repetitions of movement should be avoided.

Active and active assistive range of motion with terminal stretch aids in maintaining joint mobility and tissue pliability as well as minimizing loss of strength and preventing osteoporosis. When the patient complains of pain, exercise is discontinued briefly and the source of the pain is determined. Pain may or may not be a contraindication for exercise.

The most common complaints of pain are described by the patients as a stinging or pulling pain, originating near the wound surface, associated with stretching of the contractile healing tissues. In these instances, repetition of exercise is indicated and is performed within the patient's tolerance. At the limit of maximum achievable range, the body segment is held for a slow count of 10. If the pain decreases or subsides, the wound bed may continue to be stretched until pain recurs. Care is taken during active assistive stretching exercise since vigorous stretch, overstretching the wound to achieve full range of motion, can traumatize tissues and even cause wound separation.

When a patient complains of deep joint pain instead of pain associated with skin stretching, radiological and other diagnostic tests are indicated. If pathological conditions of the joint are verified, exercise may be contraindicated. If exercise is permitted, it is only performed within the patient's pain-free range to avoid additional joint trauma.

Coordinating administration of pain medications with the nursing staff prior to exercise sessions greatly enhances the quality of exercise and amount of cooperation offered by the patient. A patient who anticipates pain generally becomes uncooperative, resistive, and often fearful of exercise. It is helpful, for patient relaxation, to initiate the exercise treatment with nonpainful or less painful exercises and gradually progress to the more painful.

Children exhibit increased pain reactions during exercise, often due to fear and apprehension. Most young children do not understand the need for exercise and potential consequences of immobility. "Simon Says" and other play and group activities are fun and allow children increased control. Play is perhaps the best method to elicit desired active movement in young children (Fig. 6.4).

It is crucial that the therapist and patient establish a positive and effective working rapport. The patient must be carefully guided in his exercise program. Type and duration of exercises are thoroughly explained, purposes defined, and long-term benefits discussed. The patient should be an active participant in planning his exercise program, and he should be taught how to incorporate exercises into his daily activities.

Emotional support of the patient is essential from all team members. "Lending an ear" and spending a little extra time with the patient is necessary to gain an understanding of his behavior. Most patients have had no experience with burn injuries and are not always able to make decisions in their best interest. As treatment progresses, the team must be prepared to deal with the patient's denials and misconceptions about his burn injury. The therapist plays a major role in fostering positive attitudes toward exercise. Verbal praise and reinforcement are appropriate and encouraged when the patient performs adequately.

Active and active assistive exercise may provide emotional support for the patient. When the patient recognizes his ability to move and the degree to which he can move his body, he begins to develop feelings of reassurance and self-confidence.

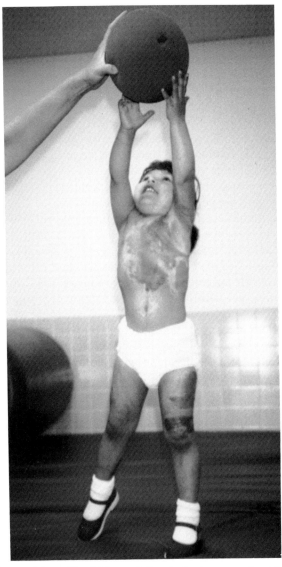

Figure 6.4. Play activity with children elicits desired range of motion and fosters positive attitudes towards exercise.

Although active and active assistive exercises are preferable during acute rehabilitation, they are not always appropriate. There are internal and external factors which influence the appropriateness and type of exercise prescribed.

Contraindications of Exercise

Some conditions preclude therapeutic exercise altogether. The use of subeschar clysis is one such condition. Any type of exercise can cause dislodging or movement of the clysis needles and interrupt flow of the lines. Positioning, as possible, should be stressed. Areas not directly involved in clysis procedures, however, should continue to be gently exercised as long as disturbance of needles is avoided and the patient is emotionally receptive.

Patients who have been diagnosed with thrombophlebitis are confined to bed. All exercise is withheld due to the increased chance of dislodging a thrombus. Exercise should be resumed only with approval from the medical staff.

Joints fixated by skeletal traction or pinning cannot be exercised. However, adjacent joints must continue to be exercised as long as fixated joints are not disturbed and medical clearance is obtained.

Indications for Passive Range of Motion

Critically ill, septic, and heavily medicated patients are often unable to cooperate in active or active assistive exercise. Depending on the medical status, passive exercise may or may not be indicated. Proper positioning continues to be emphasized.

With unresolved edema, only gentle active and passive range of motion as tolerated is implemented in conjunction with a program of elevation.

Some topical creams inhibit active motion. Pain associated with the application of some topicals such as mafenide and povidone-iodine make the patient fearful and resistive toward exercise. In deep thermal burns, povidone-iodine is sometimes used presurgically to harden eschar for easier removal. Exercise is generally inappropriate during this time period; however, in some cases, gentle passive motion is encouraged.

When energy expenditure is of major concern, passive exercise is preferred over active and active assistive exercises. When passive exercise is provided, it incorporates the principles of progressive gentle stretching of burned tissues as the joints are guided through range of motion. Care must be taken in performance of passive exercise to avoid connective tissue tears, joint dislocation, pathological fractures, and overstretch of ligamentous and capsular structures.

Patients with peripheral nervous system involvement may be physically unable to move body parts independently. In the presence of neuropathic problems, special attention to involved muscles is required. Due to absence of normal power or muscle contraction, active assistive and passive range of motion should be instituted to retain joint mobility until recovery or nerve regeneration occurs. Specialized splinting is generally required to prevent contracture formation. Appropriate timing of coordination and strengthening activities as well as use of electrical stimulation, referred to in the modalities section of this chapter, are essential. A carefully planned program is imperative early in rehabilitation in order for the neurologically involved patient to reach functional recovery.

In the presence of exposed tendons or joint capsules, exercise is implemented with caution. Exposed tendons or capsules must be protected from drying, denaturation, and potential rupture by the use of moist soaks or biological dressings. Gentle passive exercise is suggested if the tendon appears viable in order to preserve tendon glide. Splints are generally used during nonexercise periods to immobilize the involved segment, placing the tendon in a slack position. Exercise to adjacent joints is withheld when it creates excessive stress on the exposed structure. When wound closure occurs, exercise is resumed in the normal fashion.

Exercise After Graft and Under Anesthesia

Wound status directly influences an exercise program. Skin coverage directly affects the function of a joint in that, after coverage, the joint may be freely and continuously moved. The longer an extremity remains uncovered by skin, the more difficult it will be to maintain function of the joints.

Wounds that are allowed to heal spontaneously by the process of re-epithelialization need frequent gentle stretching to counteract the contractile nature of the new and underlying tissues. Care should be taken to avoid excessive tension on the fragile thin epithelial surface. Active and active assistive exercises are recommended with frequent monitoring of tissue status.

As full-thickness wounds heal, granulation tissue is formed. Since this fluid-engorged tissue can be easily traumatized, care must be taken to avoid injury during exercise. Vigorous stretch, causing undue stress and trauma to newly formed granulation tissue, is avoided as it may result in excess build up of granulation tissue and later result in increased hypertrophic scarring.

Heterografts are frequently applied to partial-thickness wounds and debrided full-thickness wounds to provide pain relief, protect wounds, debride during the healing process, and enhance growth of epithelial and granulation tissue. The method of heterograft application is a key factor when considering an exercise program. Heterografts are segmentally applied over joints when possible to allow for maximum joint excursion.

When heterografts such as pigskin are applied, adequate time must be allowed for adherence of the heterograft prior to initiating exercise. At the discretion of the attending physician, exercise can generally be resumed within two to four hours after application. Active, active assistive, and passive range of motion can all be used in the presence of heterograft (Fig. 6.5).

When all eschar has separated from full-thickness wounds and a healthy granulating wound bed is present, skin grafts are surgically applied to

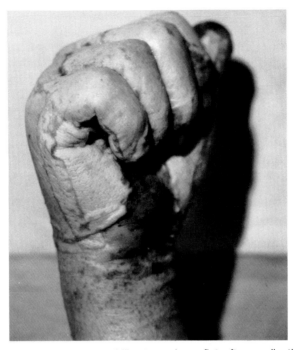

Figure 6.5. Patient demonstrates ability to make a fist after application of porcine heterograft.

achieve closure of the wound. Before surgery, joint range of motion measurements are documented and muscular function evaluated. The patient is then prepared for changes in the exercise program and the duration that changes will be in effect after surgery. If appropriate, the patient is instructed in the performance of isometric exercise for joints which will be immobilized due to graft application.

Joint range of motion exercise performed while the patient is under anesthesia is sometimes recommended as an adjunct to routine exercise sessions (18). If pain is a problem, the patient undergoing a surgical procedure to aid wound closure may have range of motion assessed in the operating room. This is a particularly beneficial procedure when assessing children if fear, apprehension, and manipulative behavior interfere with normal exercise sessions.

If pain control, relaxation, and exercise techniques have failed to maintain joint range of motion when the patient is awake, exercise under anesthesia helps determine the extent of joint restriction. Many times, the patient who appears to have joint restriction when awake does not have tightness under anesthesia. This information is often encouraging to the patient and aids his motivation to work through pain after the surgical procedure.

Exercise techniques to utilize in the operating room include passive range of motion, slow sustained stretching, and gentle joint mobilization. If the joint has had restriction for over 10 days prior to surgery, motion is completed only to the point of tightness and full range of motion is generally not attempted. Caution is necessary when performing exercises while a patient is under anesthesia as tears of soft tissue, pathological fractures and dislocations, and joint capsular damage are possible with short, abrupt, uncontrolled movements.

After range of motion is assessed, homograft or autograft are applied and secured by dressings. Sometimes the manner in which the surgeon positions the patient in dressings increases the chances for contracture formation. It is recommended that the therapist and surgeon communicate prior to the grafting procedure regarding optimal post-surgical positioning.

Following grafting, all exercise is discontinued for approximately five days to the grafted area to encourage incorporation of the graft into the wound bed. Proper patient positioning is stressed at this time. Exercise is also withheld to joints proximal and distal to the grafted area, which, if exercised, might influence graft stability. Isometric exercises, contraction of muscle groups without joint movement, are often appropriate as they are useful for maintaining muscle awareness and strength. Isometric exercises should be completed slowly and each contraction held for five seconds. Care in their use must be taken for patients with hypertension and congestive heart failure as both systolic and diastolic blood pressures may rise rapidly with sustained isometric contractions.

Active and active assistive range of motion exercises to all other non-grafted areas are continued. Upon removal of dressings, if the graft appears stable, exercise to the grafted area can be resumed with approval from the attending physician. When reinitiating exercise, gentle range of motion is encouraged for the first few days until the graft becomes adherent (Fig. 6.6). It is wise for the therapist to observe dressing changes to identify areas of graft slough and possible tendon exposure. As the graft becomes more stable, excursion of joint range of motion and repetitions of exercise increase.

It is typical that range of motion decreases during the immobilization period after grafting. A general theory is that approximately 25% of the motion is lost during the post-graft stage (1). However, the patient who maintains essentially normal range of motion during the pregrafting phase will generally survive the post-grafting phase with excellent results. With most patients, full joint motion is expected seven to ten days after grafting.

Introducing Resistive Exercise

As healing progresses, either spontaneously or after grafting, functional strengthening is introduced into the exercise program. It is important to remember that exercise is not only valuable in maintaining strength and mobility in body parts directly affected by the burn, but also in those body

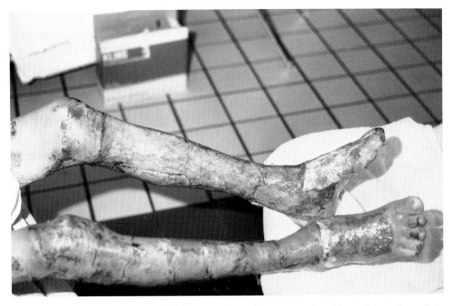

Figure 6.6. Attempting gentle active motion of knees and ankles after autograft is shown.

parts uninvolved, as muscle contracture and joint stiffness in unburned areas may occur due to prolonged immobilization.

Even if the patient has open wounds and bandages, minimal manual resistance by the therapist is begun for initial strengthening. Resistance can be applied gently as the patient contracts his muscles and attempts motion against the resistance, or the patient is asked to maintain a position and then resistance applied (Fig. 6.7). The amount of resistance used depends upon present medical status, area of burn, and patient tolerance. Occasionally, use of sandbag weights is an appropriate introduction to resistive exercise. Resistive exercise should be used judiciously with an extremely ill patient. Fatigue, muscle soreness, and joint pain are carefully monitored when using resistive exercise. A patient who is near the end of the hospital stay can rapidly progress with his resistive exercise program as the catabolic state of injury reverses.

Assessment and treatment of the body as a whole are essential for successful patient recovery. Detecting, preventing, and correcting causes for poor movement and posture during the acute phase diminish the magnitude of the problems that the patient faces in the next phase of rehabilitation.

POST-ACUTE REHABILITATIVE EXERCISE

As the patient makes the transition into the post-acute phase of burn care and is preparing to meet the added demands of functioning in the home environment, the physical treatment program escalates to accommo-

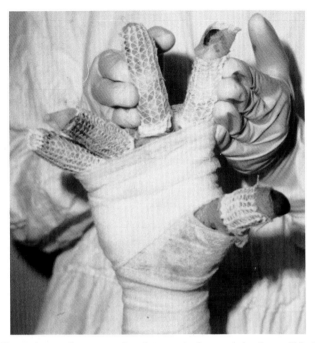

Figure 6.7. Therapist applies manual resistance to finger abduction within the patient's tolerance.

date these changes. The post-acute rehabilitative phase begins in earnest when the catabolic state reverses, the patient has few unhealed burn areas, and he/she becomes more aware and realistic regarding the impact of the burn injury on his life. This is the difficult and lengthy phase of wound contracture and hypertrophic scarring in which physical function and appearance can be altered significantly. The patient will be making psychological adaptations to his change in body image and to new social roles within his family unit. Rehabilitation ends when the patient has attained satisfactory physical and psychological adjustment to the burn injury. This usually coincides with scar maturation at 12–18 months after injury, but may extend for several years if reconstructive surgical procedures are necessary.

Settings for post-acute rehabilitation are quite variable. In acute hospitals, the patient may continue to be seen in outpatient therapy settings. Burn centers which have patients travel from great distances for acute treatment sometimes transfer daily therapy care to the patient's home setting and then follow the patient periodically in outpatient burn clinic. Some burn centers have rehabilitation beds or "step down units" which continue medical care until the patient is better able to handle the home situation. Patients with complicated injuries, amputations, large body surface area burns, or neurological involvement may need several months in a designated rehabilitation center for proper care. Careful evaluation of the patient and assignment to the most beneficial type of care facility make the difference between success and failure in rehabilitation.

Most patients require daily therapy when they make the transition into post-acute rehabilitation. Duration of sessions varies according to involvement and patient tolerance. Moderate to major burns require anywhere from one to five hours of treatment per day, including rest periods. Emphasis is placed on increased participation and responsibility by the patient during this phase. As the patient demonstrates increased independence and progresses toward his goals, sessions are reduced to two to three times a week and eventually to weekly rechecks.

In addition to formal outpatient therapy, patients and families should be instructed in home programs to be undertaken throughout the day. Although therapy is demanding and crucial during this time period, patients should also be allowed time for other activities to make the transition to a normal lifestyle.

Most patients wear some form of pressure garments during this phase. Although many activities are permitted in these garments, they are removed for the major portion of exercise sessions so that shearing action of the garment against the skin does not cause blistering and skin breakdown.

Exercise continues to be a major focal point during the post-acute rehabilitative effort. During this phase of burn care, exercise goals include:

(1) increasing joint range of motion;
(2) preventing or correcting contracture;
(3) strengthening with body reconditioning;
(4) maximizing functional abilities.

These goals are accomplished through range of motion, ADL and ambulation programs, incorporating stretching, coordination, strengthening, endurance, and conditioning.

Stretching

A patient who heals initially with full range of motion has the potential to develop severe deformities during the post-acute care as the healed skin matures and hypertrophic scarring develops. The major structures ultimately involved in burn contracture are skin, muscle, and joint capsule. In the final stages of scarring and contracture, skin is the primary source of contracture and it is the most restrictive. Sustained stretching is one of the most effective exercise techniques for lengthening bands of scar tissue and increasing range of motion (13). Maximum gains in range of motion are frequently noted if sustained stretching exercises follow paraffin application, referred to in the modalities section of this chapter. Sustained stretching exercise may be accomplished in several ways. Active assistive range of motion with the therapist applying mild manual stretching at the extremes of motion is well tolerated. Skin should be stretched to the point of blanching. Palpation of the scar tissue at this point helps in determining the "give" or pliability of the scar, indicating if further stretching will be tolerated. Holding the stretch for counts of 10 or 15 is recommended at the terminal stretch as tolerated (Fig. 6.8).

Other techniques of sustained stretching include pulley systems and weights. Nonweighted bilateral pulley systems are ideal for stretching axillae if the patient is able to maintain a sustained stretch of the involved part. Weights may be used when stretching skin or scar bands in the antecubital fossa. The upper extremity might be positioned over a table with the shoulder in 90 degrees of flexion or abduction, and the elbow in maximal achievable extension and supination. A dumbbell weight or sandbag weight secured around intravenous or similar tubing placed in the palm of the hand facilitates maximum stretch (Fig. 6.9). If the patient is unable to grasp the weight, it may be secured by elastic bandage wraps, or the padded tubing may be placed over the distal forearm. Care is taken to avoid excessive pressure or bruising at the placement site of the weight or tubing.

Specific relaxation techniques are also substitutes for passive stretching. Contract-relax exercise is beneficial when there is marked limitation of range of motion with little or no active motion available in the agonistic

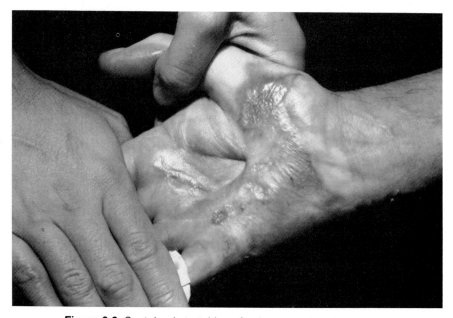

Figure 6.8. Sustained stretching of palmar scar bands is shown.

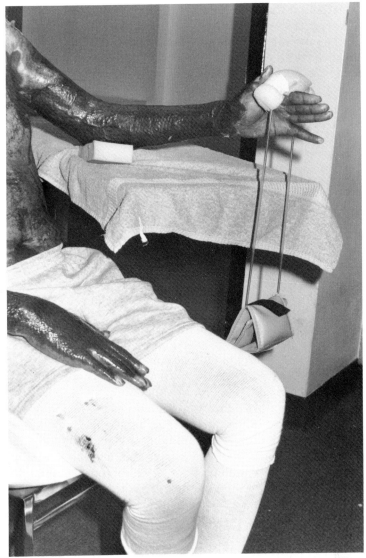

Figure 6.9. Facilitating elbow extension is shown using IV tubing and sand bag weight.

pattern. This technique involves an isotonic contraction of the antagonist, allowing range of motion in rotation against maximal resistance but no range of the other components. This short maximal contraction is followed by a brief period of relaxation after which the therapist passively increases the range of the involved joint (11). The entire procedure is repeated several times until maximal benefits are achieved.

It is sometimes difficult to stretch patients who have muscle spasm and pain. Hold-relax is an effective relaxation technique for increasing range of motion in the presence of these conditions. Hold-relax is a technique based upon maximal resistance of an isometric contraction. This technique is performed in the same type of sequence as contract-relax; however, no joint motion is implied and the contraction must not be broken (11).

Regardless of the stretching technique used, whenever possible, overall patterns of motion are emphasized as scar tissue may cause profound limitations of motion when multiple joints are involved.

Bone and joint problems directly affect achievable range of motion. Heterotopic bone, myositis ossificans, periarticular calcification and tightened joint capsules are characteristic of this phase of rehabilitation, although they can present earlier. Many of these conditions are associated with immobility and inactivity during the acute phase of rehabilitation. In the presence of these types of problems, active range of motion is encouraged and aggressive stretching avoided. Surgery may be indicated to provide relief for some of these problems.

Coordination

Coordination is defined simply as the ability to use the correct muscles at the appropriate time and with proper intensity to achieve a desired movement most efficiently. Coordinated movement patterns are those patterns in which normal neuromuscular and musculoskeletal systems act most efficiently and safely (16, 20). Normal coordinated movement is generally diminished after burn injury.

Many of the components of coordinated movement are at a subconscious level, beyond the voluntary control of the patient. Many times in burn rehabilitation, the patient is encouraged to think about the components of complex movement, but this can be detrimental, as conscious effort often fosters incoordination. It is impossible to teach coordination; rather attempts are made at establishing patterns that will eventually lead to the successful accomplishment of desired movement. It is essential that substitution patterns be recognized and altered before they become deeply ingrained as conditioned responses. This is particularly important so that when strength is regained, emphasis is directed at the most effective use of muscles.

Guidelines for performance of coordination exercises include:
(1) Select subcortical activities to facilitate coordinated movement patterns.
(2) Start with gross movements and work toward movements requiring more precision.
(3) Have the patient visually follow movement for reinforcement.
(4) Repeat the movement until it is fluid and spontaneous.

(5) Take frequent rests during training sessions.

Coordination exercises are extremely beneficial in eliminating the mechanical robot-like postures and movements frequently characteristic of burn patients (Fig. 6.10).

Strengthening

Strengthening is an essential component of the post-acute rehabilitative effort since most burn patients are debilitated and weak. Traditional approaches for strengthening, where muscle weakness has been identified, include the use of manual resistance, bar bells, bench press and sandbag weights, weighted pulleys and exercise involving resistance of body weight such as situps, pushups, and pullups (Fig. 6.11). Other approaches for

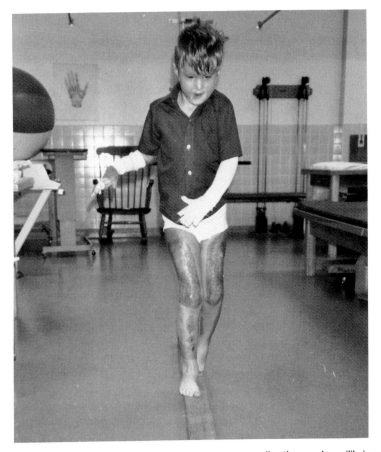

Figure 6.10. Balance beam exercise encourages coordination and equilibrium.

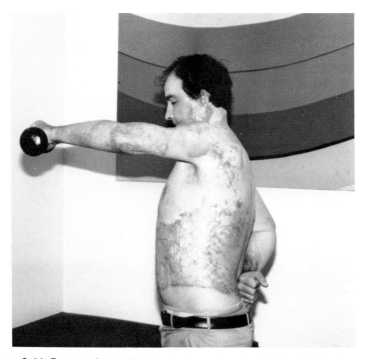

Figure 6.11. Progressive resistive exercise using dumbbell weight is shown.

strengthening include resistive exercise in developmental sequence patterns and gymnastic ball activities.

Resistance and progressive resistance are not new concepts in exercise therapy. Movement performed against resistance of sufficient degree demanding maximal effort produces an increase in strength (11, 16, 20). Many mechanical factors involving the relationship of lever systems, the axis of motion and the effect of gravity aid in determining the amount of resistance given. However, there is only one criterion for judging maximal resistance. This criterion is that the patient must put forth maximal effort while being allowed to move the part slowly and smoothly throughout a designated range of motion (11).

The needs of the patient determine the method of strengthening. Use of the progressive resistance exercise program developed by DeLorme, and the reversal of the load-resisting schedule termed the "Oxford Technique" are beneficial. The most desirable method for strengthening normal muscle which has undergone disuse atrophy, without joint pathology, is heavy resistance with weights applied directly or indirectly (16). A progressive decrease of repetitions and an increase of load are the most efficient approaches for rapid gains in strength and muscle volume. The 10 RM is the amount of weight a muscle can lift ten times. For practical purposes, the patient's 10 RM or some modification of it generally indicates the amount of weight to use to initiate strengthening. It is unwise, however, to demand maximal effort of a recently weakened muscle. For the muscle recently recovering from disease or trauma, such as burn, strengthening is initiated with loads well below the full 10 RM. Loads are gradually increased for a week or more before the 10 RM is reached. The frequency of exercise depends on the patient's response. Objective and subjective signs of fatigue are carefully observed.

Alternative strengthening methods can and should be considered for patients with known joint pathology. Initially, isometric exercises may be indicated for the patient with a painful acute joint. If this is not indicated, since cross-education strengthens the contralateral part, a similar exercise can be performed on the unaffected side until the condition improves enough to use the exercise on the affected side (16).

Endurance

Endurance is the ability of the body to withstand repetitive movements essential to prolonged activity. It can be developed using graded resistance, encouraging speed and repetition of motion. The patterns of movement to increase endurance are similar to those for strengthening except the demands on the neuromuscular system with each effort are less. A high-repetition low-resistance program usually promotes endurance rather than increased muscle bulk. Endurance exercises also increase the capillary bed in the muscle whereas strengthening exercises cause muscle hypertrophy (16).

Conditioning

Conditioning exercises promote endurance and physical fitness; both aerobic and nonaerobic exercises are important in a conditioning program. Typical conditioning exercises include bicycling, swimming, jogging, jumping rope, dancing, tennis, racquetball, and other sports. Many patients have engaged in these types of activities prior to injury, and in most instances, they can resume these activities when strength and endurance permit.

If formal aerobic conditioning programs are desirable, specific guidelines on establishing and monitoring such programs are available in the literature. For some patients, aerobic activity is inappropriate. The level and type of exercise must be prescribed according to the patient's exercise capacity. For the patient who has never been active, conditioning exercises are approached more cautiously and with careful guidance.

When possible, conditioning exercise incorporates activities enjoyable to the patient. Many times, the type of activities selected not only provides the patient with a sense of physical well-being, but also an opportunity for social interaction. Careful integration of conditioning with all other post-acute rehabilitation exercise programs enhances the patient's restoration to a normal lifestyle.

EXERCISE FOLLOWING RECONSTRUCTION

Burn scarring frequently necessitates reconstructive procedures during the post-acute rehabilitation period for improving cosmesis and increasing motion and functional abilities. Grafting procedures may or may not be necessary. Re-establishment of exercise programs for these patients is relatively easy.

For nongrafted patients, range of motion usually begins the day after surgery at the discretion of the attending physician. When grafting is involved, range of motion resumes according to routine guidelines previously addressed in this chapter, unless otherwise indicated.

Because surgical reconstruction generally occurs when scar tissue is mature, many of the problems associated with acute phase rehabilitative exercise are not encountered. Problems typical to this rehabilitative phase are pain-associated with incisions or graft sites and stiffness due to the immobility caused by a contracture, prior to release. In most instances, reconstructive surgery is elective and patients are motivated to gain optimal functional results so that the need for additional surgery is eliminated. Knowing that there is a potential for repeated contracture also provides incentive for the patient to exercise. Adjunctive splinting and positioning programs are outlined for patients when indicated.

Patients are carefully screened prior to reconstructive surgery. They must have a thorough understanding that surgery is not a "cure all" and that participation in continued rehabilitative exercises is required.

ACTIVITIES OF DAILY LIVING

The purpose of an ADL program is to train the patient to perform, within the limits of his physical disabilities. The patient is encouraged in maximal performance of activities related to daily life at home, work, and play (19). An effectively planned program of range of motion should preserve a patient's functional capability. Translating these capabilities into meaningful activity, encouraging independence, is accomplished by the second technique of exercise, ADL. Patients are encouraged to begin participating in ADL early in the acute phase of rehabilitation to avoid psychological dependency on others and to develop adeptness in necessary functional activities. The teaching method includes breaking the task into its simplest motions, selecting exercises which enable performance of the specific motions, and performing the task as a whole in a real life situation (20).

ADL in early rehabilitation are comprised of self-care tasks such as simple bed mobility, assistance with dressing changes, and the more complex tasks related to grooming, hygiene, and eating (Fig. 6.12).

ADL involves different problems for different mobility levels. For example, tasks involved in bathing are quite different for bed patients, wheelchair patients, and ambulatory patients. For most activities, the movement sequence to be practiced with the patient depends entirely on his capabilities. The patient should begin with movement components of the activity he can perform and then gradually learn the parts he cannot perform. The patient should understand that mastery of a particular exercise is a prerequisite for the accomplishment of the desired activity. Therefore, ADL are regarded as exercises, and the exercises are part of the ADL (20).

Setting reasonable goals with the patient, allowing the additional time it requires for him to perform these activities, and actively reinforcing desired behavior aid in fostering independence and preserving motor skill and coordination. For preschool and school-age children, allowing active participation in dressing changes, grooming, and other activities is extremely important to maintain ego development during the stressful period of hospitalization (8). Every effort is made to encourage patient participation in ADL. Simple things such as application of dressings in a manner to facilitate joint motion enhances patient performance and improves moti-

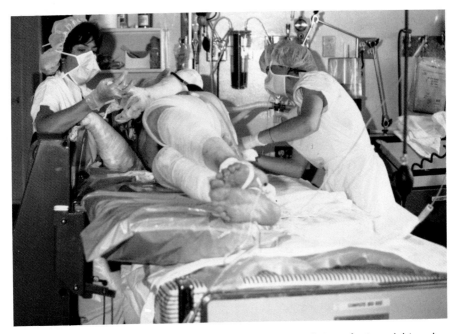

Figure 6.12. Early mobility is encouraged as patient assists in transfer to weight scale.

vation. Participation is facilitated by selection of activities in which the patient is able to achieve success rather than repeated failure.

ADL involves more than just adding one motion to another. It includes management and possible adaptations of necessary furniture and equipment. Special assistive devices are provided to aid in the performance of daily living activities. For example, an overhead trapeze during hospitalization helps the patient with bed mobility. Placing a rolled gauze or foam padding on handles of eating utensils, razors, and hair brushes facilitates independence for the individual with limited hand grasp. Other beneficial assistive devices include plate guards, special eating utensils such as swivel spoons and rocker knives, bath sponge mitts, door knob extension levers, and other long-handled devices. As mobility increases, the patient is encouraged to resume normal activities without the use of adaptive devices. Even if full range of motion is not achieved in these daily activities, the involvement of body parts and ability to coordinate movements into meaningful activity is an important part of functional recovery and the restoration of independence.

When the patient is discharged from the hospital, he continues normal ADL at home. The patient may require a period of time to readjust to daily activities he was unable to perform for himself during the emergent and most of the acute phase of treatment. Simple dressing skills may be difficult for the patient whose skin is fragile and hypersensitive. Patients sometimes shy away from clothing such as sweaters, jeans, or tight clothing that rubs or is uncomfortable. Cotton fabric and loose clothing are generally recommended for newly healed burns to prevent skin breakdown and to begin the desensitization process. Patients are discouraged from habits such as wearing pajamas during the day as this inhibits the transition into a "normal" lifestyle (Fig. 6.13).

As the patient's tolerance increases, he begins activities requiring increased strength and endurance. Household chores, outdoor activity, hobbies, and leisure activity are permitted as tolerated. Initially, the patient may require frequent rest periods. Excessive fatigue caused by "overdoing" is avoided. Work simplification and energy-conserving techniques should be included in the ADL program. Suggestions such as using two hands for lifting heavy objects, using rolling carts for transporting objects and instruction in proper body mechanics eliminate undue fatigue. Patients sometimes become easily frustrated when they are unable to accomplish formerly simple tasks, and thus, assistive equipment continues to be necessary. Bathtub grab bars, shower seats, pot handle holders and other equipment provide safety as well as personal security. Precautions must be addressed in activities that might be dangerous or harmful to patients, such as activities involving exposure to heat, sun, and sharp objects.

Patients are encouraged to attempt all activities independently. Depend-

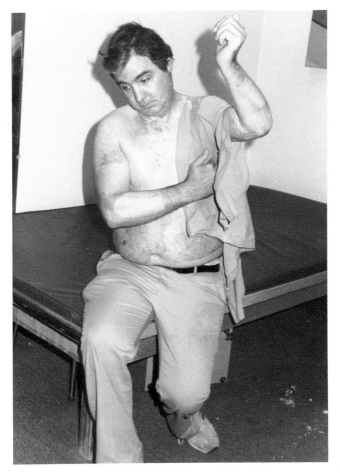

Figure 6.13. Independence in dressing is a primary goal for all burn patients.

ing on other individuals or family members for accomplishment of tasks often prolongs rehabilitative efforts and creates unnecessary interpersonal conflicts within the family. It is important that the family be educated in ADL so that they do not sympathize with the patient and foster unnecessary dependency.

Functional ability is thoroughly discussed with a patient prior to initiation of ADL so he is prepared for the fact that he will be unable to perform many tasks as he did prior to injury. This may be due to limitations of motion caused by scarring or deformity, loss of a body part, pain or hypersensitivity, weakness or lack of endurance. A clear understanding of possible limitations eliminates undue frustration and the attitudes of failure frequently associated with lack of success in completing tasks.

Successful rehabilitation in terms of ADL is not something that merely happens or that is naturally learned. It must be carefully planned and practiced. In conjunction with range of motion exercise, incorporating movement into purposeful activity through ADL directs the patient towards independence.

AMBULATION

In conjunction with range of motion and ADL, the third physical treatment related to exercise is ambulation. The ability to move about freely has a significant impact on the restoration of independence. The debilitating effects of immobility are counteracted by a program of ambulation. Although emphasis shifts throughout the phases of rehabilitation, the primary goals of ambulation include:

(1) maintaining lower extremity range of motion;
(2) reducing the risk of thrombophlebitis;
(3) preventing decubiti;
(4) providing mild cardiovascular conditioning;
(5) maintaining or increasing strength and endurance;
(6) increasing appetite.

The following are considered prior to initiating a gait program: (1) patient's prior level of activity, (2) location of burn, and (3) tolerance of sitting and standing. Patients begin ambulation as soon as the physical condition warrants, usually by 48–72 hours after injury, when vital signs are stable and fluid resuscitation is complete.

If lower extremities are not burned, the patient is encouraged to achieve early independence in ambulation and to be up throughout the day. Generally patients wear antiembolic stockings for initial gait sessions. As the patient accommodates to being up and around, these stockings are no longer necessary.

Patients with burns to the feet and legs must be carefully evaluated prior to initiation of the gait program. For nongrafted lower extremities, ambulation is initiated once the patient is medically stable unless tendons or joint capsules are exposed, severe swelling or cellulitis is present, or if the soles of the feet are severely burned. Mild to moderate burns of the feet do not preclude early ambulation. Dressings with extra padding and foam-soled slippers will protect the wounds and aid in reducing the discomfort of weight-bearing. Burns of greater involvement necessitate an ambulation program of partial weight-bearing with crutches or walkers to decrease the risk of wound trauma. The patient progresses to full weight-bearing as the area heals and tolerance increases on the painful extremity.

Stasis or pooling of blood in the lower extremities is a common problem for patients who have sustained lower extremity burns. When extremities are dependent, excessive pooling of blood occurs in the feet and legs resulting in swelling and pain generally described as throbbing, stinging, or tingling. To avoid venous stasis in lower extremities, and discomfort associated with upright positions, elastic bandages are applied from toe to groin before standing (Fig. 6.14). A figure of eight wrap is used, as this provides an even distribution of pressure and better support for the extremity than circular wraps (1, 8).

For all patients with lower extremity burns, gait sessions are an integral part of the exercise program, along with lower extremity range of motion and ADL. Assistive devices such as canes, walkers, braces, and use of parallel bars which facilitate independence or improve gait patterns are

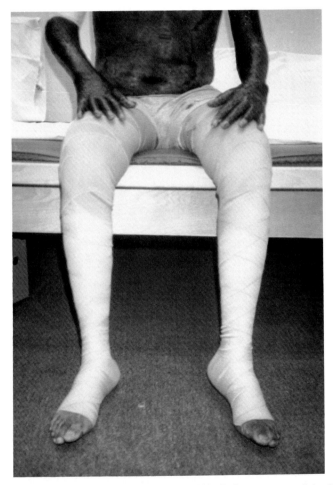

Figure 6.14. Vascular support of lower extremities is best accomplished using an elastic bandage with a figure of eight wrap from toe to groin.

encouraged. As mobility improves, however, the use of assistive devices is discouraged so that patients do not develop unnecessary dependencies.

Once the patient is ambulatory, emphasis is initially placed on brief and frequent gait sessions rather than prolonged periods of standing. Training in early walking sessions emphasizes proper posture and gait patterns. Every effort is made to evaluate and correct walking deviations (Fig. 6.15). Burns of the lower extremities can cause changes in step length and heel-toe gait pattern as the patient tries to avoid weight-bearing on the affected extremity. Burn wound pain and positioning of the upper extremities can also change normal patterns. If the patient must elevate burned hands due

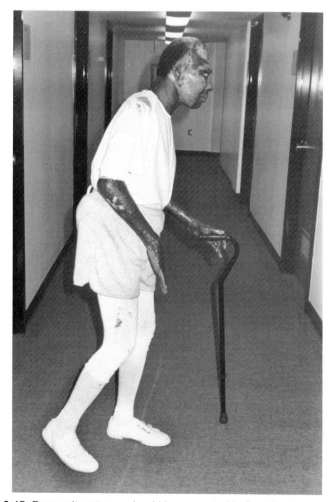

Figure 6.15. Poor gait patterns should be corrected before they become habit.

to discomfort when they are dependent, normal arm swing is impossible. Burns of the anterior neck and trunk often contribute to posturing characterized by a forward head and elevated and protracted shoulders. Regardless of the problem, patients must be made aware of abnormal gait patterns early, before they become habit. Having the patient view himself in the mirror as he ambulates provides a feedback system whereby he too can recognize gait abnormalities. The therapist must implement specific exercises on a subcortical level as well, which aid in correcting gait deviation.

Children require special attention in a gait program. Play activity, circular walkers, bicycles, tricycles, and group activities provide incentives for walking. Children have a greater tendency for assuming comfortable positions and need additional guidance in correct posture and movement patterns.

Early ambulation is not possible for all patients. Critically ill patients and patients with thrombophlebitis, deep or circumferential burns to lower extremities, are not candidates for ambulation until the medical status improves or until grafting procedures have been completed. When homografts or autografts are surgically applied to lower extremities, ambulation is suspended for approximately six days. When grafts are applied over open joints, tendons or bony prominences, ambulation is often suspended for as long as 10–14 days due to decreased vascularity in these areas.

If ambulation is begun too early after grafting, risk of graft slough increases. The graft could become dislodged and loosened if blood is allowed to accumulate in the area before the venules have developed to provide proper drainage (12).

Prior to ambulation after grafting, range of motion exercises are performed at bedside. If the patient demonstrates excessive limitations of motion, ambulation is inappropriate until range of motion increases. Toes, ankles, knees, and hips receive active and active assistive exercise in all directions permitted by each joint; however, undue stress to grafted areas is avoided.

Some patients are extremely weak from prolonged bedrest or post-graft immobilization. Although a patient desires to get out of bed he may not have the strength to accomplish this, or the endurance to stay up for long periods. For these patients, transferring to upright positions must be carefully monitored since the ability for the vasomotor mechanism to maintain blood pressure decreases with bedrest. Tilt tables are often used to progress a patient to the upright position if the problem is irregular blood pressure. Other patients require several periods of sitting on the bedside or in a chair to prepare for ambulation. Pallor, diaphoresis, weakness, dizziness, and elevated or diminished blood pressure and pulse, associated with upright positions, indicate that the patient is not yet ready for ambulation.

When normal reactions to being upright are established, the gait program is initiated in the appropriate manner. Many patients are eager to resume walking after grafting while others are hesitant due to pain or fear of movement and falling. Reassurance and encouragement by all medical team members and family are essential. Appropriate dressings and figure of eight elastic support wraps are always applied before ambulating the patient with recent grafts and donor sites to the lower extremities. Modified weight-bearing is prescribed according to graft location and integrity. Otherwise, short distance walking is permitted within the patient's tolerance. Observation of grafted sites is important during the first few days of ambulation. Minor graft slough and open areas do not usually affect ambulation whereas excessive bleeding may hinder progressive ambulation. Medical staff are consulted in the presence of "problem" graft sites.

As the patient's tolerance increases, ambulation is encouraged for longer time periods and distances. With the transition into the post-acute phase of rehabilitation, ambulation becomes more than forward walking. Equilibrium exercises, stretching, strengthening, and coordination are emphasized until walking is a fluid, coordinated body movement (19). Mat exercises aid stretching and equilibrium of the trunk. Dance exercises stretch and coordinate muscular activity as well as increase endurance. Markers are placed on the floor to provide proper step length, and a metronome directs walking rhythm. Stair climbing, changing walking velocity, turning, walking on uneven surfaces, walking sideways, and crossover walking strengthen the patient and improve coordinated walking skills.

When the lower extremity burns are in final healing stages, correct ambulation is dependent upon proper shoes and leg support. Elastic bandage supports are usually replaced with tubular elastic supports or commercial support stockings or garments. These generally allow more freedom of movement as well as better control for anticipated scarring.

A variety of footwear is appropriate for ambulation. Some patients with severe foot burns tolerate slippers with nonskid soles, or customized total contact sandals are often prescribed until healing is complete and the feet are desensitized. Most other patients easily adapt to tennis shoes until the burn scar and foot size are stable. Then the patient progresses to regular shoes. In some cases, extra depth shoes are recommended to accommodate molded inserts which provide even distribution of weight and extra padding for hypersensitive feet. Care is taken in the choice of any shoe to avoid rubbing by the shoe on the immature burn scar.

For patients with peroneal neuropathy, a temporary polypropylene ankle-foot orthosis (AFO)can be worn in the shoe to prevent dropping of the foot on heel strike. If there is a permanent peroneal paralysis, a permanent custom-fitted AFO is needed for walking.

The patient with deep leg burns can walk too much. Signs of compromised circulatory status are throbbing pains lasting more than one-half hour after exercise, abnormal color changes lasting longer than usual, and increased skin breakdown. If these symptoms appear, walking is reduced, then gradually increased again as symptoms subside. In deep leg burns, the legs are elevated at all times when not ambulating. In the presence of circumferential, full-thickness leg burns, support stockings are needed throughout life to provide vascular support which has been compromised.

The therapist incorporates ambulation early in the burn patient's rehabilitation program. The ambulation program is closely monitored and adjusted to meet the needs of the patient as he progresses with his rehabilitative exercises. The functional orientation of gait as a form of exercise fosters physical as well as psychological independence for the patient (Table 6.1).

Modalities

Numerous modalities, each having a specific physiological effect, are available in rehabilitation today. The physician and therapist should base

Table 6.1.
Specific Exercises for Common Problems

Face

Common Problems

A. Tight skin, especially forehead, cheeks, chin (use exercises 1–3, 6–9, and 11–14)
B. Eyelid contractures (use exercises 4–5)
C. Microstomia (use exercises 9–10)
D. Poor lip closure (use exercises 15–17)
E. Flat nose/closed nostrils (use exercises 18–19)

Exercise Suggestions

1. Wrinkle forehead and raise eyebrows
2. Frown, drawing eyebrows down and together
3. Look side to side raising eyebrows
4. Shut eyes tightly and open widely
5. Wink
6. Fill cheeks with air, keeping mouth shut
7. Blow air out of cheeks until lips pucker
8. Suck cheeks in
9. Smile and frown
10. Open mouth widely
11. Shift lips from side to side
12. Protrude lower lip like pouting
13. Thrust jaw from side to side
14. Move lower jaw forward
15. Draw lips into mouth
16. Pucker lips
17. Press lips together

Table 6.1—*Continued*

18. Squint or wrinkle like sniffing
19. Flare nostrils

Tips

1. Use fingers to massage tight areas and stretch, especially lips
2. Use mirror for visual feedback
3. Exaggerate speech
4. Whistle
5. Blow balloons
6. Sing
7. Chew food vigorously

Neck

Common Problems
A. Forward flexion contracture (use exercises 1 and 5–6)
B. Lateral flexion contracture (use exercises 2–3 and 5–6)
C. Posterior neck tightness (use exercises 3–6)

Exercise Suggestions

1. Look up at ceiling
2. Tilt head and touch ears on shoulders
3. Turn head to side, looking over shoulder
4. Touch chin to chest
5. Rotate head in a circular motion
6. Combine any of the above motions

Tips

1. Neck movement affects facial movement, so combine with facial exercises, stabilizing face to achieve maximum stretch
2. Work on neck motions in the back lying and sitting positions
3. Neck motions should be active and active assistive
4. Manual resistance may be used for strengthening neck musculature
5. Avoid prolonged neck hyperextension to minimize orthopedic complications

Trunk—Abdomen—Back

Common Problems

A. Immobile trunk/robot posture (use exercises 3–7)
B. Tight chest/anterior banding (use exercises 1, 9, and 11)
C. Tight back (use exercises, 2, 8, and 10)

Exercise Suggestions

1. Inhale deeply and arch backward to expand chest
2. Exhale deeply, rounding shoulders forward
3. Lying on back, bend hips and knees, rotate both knees to same side

Table 6.1—*Continued*

4. Windmills—standing, feet apart, arms straight out at sides at shoulder height, bend at waist and touch right hand to left foot and vice versa
5. Standing, feet apart, arms straight out at sides at shoulder height, twist upper trunk to the right and then to the left
6. Teapots—raise right arm sideways and upward, reaching overhead, while bending at waist to left, reaching with left hand down toward the left knee; repeat, changing sides
7. Bolster activities—backbends, sidebends
8. Hugs—reach hands around head to opposite shoulder
9. Arms down at sides, clasp hands behind the back, elevating arms
10. Shoulder shrugs
11. Stretch the chest, lie on back on narrow bench, arms out at side, palms up; place weights on forearms or in hands for extra stretch

Strengthening Activities

A. Situps
B. Developmental mat activities with emphasis on trunk stability and mobility
C. Gymnastic ball activities with emphasis on trunk stability and mobility
D. Universal gym
E. Progressive resistive exercises for posterior shoulder girdle

Tips

1. It is easy to compensate when doing trunk exercises; therefore, close supervision is necessary
2. Lack of trunk mobility and stability decrease balance and equilibrium reactions which affect overall quality of movement

Shoulders

Common Problems (axillary banding limits shoulder range of motion)

A. Limited flexion (use exercises, 1, 6, and 8–12)
B. Limited abduction (use exercises 2–3, 7–8, and 11)
C. Limited internal/external rotation (use exercises 3, 5, and 11)
D. Limited horizontal abduction/adduction (use exercises 4, 7–8, and 10–11)

Exercise Suggestions

1. Clasp hands in front of body, raise straight arms toward ceiling
2. Arms at sides, raise arms sideways and upward until palms touch
3. Arms at sides, shoulder height, rotate arms in circles
4. Arms at sides, shoulder height, cross arms in front and return to starting position
5. Lying on back, arms shoulder height with elbows bent, raise forearms so that back of hands touch bed; lower forearms so that palms touch bed
6. Grip cane with both hands and raise above head
7. Hold one end of cane in each palm and push hand upward and sideways to stretch underarm, keeping elbows straight
8. Use pulleys, overhead and wall

Table 6.1—*Continued*

9. Reach hands over top of door or up stall bars; hang, letting body weight stretch underarms
10. Lying on stomach over a bolster or mat, extend arms forward
11. Proprioceptive neuromuscular facilitation diagonals, active, active assistive, and active resisted
12. Lying on back, hold opposite elbows in hands and raise arms up and behind head

Strengthening Activities

A. Progressive resisted exercises with sandbag weights and dumbbell weights
B. Universal gym
C. Gymnastic ball activities—lying on stomach, ball under chest, lift feet and walk forward on hands rolling ball toward knees and ankles; walk backward on hands returning to starting position
D. Developmental mat activities—rolling, prone on elbows, hands and knees

Tips

1. Prescribed ultrasound is often beneficial for axillary bands and tight joint capsules
2. Joint mobilization techniques are helpful for loosening tight joint capsule; DO NOT FORGET TO MOBILIZE THE SCAPULA
3. Releasing of tight skin in axillae may occur with stretching exercise which may eliminate the need for surgical release; exercise should be continued to maintain increased range of motion
4. Begin exercise early to avoid capsular problems
5. Many sports emphasize shoulder motions—swimming, basketball, tennis, rowing, etc.

Elbows

Common Problems

A. Flexion and pronation contractures (use exercises 1–11)
B. Heterotopic bone (use exercises 1–16)
C. Tight posterior elbow-joint capsules (use exercises 11–16)

Exercise Suggestions

1. Wheelbarrow walks with straight elbows, on flat hands
2. Gymnastic ball activities lying on stomach, reaching
3. Developmental activities stressing positions on straight elbows
4. Diagonal I extension—contract, relax (PNF pattern)
5. Pushups, the push part
6. With straight elbow, carry a container filled with sand or gravel
7. Forearms on table with elbows close to body, rotate forearms turning palms up and down
8. Wring out wet towels
9. Open door knobs with bent elbows
10. Turn on faucets with bent elbows
11. Pulley activities

Table 6.1—*Continued*

12. Hugs
13. Hold a wand or cane, keep palms up, bring to chest
14. Mat activities in the prone on elbows position
15. Diagonal I flexion—contract, relax
16. Wall or mat pushups

Strengthening Activities

A. Universal gym
B. Progressive resisted exercises with sandbags or dumbbell weights
C. Resistance throughout the developmental activities
D. Arm wrestling

Tips

1. Use ultrasound to aid in the treatment of heterotopic bone
2. Forcing an elbow to bend in the presence of heterotopic bone will proliferate the deposits of bone; DO NOT BE AGGRESSIVE
3. Emphasize overall patterns of motion; supinated forearms with elbow, wrist and finger extension; neutral forearm with elbow extension, wrist in ulnar deviation and thumb opposed to base of little finger
4. Some elbow exercises can be fun—eating, ball activities, fishing, etc.

Wrist

Common Problems

A. Flexion contracture (use exercises 1–3)
B. Deviation contractures (use exercises 4–5)
C. Dorsal skin tightness (use exercises 6–7)

Exercise Suggestions

1. Keeping hand with palm flat on table or chair, bend forearm up (hand pushup)
2. Place palms together, raise forearms up in air stretching underside of wrist
3. Place forearm on table with hand off edge, palm up; place dumbbell weight in palm to provide stretch
4. Move wrist from side to side
5. Move wrist in giant circles
6. Keeping back of hand on table, bend forearm toward you
7. Place back of hands together, bend forearms down stretching tops of wrists

Tips

1. Since wrist motion is often affected by elbow motion, particularly supination, it is good to combine exercises for both joints
2. Fun activities providing wrist movements may include crawling, pushups, jumping rope, tennis, ping-pong, and hammering

Table 6.1—*Continued*

Hands—Fingers

Common Problems

A. Claw hand deformity (use exercises 1–2 and 4)
B. Finger deformities (use exercises 1–2 and 8)
C. Web space contractures, fingers and thumb-index (use exercises 3–5, and 7)
D. Palmar scar banding (use exercise 6)
E. Little finger flexion, external rotation and abduction contracture (use exercises 1 and 3)

Exercise Suggestions

1. Straighten fingers and thumb, all joints
2. Make fists touching fingers to base of palm near wrist, middle of palm, and then upper palm near base of fingers
3. Spread fingers apart and bring back together
4. Interlock fingers
5. Wedge a bottle between fingers, forcing spread
6. With hand flat, stretch thumb sideways, away from the palm
7. Stretch thumb away from the palm like holding a canned drink or stretch the same way around a large jar
8. Touch thumb to each fingertip and to base of the little finger

Strengthening Activities

A. Therapy putty
B. Hand helper/hand grip squeezers
C. Stacking cones
D. Nuts and bolts
E. Bend fingers against resistance of sandbag weights hung on IV poles
F. Turn faucets and doorknobs
G. Open bottles and jars
H. Use tools such as hammers and pliers

Coordination/Dexterity Activities

A. Dealing and playing cards
B. Pegboard
C. Lacing activities
D. Shooting marbles, playing jacks, etc.
E. Cutting with scissors
F. Tearing tape
G. Turning pages
H. Crafts—painting, drawing, ceramics, making models
I. Typing

Tips

1. Use an ace bandage wrap to facilitate finger flexion
2. Metacarpal mobilization increases palm mobility and improves hand function

Table 6.1—*Continued*

3. Do not forget intrinsic stretching with wrist and metacarpals in neutral extension while flexing interphalangeal joints
4. Hands require desensitizing and tactile input; incorporate activities to provide these
5. Emphasize activities of daily living as hands are essential in most of them
6. Exercises forcing motion in the presence of joint pain may traumatize capsules and ligaments thereby decreasing motion and possibly increasing internal scarring

Hips—Knees

Common Problems

A. Hip flexion contracture (use exercises 2, 5, 7, and 8)
B. Hip abduction/external rotation contracture (use exercises 1 and 7)
C. Hip adduction/internal rotation contracture (use exercises 1 and 7–9)
D. Knee flexion contracture (use exercises 1–2 and 4–8)
E. Knee extension contracture (use exercises 3–8)

Exercise Suggestions

1. Long sit, straighten legs; with legs straight, turn feet in and out; spread straight legs apart and bring them together
2. Lying on stomach, raise straight leg in air toward ceiling; alternate legs
3. Lying on stomach, keeping hips straight, bend knees and point feet toward buttocks
4. Lying on back, straighten legs, bend and pull one knee up toward chest, return to straight position; repeat with other leg
5. Practice standing and sitting, using a straight back chair
6. To increase knee motion, progress sitting and standing from chairs of decreasing height, like progressively deeper knee bend
7. Developmental sequence activities—rolling, crawling, creeping, kneeling, and standing
8. Stationary bicycle for increasing range of motion
9. Sit with bolster between legs

Strengthening Activities

A. Resistance to activities in developmental sequence for hips and knees
B. N-K table for knee flexion/extension
C. Orthotron for knee flexion/extension
D. Progressive resistive exercise for hips and knees using sand bag weights

Tips

1. Most patients with lower extremity burns require some type of elastic support on the legs when performing upright activities
2. Some exercises may be performed best without support garments to avoid shearing of garments against the skin and to aid in monitoring stretch
3. Lower extremity contractures alter gait pattern

Table 6.1—*Continued*

Ankles

Common Problems

A. Plantar flexion contractures/tight heelcords (use exercises 1–4)
B. Inversion contractures (use exercises 1 and 3–4)

Exercise Suggestions

1. Sit with leg straight and loop a belt around the ball of the foot; using the ends of the belt, pull foot up and out; hold for count of five and relax
2. Stand facing wall about two feet away; place involved foot slightly behind and lean upper body toward wall; keep heels on floor; stretch slowly; use heel wedge to increase stretch on involved heel
3. Rotate feet in giant circles; emphasize upward and outward motions (dorsiflexion with eversion)
4. Practice stair climbing, up, down, sideways and backwards

Strengthening Activities

A. Walk on heels
B. Long sit, with feet flat against wall; push one foot into wall; hold for count of three and relax; repeat with other foot
C. Loop a wide elastic band around a stationary post; place foot inside loop in a manner to offer resistance to the upward and outward motion (dorsiflexion and eversion)
D. For ankle stability, from a sitting position in a straight back chair with hips and knees at a 90-degree angle, feet apart with uninvolved foot slightly forward, stand; do not assist with arms

Tips

1. Low heeled shoes encourage stretch on heelcords
2. The calf muscle is a two-joint muscle so the heelcord must be stretched with the knee straight and with the knee bent
3. High top tennis shoes provide additional ankle stability
4. Peroneal neuropathy:
   a. Observe for skin breakdown when using AFO
   b. Encourage patient independence on electrical stimulation and passive range of motion programs
   c. External dorsiflexion assists may be sufficient support and do not cause skin breakdown
5. Use tilt table to stetch heelcords

Feet

Common Problems

A. Toe hyperextension with metatarsal subluxation (use exercises 1–3 and 5–6)
B. Toe webbing (use exercises 4–5)

Table 6.1—*Continued*

Exercise Suggestions

1. Bend toes up and down
2. Curl toes over dowel rod
3. Pick up small objects with toes
4. Spread toes apart
5. Wiggle toes
6. Standing, elevate up and down on forefoot and tips of toes

Tips

1. Hypersensitive feet affect walking; therefore, incorporate desensitization into the exercise program
2. Like fingers, toes need to be stretched in adduction and abduction as well as flexion and extension
3. Molded insoles may foster earlier ambulation
4. Mobilize metatarsals

the choice of a specific modality on the following criteria:
  (1) patient's problems and goals to be achieved;
  (2) modality's indications and contraindications;
  (3) physiological effects and patient tolerance;
  (4) cost-effectiveness for the patient and provider.
Due to the unique problems inherent to the burn population, care must be taken in prescribing therapeutic modalities. Although the use of modalities is sometimes more limited with burns, the correct choice and application of a specific modality fosters the patient's achievement of a functional goal. The modalities to be addressed have proven effective for the management of problems existing in the burn population.

ELECTRICAL MUSCLE STIMULATION

Nerve and muscle stimulating currents are often useful with any disorder in which the patient has lost adequate voluntary control over skeletal muscle (6). In the absence of voluntary muscle control, electrical stimulation provides a stimulus to the involved muscle producing active joint motion. This is beneficial until the patient regains functional voluntary muscle control. There have been a number of machines designed to meet the patient's needs for electrical stimulation. Each unit delivers a type of alternating or direct current with variations in frequency and wave form. Some units contain special modifications such as electrodes that can be used under water or channels that can be programmed to elicit a response from a muscle in an appropriately timed sequence. The therapist should be knowledgeable of the types of machines available.

In the burned patient, decreased range of motion, or insufficient voluntary control of muscle, may be a result of lacerated, compressed, or overstretched nerves. Monopolar or bipolar alternating or direct currents assist in effectively managing the types of problems found in the thermally injured patient.

The use of bipolar or monopolar direct current muscle stimulation preserves the muscle elasticity prior to muscle reinnervation (6). Electrical muscle stimulation is usually begun as soon as possible after the diagnosis of denervation has been established. Two or more sessions per day of electrical stimulation at an intensity high enough to cause a visual contraction of the involved muscle are beneficial. With proper guidance, the patient can learn to do his electrical stimulation program himself (Fig. 6.16).

Bipolar, pulsed, or surged alternating current helps reduce edema and increase joint range of motion. The patient is positioned to aid in reduction of edema and electrodes placed on the skin in close proximity to the edematous area. In the case of an edematous extremity with open areas or fragile skin, the therapist might consider using the electrical stimulator with underwater electrodes to avoid direct skin contact. Since edema will increase the impedence of the tissues, a higher stimulating intensity must be employed. Two 15- to 20-minute sessions per day are advisable. The therapist should evaluate the edematous extremity with respect to range of

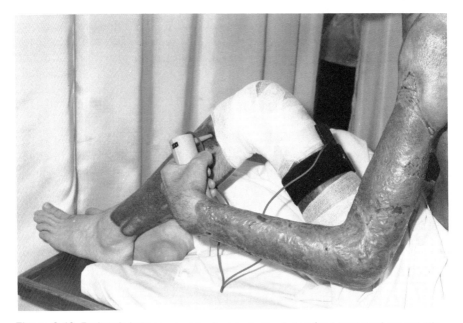

Figure 6.16. Patient is independent in electrical stimulation for a peroneal neuropathy.

motion and circumference to document the effectiveness of this modality. Alternating current, pulsed or surged, is used to free adhered tendons or break up calcium deposits to increase joint range of motion. Careful evaluation of the extremity by the physician and therapist must be made to document the problem as being one of adherence. When using electrical stimulation for increasing range of motion, the extremity is positioned at maximal stretch and all proximal joints are stabilized. The intensity of the current should be sufficient to cause a visable contraction in the agonistic muscle or muscle group associated with the adherence.

Alternating current at an intensity high enough to elicit a muscle contraction through the greater part of the available range of motion is indicated for use in muscle re-education and to increase functional range of motion (6). The movement of the extremity through the range provides kinesthetic feedback to the patient regarding the desired motion. This type of electrical stimulation is a viable adjunct to the patient's program of active and active assistive exercises.

Caution must be taken when stimulating over scar tissue because it offers increased impedance to the electrical current. A higher intensity current is required to depolarize the underlying nerve effectively. Because of this, there is risk of damaging tissue, especially with prolonged use of direct current. The use of electrical muscle stimulation should also be avoided over newly healed areas or recent grafts because of decreased skin impedance to the current and the apparent possibility of reburning the patient. Whenever possible, dispersive and active electrodes are placed on nonburned tissues. As soon as the patient regains voluntary control of the muscle, active exercise is both physiologically and psychologically superior to the externally applied stimulating current (6).

TRANSCUTANEOUS ELECTRICAL STIMULATION

Transcutaneous electrical nerve stimulation (TENS) has been used in physical therapy for the control of both acute and chronic pain in many types of disabled patients. The mechanisms by which TENS counters painful afferent stimuli are complex and careful patient evaluation is essential prior to the use of this modality.

TENS is simply defined as the placement of electrodes at various locations on the surface of the skin; the electrodes are connected to battery-operated generators to deliver a low intensity current of various wave forms. This current acts to provide counterirritation to block certain afferent fibers, to jam pain pathways, or to interfere with the patterns of impulses that arrive at the somatosensory cortex. Low frequency TENS is thought to facilitate the release of endogenous opiates, which produce an analgesic effect similar to that of morphine. Patients with dull, chronic, less localized pain tend to demonstrate relief from low frequency TENS (17).

The thermally injured patient with associated injuries such as bursitis, tendonitis, peripheral nerve injury, or phantom limb pain often benefits from the use of TENS. Donor-site and scar-tissue pain may also be reduced with the TENS unit.

Stimulators generally have either two or four electrodes, which are placed on trigger or acupuncture points, points directly around the area of pain, or in the myotonal or dermatonal distribution. Electrode pairs are applied either in a crisscross or linear pattern over the painful area. The conductive gel and electrode tape used to apply some surface electrodes, however, often irritate newly healed skin, and they cannot be used over open areas. Disposable, self-adherent electrodes sometimes solve the skin irritation problems. Since it is difficult to keep the electrodes in place on well-lubricated skin, all lotion and oil should be removed from the electrode sites prior to application. If the therapist achieves the desired results by placing the electrodes on nonburned skin, problems associated with electrode application may be alleviated.

Most TENS units have a variety of changeable stimulus parameters. Changes in pulse width, stimulus rate, and intensity can be made according to the patient's tolerance, type of pain and desired results. The length of treatment time varies. Many patients leave the unit in place all day except for times of personal hygiene activities. Some burn patients, however, do not tolerate long durations due to skin and scar sensitivity. It is essential that the skin underneath the electrodes be checked frequently for evidence of electrical irritation.

BIOFEEDBACK

The use of biofeedback is often effective with patients who have not experienced success with traditional modalities. The self-feedback supplied by audio or visual means gives the patient a better understanding of his problem and the goal he is trying to achieve.

Biofeedback is a useful modality for muscle relaxation and muscle re-education. For the burn patient, biofeedback is beneficial in treating neurological deficits, increasing wound healing, facilitating normal movement, and promoting general patient relaxation.

The electromyographic (EMG) biofeedback unit should be considered as a modality when the goal for the patient is either recruitment of more motor activity or achievement of muscle relaxation. To use the EMG biofeedback, three electrodes, two active and one ground, are placed on the patient's skin over the appropriate muscle belly with electrode gel and tape. To maximize electrode sensitivity, the patient's skin must be thoroughly scrubbed prior to electrode application. This preparatory procedure precludes the use of this modality with newly healed burns or in the presence of open areas.

Once the electrodes are in place, the therapist must give the patient time to accommodate to the audio and visual mechanics of the modality and then educate the patient as to the specific goals while on the machine. The specific effect of the EMG biofeedback presumes that the added information provided by the feedback enables the patient to attain a degree of strength, control, or relaxation that would not have been possible without this additional information. Using EMG biofeedback teaches the patient muscle relaxation or re-education faster than traditional methods and allows for longer retention of the skill (2).

Thermal biofeedback may be used to increase peripheral blood flow, as demonstrated by increases in skin temperature. Instructing the patient in how to raise his peripheral body skin temperature helps alleviate muscle and/or joint pain and facilitates healing of damaged tissues. It has been hypothesized that thermal biofeedback with relaxation stimulates passage of metabolites and electrolytes down the adrenergic neurons that innervate skin blood vessels. The alteration in the metabolic process leads to improved nerve excitability, synaptic transmission, or function of muscle cells (3).

A monitoring device with a thermal sensor electrode comprise the machine. The thermal electrode is small, and, if possible, is taped distal to the open wound or directly over the painful area. The unit provides audio and/or visual feedback regarding changes in the skin temperature. Educating the patient in techniques of imagery and deep breathing to use while undergoing treatment with the modality facilitates an increase in peripheral blood flow.

An enclosed or private area with a comfortable chair or plinth is recommended when using biofeedback, due to the total patient concentration required for success. Average treatment sessions are 30 minutes and a minimum of three treatments per week is recommended.

AUTORANGE

Grafting procedures, hypertrophic scarring, orthopaedic complications or neurological impairment contribute to joint immobility in the thermally injured patient. Joint immobility leads to contractures which limit the functional ability of the patient. To restore a joint's range of motion, it is necessary to stretch soft tissue and break down any scar tissue or adhesions that have formed. The autorange is a mechanical device designed to increase joint range of motion with passive manipulation or passive stretch to the joint. The mechanics of the unit are such that it can be calibrated to deliver a specific arc of motion at a specific speed. The constant control of rate and the degree of motion provided by the machine often lessens the patient's apprehension and allows increases in range of motion to be made simply by fostering patient relaxation (Fig. 6.17).

The machine is adjusted by the therapist so that when it starts, the motion is within the patient's pain-free existing range. As the patient

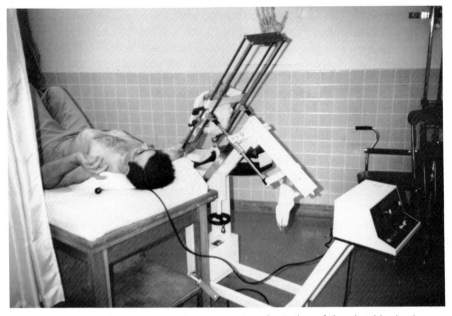

Figure 6.17. Use of autorange to increase external rotation of the shoulder is shown.

becomes accustomed to the motion of the machine, small adjustments are made to increase the arc of motion. The autorange can be adjusted to maintain the contracted extremity at the end of its available range for a regulated amount of time. The modality's ability to maintain an extremity in a position of sustained stretch for a specific time period increases its usefulness in the treatment of the thermally injured patient. The number and length of treatments with the machine vary according to the patient's tolerance and desired results.

Thorough evaluation of the joint and the etiology of its limitation must be made prior to treatment with the autorange. The use of the machine is contraindicated when there is a question of the joint's stability, regardless of the etiology. The autorange should be used as an adjunct to, and not a replacement for, the traditional manual therapy techniques. Goniometric measurements are necessary pre- and post-treatment on the autorange to document the effects of this modality.

INTERMITTENT COMPRESSION

An intermittent compression unit aids in the reduction of persistent edema in a healed burn extremity. The trauma of the burn often destroys the lymphatic channels causing edema to form around and distal to the injured tissues. Distal swelling in an extremity is fairly common following second and third degree circumferential burns due to the compromised venous return.

The intermittent compression unit provides a type of mechanical massage to the edematous extremity. The unit consists of a pressure generator and a pneumatic appliance. The pneumatic appliance or pressure sleeve is available in a variety of sizes to accommodate children and adults. It is designed in such a manner to supply a graded amount of mechanical pressure to an edematous extremity.

Prior to treatment, the patient's blood pressure is taken, and he is positioned supine with the edematous extremity elevated. The pressure sleeve is then applied and the pressure generator set to deliver 10–15 mm Hg of pressure less than the patient's diastolic reading. In some instances, it is desirable for the patient to wear a stockinette or commercial pressure garment such as a glove under the pneumatic device to maximize venous return. Normal treatment duration is approximately 60–90 minutes twice a day.

To document the effectiveness of the compression unit, the therapist records circumferential measurements of the edematous extremity before and after treatment. The treatment is terminated if the patient feels any numbness or tingling in any part of the extremity while on the machine. The unit is contraindicated when a systemic infection is suspected or when open areas are present on the edematous extremity.

PARAFFIN AND SUSTAINED STRETCHING

Burn scar is characterized by dryness and inflexibility. Paraffin, which provides superficial heat and lubrication, is best applied to the healed burn scars in conjunction with static stretching prior to active exercises. The combination of paraffin with sustained stretch usually begins late in the acute phase of rehabilitation after major healing has occurred and it is generally continued throughout the patient's rehabilitation. The use of paraffin is particularly indicated when a painful and contracting scar limits joint range of motion. The superficial heat and lubrication reduce scar pain and improve scar extensibility. A standard paraffin machine is usually available in physical therapy departments; small paraffin machines are also available and are frequently prescribed by physicians for home use. If commercially available premixed paraffin is not selected for use, a mixture of two and one-half ounces of mineral oil to one pound of paraffin can be used (7). Routinely, paraffin is maintained at a temperature of 51.7–54.4° C (15). However, the use of paraffin at this temperature is contraindicated on newly healed, fragile, or insensitive skin. With burn patients, the paraffin should be used at lower temperatures, approximately 46–50° C or 118° F (18). Paraffin cooler than 46° C is advised for the treatment of children and all patients with newly healed areas. The required amount of paraffin is either removed from the machine to cool prior to application, or paraffin with a low melting point is used, if available, and the paraffin machine adjusted to maintain the proper temperature. Hot packs must not be used as a substitute for paraffin because they retain a higher degree of heat than paraffin and could reburn the patient. When paraffin is not available, an alternative method for achieving the benefits of superficial heat is to (1) apply a generous layer of Vaseline to the involved extremity; (2) cover with a moist warm towel no warmer than 118° F; (3) cover the towel in plastic to retain the heat; (4) wrap the plastic in a towel or elastic bandage for additional heat retention and to facilitate positioning; and (5) leave in place for 20 minutes.

The paraffin should be applied in such a way as to maximize the combined benefits of heat, lubrication, and sustained stretch. Prior to application, the patient is positioned with the involved scars on maximal stretch. If a joint or multiple joints are involved in the wound, the contractile nature of the scar must be considered and body positions devised that provide stretch along the entire length and width of the involved area. Hands, elbow, and feet may be dipped into the paraffin 8 to 10 times or until they are thickly coated. For areas such as knees, shoulders, and chests, better results are achieved by having the patient lie down and then pouring or patting the paraffin in place until there is a thick coating (7). The area should then be covered with plastic and wrapped in a towel or elastic bandage to minimize heat loss. Sandbag weights, splints, and restraining ties assist in maintaining the stretched position (Fig. 6.18). Normal treatment time in paraffin is 20 minutes.

Modifications in the application of paraffin with sustained stretch and length of treatment time are made according to the newness of the healing, the age and size of the patient, and the patient's tolerance for sustained positioning. Small open areas are protected by covering with gauze prior to the paraffin application. If hypertrophic scars are aggravated by paraffin usuage, it is discontinued or reduced in frequency. When using paraffin as a modality, all contraindications for superficial heat are followed. The majority of thermally injured patients respond favorably to paraffin from a physical and psychological standpoint.

FLUIDOTHERAPY

The fluidotherapy unit must be considered when seeking a thermotherapeutic agent to decrease pain and/or increase range of motion in a body part, particularly a foot or a hand.

This high intensity superficial heat modality consists of a dry whirlpool of finely divided solid particles suspended in a heated air steam. The mixture

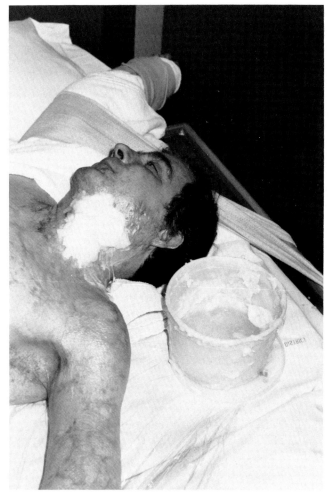

Figure 6.18. Paraffin application is in progress: note positioning of right shoulder in sustained stretch.

has the properties of a liquid, and the temperature can be regulated between 95–130° F. The solid particle medium used in the unit is self-sterilizing, making one unit suitable for the treatment of a variety of diagnoses without the risk of infection and contamination (5). This unit delivers more heat to the body part during a 20-minute treatment than the dip method of paraffin or hydrotherapy (4). Fluidotherapy provides the patient with the benefits of massage and allows the patient to exercise actively while receiving heat to the specific body part. Some of the larger units have an additional entrance for the therapist so the patient can be assisted with active exercise.

To use the unit, the body part is positioned horizontally into the medium thereby decreasing the tendency for the part to swell. By protecting small open areas, treatment can be continued with this modality. Contraindications for fluidotherapy are those associated with any type of superficial heat.

The use of fluidotherapy with burns is not well documented. The burn patient's skin durability and sensation must be evaluated prior to emergence in the unit. Periodic monitoring of the patient's skin responses while undergoing each treatment is imperative. The combination of the dry heat with the massaging solid particles, the allowance for active exercise while undergoing each treatment, and the fact that this unit can be used in the presence of open wounds make it an attractive modality to consider for the management of problems in the adult burn patient.

LASER

A new development in modalities is the use of the low power laser for biostimulation. Marketed as a "cold beam" laser, this type of unit gives the therapist access to monochromatic light generated by a helium-neon glass tube. The power output is minimal, well below the threshold required to cause tissue warming. The laser is claimed to provide a biopositive stimulation, creating cellular microoscillation which leads to a host of reactions, possibly even DNA repair (10).

The applications of the laser for the treatment of the thermally injured patient fall into two main areas, tissue healing and pain management. Stimulation provided by broadcasting the laser light over the open wounds is stated to accelerate the rate of tissue regeneration. Marked activation of phagocytosis, increases in tissue granulation rate, and faster epithelization of wounds have all been reported with the laser treatment (13). Clinical experience supports using the laser with burn patients to facilitate healing of chronic open areas less than one inch in diameter that have been open for an extended period of time. Areas of sloughed graft, open areas in web spaces, chronically draining areas and other similar conditions are also appropriate for laser application. Laser use in wound healing requires a stroking technique with the wand held one-half mm from the recipient tissue for a 15-second time duration per mm of tissue stimulated. The entire wound may be treated with the laser or the therapist may choose to stimulate only those points on the perimeter of the wound. When treatment is performed on a daily basis, evidence of tissue healing is usually apparent after the second or third session. The laser should not be used for promoting tissue healing in the presence of cellulitis or any other type of systemic infection.

The cold beam laser is sometimes effective in the management of pain. The effect of applying laser energy to trigger and acupuncture points is believed to be similar to that of electrical or mechanical stimulation (10). Due to the small diameter of the laser beam, auricular points can be accurately identified and stimulated. The laser is held directly on the trigger area and each identified point stimulated for 20 seconds. Most patients demonstrate some relief from pain within three treatment sessions.

The use of the laser as a healing and pain management tool is relatively new in the United States. Specific contraindications for use of the cold beam laser are not well documented. Adherence to safety precautions and treatment guidelines should, however, ensure proper use of the laser with the burn population.

ULTRASOUND

Ultrasound is any vibrational energy of a frequency too high for stimulation of sensory receptors of the human ear. Therapeutic ultrasound, using the direct contact or underwater method, is administered at intensities no higher than three watts per cm^2 (6). Using ultrasound under water is indicated for small areas with irregularly shaped surfaces such as fingers and ankles. Due to water's conductive properties, lower wattages of ultrasound are effective when using this technique. The thermal and nonthermal effects of ultrasound combined with its depth of penetration make it a useful modality in the management of many physical problems associated with the thermally injured patient. Its use is supported in the literature and by clinical experience for the management of pain and decreased range of motion.

Ultrasound at one-half to one and one-half watts per cm^2 decreases the conduction velocity of peripheral nerves. Due to this physiological effect, ultrasound is an effective modality for decreasing pain associated with peripheral neuropathies or neuromal pain following amputation. When pain is due to increased proliferation of connective tissue as in severe scarring, polypeptides absorb ultrasonic energy and cause a relaxation of these bonds, decreasing painful symptoms (6). The patient usually experiences a greater decrease in pain if the therapist treats the involved scar tissue with ice massage prior to the application of ultrasound.

There is a 1 to 2° C increase in temperature of the underlying muscle tissue when a continuous moving technique is used with the ultrasound head. The increase in tissue temperature facilitates increased blood flow to the area, causing decreased pain with a general relaxation of the tissue. The effects of increased blood flow to the area last up to an hour after a five-minute exposure to ultrasound (6).

Ultrasound increases the elasticity of tendon, muscle, connective fascia, and most scar tissue, thus allowing for an increase in range of motion (Fig. 6.19). Although difficult to document, the use of ultrasound is advocated for increasing joint range of motion in long standing conditions of bursitis

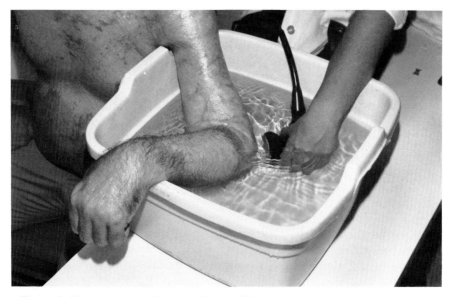

Figure 6.19. Underwater ultrasound is beneficial in treatment of heterotopic bone.

or tendonitis. This increase in range of motion may be due to the absorption of calcium deposits or the increase in elasticity of the ligamentous tissues. Goniometric measurements of the involved joint should be made to document progress towards the desired goal (6). Application of ultrasound for at least five consecutive days is advisable for achievement of maximum benefits.

All clinically accepted contraindications of ultrasound should be observed. Healed burned areas often have compensated sensation; therefore, a sensory evaluation of the scarred area is advisable prior to the application of this modality.

Summary

It is necessary that professionals involved in burn care have a thorough understanding of the current information in their respective medical specialties to provide optimal care and make decisions which are in the patient's best interest. All team members must work together with an awareness of and mutual respect for all facets of burn care. In the physical treatment of burns, there is no single best treatment method. As each patient presents with unique problems, specific treatment techniques are incorporated into his individualized rehabilitation program.

As stated in this chapter, the therapist must carefully integrate the exercise techniques with the appropriate treatment modalities to meet the patient's constantly changing needs. The suggestions offered represent successful and current therapeutic techniques. Ultimately, the patient's successful rehabilitation is not only dependent upon his commitment to the program, but also upon the knowledge and skill of the professionals in utilizing these techniques.

REFERENCES

1. Artz C, Moncrief J, Pruitt B: *Burns: A Team Approach.* Philadelphia, W.B. Saunders Company, 1979.
2. Basmajian J, Fernando C: Biofeedback in physical medicine and rehabilitation. *Biofeedback Self Regulation* 3:435–450, 1978.
3. Bird E, Colbourne G: Rehabilitation of an electrical burn patient through thermal biofeedback. *Biofeedback Self Regulation* 5:283–286, 1980.
4. Borrell RM, Henley JE: Fluidotherapy in a hand clinic. *Arch Phys Med Rehabil* 60:536, 1979.
5. Fuentes L, Lopez D: An evaluation of a new heat modality: Fluidotherapy. Presented at the National Meeting of the American Physical Therapy Association, Atlanta, GA, 1979.
6. Griffin J, Karselis T: *Physical Agents for Physical Therapists.* Springfield, IL, Charles C Thomas, 1978.
7. Head M, Helm P: Paraffin and sustained stretching in the treatment of burn contracture. *Burns* 4:136–139, 1977.
8. Helm P, Kevorkian C, Lushbaugh M, et al: Burn injury: Rehabilitation management in 1982. *Arch Phys Med Rehabil* 63:6–16, 1982.
9. Hummel R (Ed): *Clinical Burn Therapy: A Management and Prevention Guide.* Boston, John Wright, 1982.
10. Kleinkort JA: Clinical use of laser in chronic pain and tissue healing. *Stimulus* 7:1, 1982.
11. Knott M, Voss D: *Proprioceptive Neuromuscular Facilitation.* New York, Harper and Row, 1969.
12. Koepke G: The role of physical medicine in the treatment of burns. *Surg Clin North Am* 50:1385–1399, 1970.
13. Kovinskii IT: The treatment of burns by laser. *Zdravookhr Kaz* 3:46, 1973.
14. Larson D, Abston S, Evans E, et al: Techniques for decreasing scar formation and contracture in the burned patient. *J Trauma* 11:807–823, 1971.
15. Lehman J (Ed): *Therapeutic Heat and Cold.* Baltimore, Williams & Wilkins, 1982.
16. Licht S (Ed): *Therapeutic Exercise,* 2nd ed. Baltimore, Waverly Press, 1961.
17. Mannheimer J: Neurophysiology of pain. Presented at the Conference on Pain Management, Chicago, IL, 1977.
18. Nicosia J, Stein E, Stein J: The advantages of physiotherapy for burn patients under anesthesia. *Burns* 6:202–204, 1979.
19. O'Sullivan S, Cullen K, Schmitz T: *Physical Rehabilitation: Evaluation and Treatment Procedures.* Philadelphia, F.A. Davis Company, 1981.
20. Rusk H: *Rehabilitation Medicine.* St. Louis, C.V. Mosby Company, 1971.
21. Wenger N: *Coronary Care: Rehabilitation After Myocardial Infarction.* New York, American Heart Association, 1973.

ADDITIONAL READINGS

1. Artz C (Ed): *Research in Burns.* Philadelphia, F.A. Davis Company, 1962.
2. Feller I, Jones C: *Nursing the Burned Patient.* Ann Arbor, MI, Institute for Burn Medicine, 1974.
3. Stone N, Boswick J: *Profiles of Burn Management.* FL, Industrial Medicine Publishing Co., 1969.

7

Wound and Skin Care

MARJORIE D. HEAD

Infection is the major problem in patients who survive the resuscitation phase of burn injury. Destruction of the normal skin barrier to bacterial invasion and the presence of a large necrotic tissue mass, acting as a bacterial incubator, are the most obvious bases for burn wound infection. This can seriously interfere with healing, and convert a partial-thickness burn into a full-thickness wound (1, 9, 24). Increased tissue damage may also occur due to the loss of water vapor through the injured surface causing dehydration of the exposed dermis. This may increase the depth of the burn and thus delay healing (1).

The scope and importance of wound care, débridement, and subsequent skin care during the course of treatment cannot be overemphasized, and indeed, are the most important considerations for functional and cosmetic outcome. After resuscitation is initiated, the burn wound should be thoroughly cleansed and debrided of all nonviable tissue. The care begins in the emergent phase and continues through acute and convalescent phases for both inpatients and outpatients. With meticulous treatment, large partial-thickness burns may require no surgical intervention, or only limited procedures.

Early surgical excision is one of the most important advances in decreasing the morbidity and mortality in burns; still there are many times when this procedure is impractical or contraindicated early in the course of burn care. Aggressive and thorough wound care becomes even more important to help delineate wounds prior to early surgical intervention, to protect and promote good granulation tissue until grafting, or to promote rapid healing in those moderate to deep partial-thickness wounds which tend to have prolonged healing times and subsequently increased scarring.

Wound Care

Wound care is best provided in areas designed specifically for that purpose, either on the nursing unit or in the hydrotherapy section of a Physcial Medicine Department. It must be provided in a clean area using sterile techniques to protect the patient from bacteria. The goals of wound care are:

(1) preventing and/or controlling infection.

(2) preserving as much tissue as possible, and preventing destruction of remaining viable epithelium.

(3) preparing a wound for the earliest possible closure either by primary healing or by grafting.

CLEANSING TECHNIQUES OF OPEN WOUNDS

There are three types of cleansing techniques: local care of a particular wound or area, spray hydrotherapy or nonsubmersion, and submersion, which may or may not include agitation of the water. The choice depends upon the depth of injury, extent and location of the wound, and the medical condition of the patient. Hydrotherapy is generally discontinued for three to five days following autograft or homograft, but can be continued daily when a heterograft is applied. Dressings should be removed, if possible, prior to moistening, since this aides in débridement of the area by removing devitalized tissue stuck to the bandage. If the dressing cannot be removed without undue pain or damage to the tissue underneath, the dressing should be moistened prior to removal. In extreme cases, it may be necessary to let the bandage soak for a few minutes before removing it. All areas should be scrubbed gently, but thoroughly, with a mild detergent to remove all loose tissue, medications, and exudate. Commercial brushes impregnated with surgical scrub are available; a piece of sterile fine mesh with soap applied to it may also be used for washing the wound. Agents such as hexachlorophene or povidone-iodine surgical scrub can be routinely used for the washing process (11). However, the clinician should be aware of the reported complications of hexachlorophene (21) and the large percentage of patients who have a sensitivity to iodine products. In these cases, an alternate agent is a soap without perfumes or dyes, such as Calgon Lotion Soap, or water without a cleansing agent. A new sponge or piece of sterile gauze should be used for each area of the body treated, washing from least contaminated to most contaminated area. When mechanical débridement is indicated, it immediately follows the cleansing process.

Local Wound Care

Local wound care generally involves the care of small wounds using a sterile container of water and cleansing agents. This can be accomplished at bedside or in any convenient area. Local wound care is also indicated for areas of the body which are difficult to treat in submersion hydrotherapy, such as the ears and face.

Spray Hydrotherapy or Nonsubmersion

Spray hydrotherapy or nonsubmersion wound care involves the use of a hose or shower head to allow the water to run intermittently or continuously over the burn wounds. Preferrably, this is accomplished by placing the patient on a stretcher which is suspended over a tank or tub. The water temperature is 100° Fahrenheit which allows for some cooling as it is sprayed on the wounds. In some cases, the patient is treated in a conventional shower, but this does not allow the treating personnel easy access to the wounds, and thus, the patient is responsible for much of the cleansing and scrubbing.

Spraying allows for easier protection of trachiostomies, intravenous catheters, and cutdowns. It is indicated for areas of severe swelling, such as lower extremities where dependent positioning and submersion in warm water would increase edema. Areas that are especially moist and purulent do not require soaking for adequate cleansing and can be easily cleansed and debrided by using the spray technique. Burns to the perineum are easier to treat using the spray as the area is difficult to reach when the patient is submerged. The spray rinses extraneous material from the wounds, loosens eschar and dead tissue, and is helpful in decreasing the pain of scrubbing and débridement. Submersion is usually limited to 20 minutes or less, whereas the spray may be used for longer periods of time, depending upon the patient's condition and tolerance. Débridement can thus be more extensive.

Submersion

Submersion hydrotherapy consists of filling a tub, tank, or whirlpool with water at a temperature of 96–98° Fahrenheit. The patient or burned extremity is placed in the water and submerged for a period of usually 10–20 minutes. Extended submersion of moderate to large burns should be avoided due to the loss of electrolytes (13) that may result in respiratory complications.

Submersion is indicated for wounds that are dry and have thick adherent eschar to help soften the dead tissue and allow for easier débridement. Most tanks and whirlpools are equipped with agitators that assist in removing creams and debris, softening eschar, irrigating wounds, and adding to patient comfort. Agitation is not recommended for new or tenuous grafts. With submersion hydrotherapy there is the potential for wound contamination from normal body flora and from one wound site to another.

There is always some risk of contamination with any type of wound care but this can be minimized with proper attention to asceptic techniques (34), careful selection of the wounds to be submerged, proper scrubbing and rinsing of the wounds following submersion, and thorough cleansing of the hydrotherapy unit between patients (8, 10, 23, 32, 33, 37).

Débridement

Débridement is the removal of any devitalized or contaminated tissue. It can be divided into five broad categories: surgical, infection, natural enzymatic, commercially prepared enzymatic, and mechanical. Surgical débridement including full-thickness and tangential excisions will be addressed in another chapter. When surgical débridement is not indicated, conservative techniques are employed.

In infection, bacteria and inflammation hasten the separation of devitalized tissue (1); however, the infection also destroys epidermal vestages and, in effect, deepens the wound. Topical antibacterial agents can help control the infection and thus lead to slower natural separation of dead tissue (35). Decreasing infection produces a more superficial burn with a higher percentage of spontaneous healing.

Natural enzymatic cleavage of collagen can produce separation of dead tissue in a very slow process (19). However, this is too slow a process to be advantageous and is dangerous in large burns, when infection may jeopardize the patient's life. Commercially prepared enzymes work in much the same way, but more quickly. They are used for rapid eschar removal, permitting earlier grafting. Treatment with topical enzymes has been used with only varying degrees of success (1, 2, 13, 31).

Rapid separation of eschar is also possible by a more aggressive program of mechanical débridement. It is usually the treatment of choice because of the disadvantages of the other methods.

Nonsurgical débridement involves the use of sterile scissors and forceps, a straight-edged blade, safety razor, or a scalpel. Shaving a small margin of normal skin around the wound is generally recommended to prevent contamination from hair follicles (17, 27). Forceps are used to remove loose necrotic tissue from the wound bed (Fig. 7.1). The end of the forceps or the blunt end of the scissors may be used to probe under the edge of the eschar, using careful sweeping motions, to separate parts of the eschar and allow it to be trimmed. Only dead tissue should be removed.

When using local wound care or nonsubmersion hydrotherapy techniques, saline-soaked sterile mesh can be applied to open areas to keep them from drying. Drying causes dead tissue and eschar to adhere to the wound, makes removal painful, and may cause excessive bleeding. Dry sterile mesh is applied to all areas that tend to remain moist with excessive exudate. It is allowed to adhere for two to five minutes and then gently pulled from the wound, removing much of the exudative material. This can be repeated until the area is fairly clean and dry and allows individual pieces of dead tissue to be identified and removed with forceps.

It is well worth noting that there is a basic cellular inflammatory reponse to trauma (25, 26), and the very act of removing bandages, cleansing the wound, and debriding can constitute daily repeated traumas to an existing wound. Daily hydrotherapy and wound care, which must be aggressive and vigorous to be effective, should always be done in a manner to inflict as little trauma as possible to the wound and the granulating bed.

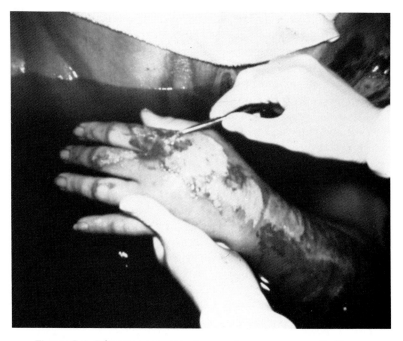

Figure 7.1. Débridement using forceps to remove necrotic tissue.

Anatomical Considerations

HEAD

This is not an area which can realistically or practically be submerged or sprayed. Burns to the head and face can be covered with saline soaks for 20–30 minutes prior to cleansing and debriding to obtain the softening effects of submersion.

Care must be taken to avoid excessive trauma or overdébridement to an area that can easily develop hypertrophic scarring. Due to the highly vascular state and the preponderance of hair follicles, the majority of facial burns will heal spontaneously with varying degrees of scarring. For men suffering burns over the cheeks, jaw, and neck, shaving with a safety razor offers a surprisingly well-tolerated method of wound care and débridement. This is especially useful for outpatient burns, which secondarily gives the patient a feeling of control over his treatment. Hair which comes in contact with facial burns should be trimmed or shaved. Even when hair does not come in contact with the burn, it should be kept clean with daily washings, to decrease bacterial fallout into the wounds. For outpatients, this can easily be accomplished by simply showering, washing hair and face, and shaving in the routine fashion.

Eyelids and Lips

Except in severe burns where early surgical intervention is indicated, these areas are unlikely to be full-thickness and will not form a true eschar. More likely, there will be the formation of an exudative coagulum and drying of the crust exposing the healed epithelium. Burns to the eyelids and lips should not be debrided. Rather, the areas should be gently washed, allowing the crust to remain until it separates naturally. The application of an antibacterial ointment or Vaseline may help prevent cracking and repeated trauma to the lips.

Ears

After burn injury, the ears are prone to trauma and infection. Because of minimal subcutaneous tissue, cartilage can easily be exposed. Wound care should always be done with a gentle hand, avoiding débridement to expose cartilage except in areas of obvious nonviability when separation is occurring (27). Prolonged pressure to the ear with equipment, supplies, and positioning can lead to necrosis. The area should be closely watched for signs of increased swelling, redness, pain or drainage which may indicate chondritis or infection.

Scalp

Even though the scalp is highly vascular with an abundance of hair follicles, it can still be a relatively difficult area to heal, and is prone to delayed healing and repeated breakdown. The skin on the scalp is the thickest of the body; the subcutaneous fascia and epicranial aponeurosis are bound firmly together acting as an inelastic covering with the skin fixed to the subcutaneous tissue (9). Scalp burns are treated by shaving the involved areas as often as necessary to keep growing hair from interfering with the healing process. Shaving too often, however, can traumatize the thin healing skin, and thus is reserved for use only when necessary. Repeated vigorous aggressive débridement and scab removal delays healing. The scalp should be washed once or twice daily, but shaved only when hair growth reaches the point where it prevents adequate cleansing by trapping nonviable particles and debris on the wound. Scabs should be removed only when they are loose or purulent and draining.

PERINEUM

Partial-thickness burns to the perineum, especially involving the penis and scrotum, generally respond to submersion, with mild agitation, to soften crust and eschar, followed by gentle but thorough washing. Forceps can be used to remove debris, but débridement should be avoided. The scrubbing motion using sponges or mesh is usually adequate to remove necrotic tissue as it separates from the wound. Often the patient can more effectively scrub the area, using forceps to remove loose necrotic tissue.

Special Concerns

PAIN

Physical and emotional limitations of the patient, in regard to his level of pain tolerance, have a vital effct on the duration and degree of wound care that can be rendered. As opposed to surgical intervention, daily wound care cannot be preceded by anesthetization of the patient. The patient's response to and tolerance of treatment can sometimes be enhanced by using techniques such as relaxation, biofeedback, self-hypnosis or mind-altering drugs. Administration of pain medication prior to dressing changes varies from center to center. Still, pain during wound care and dressing changes remains a constant dilemma, yet to be resolved.

BLISTERS

There are differences in opinion as to whether or not blisters should be removed (see Chapter 4). Some advocate removal (11, 16), except in areas of thick calloused skin as on the palms of the hands. Others believe that as long as blisters are intact, they represent a sterile field (18). However, it is impossible to be certain that some minute opening does not exist, allowing bacterial invasion; also, wound infection can occur from bacteria harbored within skin appendages in intact blisters. As large blisters continue to fill with fluid, they are subject to rupture, causing additional trauma to the wound. Topical antibacterial agents do not effectively penetrate intact bullae. Blister formation may limit the amount of exercise or functional activity that the patient can accomplish. Small blisters, not in danger of rupturing or limiting motion, can be left intact with close monitoring for possible enlargement. Small and moderate-sized blisters may be drained and the blister roof flattened for use as a biological dressing (29).

EXPOSED TENDON AND BONE

Exposed bones and tendons must be kept moist to prevent dehydration, so that they can be adequately covered when a good granulation bed has formed. Granulation tissue in and around the wound should be stimulated to encourage growth, which is accomplished by gently rubbing with a semirough material such as a sponge or gauze, or by gentle pin prick with a sterile needle. Granulating islands should be covered with coarse mesh to stimulate growth (Fig. 7.2). Wet-to-wet dressings with saline or triple-antibiotic solution (polymyxin, bacitracin, and neomycin) can be used to prevent drying of the bone or tendon. Care must be taken to avoid maceration of the surrounding area. To protect the surrounding skin from maceration it should be washed, thoroughly dried, and then coated with a thin

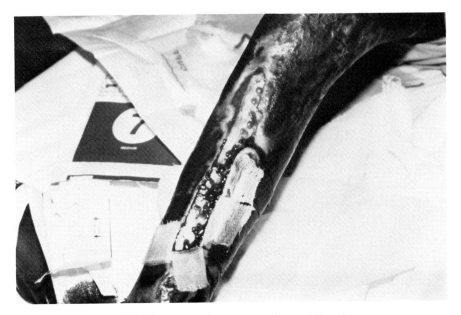

Figure 7.2. Coarse mesh on areas of granulation tissue.

layer of Vaseline prior to the application of a wet dressing. The dressing over the wound should be kept moist and changed two to four times a day. A simpler method to prevent drying of tendons and bone, especially on outpatients, is the use of Second skin (Spenco Medical Corp., Box 8113, Waco, TX 76710) (Fig. 7.3), a synthetic gel-like plastic-coated material. The product is coated on both sides with a thin sheet of plastic. One side of the plastic is peeled and the gel is placed directly on the wound. (Figs. 7.4 and 7.5). The plastic is left intact on the opposite or outer side. When applied to the wound and covered with a light dressing, it requires changing only every 12 hours to prevent drying. It has worked effectively to prevent dehydration of these structures for a period of several months (Figs. 7.6 and 7.7).

DELAYED HEALING

Patients who are discharged early with significant open areas can generally be treated adequately as outpatients. Healing should proceed with the proper selection of topical agents and dressings. However, patients who are discharged with areas that have been open for extended periods of time and which show evidence of delayed healing or graft rejection, present special wound care problems.

Vigorous mechanical débridement of the wound at this time is generally not indicated. Rather, the emphasis is on cleaning the area, protection, and stimulation of the granulation tissue to maintain a healthy vascular bed.

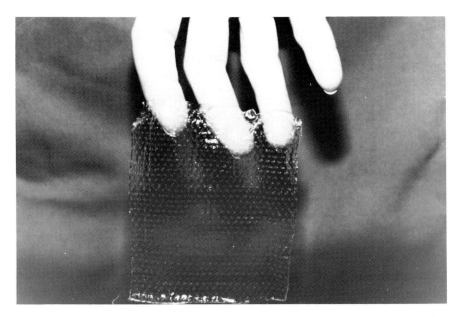

Figure 7.3. Second skin.

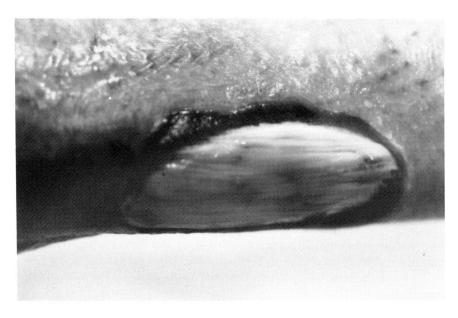

Figure 7.4. Exposed Achilles tendon.

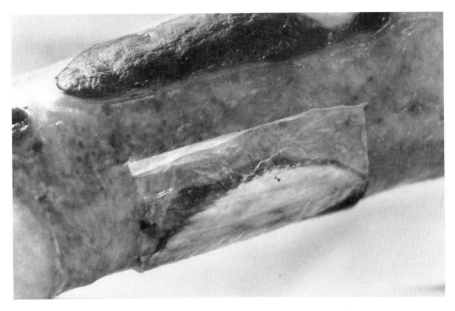

Figure 7.5. Exposed tendon with second skin in place.

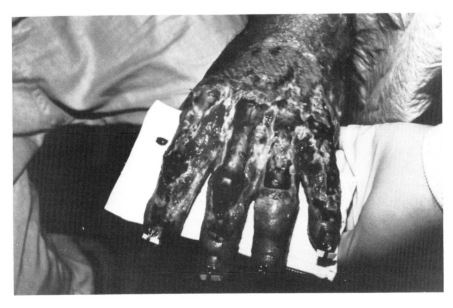

Figure 7.6. Exposed bones.

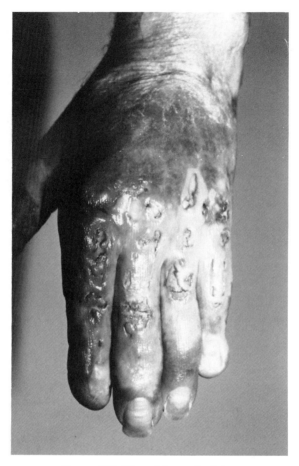

Figure 7.7. Wound 5 months later.

Wounds that have been open for prolonged periods tend to develop hypertrophic granulation tissue or slick avascular layers of granulation over the wound. They tend to repeatedly slough pigskin and do not respond well to silver sulfadiazine dressings. Coarse-mesh patches stimulate growth of granulation tissue in small deep wounds, while fine-mesh patches will help control or decrease overgranulated areas. Patches are applied wet and allowed to dry on the wound. Areas which are more difficult to control may require cauterization with a few applications of silver nitrate daily for one to three days, or until the excessive tissue is under control. The avascular wound seems to develop healthier granulation tissue when stimulated by a variety of agents. Sometimes a dry dressing or wet-to-dry dressing with saline or triple-antibiotic solution improves the wound. If not, this can be alternated with days of barrier type dressings, or a trial of Sulfamylon.

Ulceration of scar tissue in the popliteal and cubital fossas is another problem that easily becomes chronic and requires special attention. Areas of breakdown over elbows and knees are treated by limiting motion and keeping the joint slightly flexed. Neomycin ointment will help prevent drying and further cracking of the granulation tissue.

Dressing and Bandages

A dressing includes any agent or medication applied directly to the wound. A bandage is the outer gauze or mesh wrap applied over the dressing. Following wound care and débridement, the wound must be redressed, or at least protected until it can be redressed. Dressing wounds on inpatients can be a time-consuming procedure, but a variety of options are available for dealing effectively with this aspect of treatment. In some institutions, wound care and dressing changes are done on the nursing unit; in others, wound care and dressing changes are provided in the hydrotherapy area. Some burn units have dressing teams available following hydrotherapy, with the patient being returned to the unit for dressing application. Any of these methods can work effectively, depending upon the institution's environment, staffing patterns, and rapport between services. The goal is an efficient and effective method to best provide for the patient's needs.

If the patient is to be transported elsewhere for dressing, the wound must be protected while the patient is being moved. A single layer of sterile mesh can be gently laid over the wound, but must not be allowed to adhere because of pain with removal later. All exposed tendons, joints, bones, and cartilage should be covered with multiple layers of saline-soaked mesh to prevent drying until dressing is applied. The patient should also be covered with sheets or blankets to prevent chilling. Outpatients are usually more easily dressed in Physical Therapy, or where hydrotherapy is provided.

DRESSINGS

The type of dressing and manner of application for inpatients is critical. For outpatients, the selection is less crucial because most small partial-thickness burns will heal regardless of the type of dressing (30); however, the daily wound care can either enhance or hinder the healing process (36).

A multitude of topical agents and dressings is available and all are used with varying degrees of success. Dressings include topical agents, biological, and synthetic or barrier. Biological dressings play a major role in the treatment of outpatient burns. New, but effective in selected cases, are the barrier type of dressings. The proper mode of treatment is based upon the patient's age, activity level, and home environment. The agent is selected according to the location, extent, and type of burn. Healing time can be enhanced by alternating dressings as the wound changes. Wounds should be evaluated frequently and agents and dressings changed as needed (15, 31).

Topical Agents

Creams and ointments can be applied with a sterile tongue blade with care not to contaminate the container by putting the used blade into it. Cream is applied in a thin layer over the wound, allowing enough extra for absorption by the bandage. It is not necessary or desirable for the cream or ointment to be applied in a thick coat as heavy layers of cream encourage maceration and can harm regenerating epithelium.

Topical agents are applied to the wound one to three times a day on inpatients, while once or twice daily is usually sufficient for outpatients.

Silver sulfadiazine is by far the most commonly used topical agent (4, 15, 31). It is a broad spectrum antibacterial agent, is not associated with metabolic disturbances, and is relatively painless (24). It does not dry the wound; it keeps the eschar and granulating bed soft, and thus, facilitates exercise and normal daily activities. It is only mildly effective in penetrating eschar. It is less effective in purulent wounds and in maintaining a good bed of granulation tissue in wounds with delayed healing; granulation tissue is best stimulated by a more drying type agent.

Sulfamylon has a wide antibacterial spectrum and penetrates eschar very effectively (15, 20, 24). However, it is extremely painful on application, is drying to the wound and, when used under bandages, can cause maceration of the skin and contact dermatitis (29). Because it produces pain and has a drying effect on the wound, it also interferes with the exercise programs. Therefore, it is seldom used in outpatient treatment, except in selected instances. It is, however, effective in treating burns of the ears, as it will rapidly penetrate the cartilage, does not dissolve, and adheres to the surface. It is sometimes the agent of choice for small full-thickness burns with thick eschar formation, being treated on an outpatient basis until ready for grafting.

Povidone-iodine ointment is another of the agents which is effective against a broad spectrum of organisms (4, 20), has good penetration of eschar, and has no serious metabolic consequences (15). However, many patients report a moderate degree of pain with its use and it is extremely drying to the wound. It is commonly used prior to excision to dry the eschar to better delineate the area for surgical intervention.

Many antibacterial ointments are available, including neomycin and bacitracin, which are effective in managing small burns. They are painless, easy to apply, and keep the wound bed from drying. They are especially useful for facial burns and where burns are prone to drying and cracking. However, the antibacterial effectiveness of such agents is short-lived in the presence of proteinaceous exudate (29), and less effective on moist wounds. Gentamicin cream is used cautiously because of early development of resistant strains of microorganisms, especially *Pseudomonas* (4, 14).

Biological Dressings

The easy availability and relatively low cost of heterograft (xenograft or pigskin) in recent years has made it a valuable and realistic option for outpatient treatment, while the scarcity and expense of homograft (allograft or cadaver skin or fetal membranes) (28) make it impractical for use with relatively minor burns. The most common use of the biological dressing has been for the protection and promotion of granulation tissue, and for its effectiveness in indicating the readiness of a site for grafting (38, 39). For inpatients, this becomes extremely valuable following early surgical excision in preparing the wounds for final grafting. Some hospitals have used biological dressings for mechanical débridement with frequent removal and reapplication. This can be achieved equally well at less cost with conventional wet-to-dry dressings (39).

Commercial pigskin is an effective biological dressing, and is one of the most commonly used. When applied early in the course of burn treatment, it effectively seals the burned area, decreasing water loss (31) and preventing dehydration of the injured skin. It can be applied to burns that are moderate to deep partial-thickness following initial cleansing and débridement. These wounds characteristically appear red to whitish in color, are dry with little or no exudate, and have minimal or no blister formation. Similarly, superficial partial-thickness burns may be covered early with pigskin, once initial débridement is accomplished and the blisters removed. The wound should appear cherry red and moist, but without drainage or exudate.

Once pigskin is applied, it is usually left in place as long as there is good "take" and healing is occurring underneath. In moderate to deep burns, this should occur in two to three weeks; in light to moderate burns, the wound should be healed within seven to ten days (Tables 7.1–7.3). A take is defined as adherence of the pigskin to the wound, strong enough to resist some sheer force, and uniform in appearance without fluid-filled pockets (35).

Table 7.1.
Mean Healing Time by % of Burn, Nondelayed Treatment—2° Burn, 85 Patients

%	No. of Patients	Mean Healing Time (Days)	Standard Deviation	Range in Days	
				Min.	Max.
1% or less	28	12.9	±5.06	4.0	24.0
2–4%	30	13.2	±5.81	6.0	29.0
5–10%	20	14.6	±6.31	5.0	27.0
11–18%	7	17.4	±9.71	7.0	36.0
Total	85				

Table 7.2.
Mean Healing Time by Type of Burn, Nondelayed Treatment—2° Burn, 85 Patients

Type Burn	No. of Patients	Mean Healing Time (Days)	Standard Deviation	Range in Days	
				Min.	Max.
Flame	15	15.5	±6.00	7.0	27.0
Scald	36	11.8	±6.41	4.0	36.0
Grease	15	15.7	±5.19	7.0	29.0
Chemical	5	14.2	±5.54	8.0	20.0
Thermal	13	15.0	±5.86	6.0	26.0
Electrical	1	11.0	±0.00	11.0	11.0
Total	85				

Table 7.3.
Mean Healing Time by Location, Nondelayed Treatment—2° Burn, 85 Patients

Location	No. of Patients	Mean Healing Time (Days)	Standard Deviation	Range in Days	
				Min.	Max.
Head and Neck	8	9.3	±4.13	4.0	18.0
Upper ext.	20	12.4	±4.37	7.0	22.0
Hand	14	15.1	±5.78	2.0	24.0
Trunk	23	13.6	±8.23	5.0	36.0
Thigh	8	16.0	±6.14	9.0	29.0
Leg and Foot	12	16.0	±5.43	7.0	24.0
Total	85				

The wound should appear dry without drainage or exudate and should be able to withstand daily bandage changes and gentle washing.

Small pockets of fluid can sometimes be effectively drained and flattened without removing the pigskin. In the presence of considerable drainage, multiple pockets of fluid or slippage of the pigskin over the wound, the xenograft should be removed, the area scrubbed, and new pigskin applied. It is sometimes necessary to make several such applications to achieve a good take. If, however, a good take does not occur within three to four days, other agents are indicated.

When applying pigskin, care should be taken to avoid crossing joints with a single piece. Instead, the pigskin should be trimmed to fit the burned area but stopped at the joint. An additional piece is used to hinge across joints, especially over the multiple joints of the hand (Fig. 7.8). This allows greater freedom of motion when the pigskin has "taken."

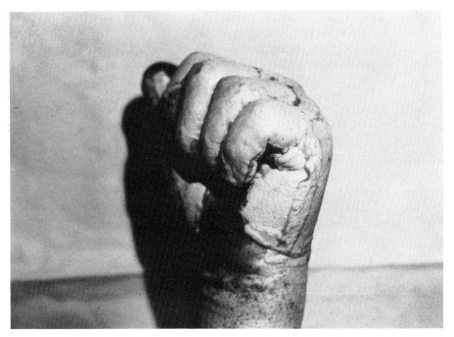

Figure 7.8. Heterograft in place allowing for functional use of hand.

Daily cleaning of the area should continue; but, as long as the pigskin is dry and adherent, it need not be removed. For outpatients, a light bandage applied over the pigskin will prevent slipping and absorb minor drainage. However, on the face, the pigskin may be treated by the open method, unless the patient desires otherwise. On partial-thickness wounds, healing can be observed under light-colored pigskin as it will become translucent and parchment-like, and begins to curl at the edges. It can be gently trimmed as healing occurs. Generally, incorporation into the healing wound does not occur.

When pigskin is the dressing of choice, consideration should be given to matching, as closely as possible, the color of the pigskin to the color of the patient's skin. This is especially important for areas of the body such as hands and face, which are not usually concealed. With the darker colors of pigskin, however, the wound underneath cannot be viewed.

Outpatients who are having pigskin applied for the first time should be warned about the possibility of allergic reactions and infection under the heterograph. With any sudden increase in pain, swelling, or purulent drainage from the wound, the patient is instructed to return to the hospital for evaluation. In any case, the patient should always return to the hospital the day following application for inspection and evaluation of the wound. In the presence of a good take, the patient need only to be checked every two to three days to be certain healing is occurring.

One of the chief advantages of pigskin is the relief of pain and this facilitates the exercise programs. While patients often report that the pigskin stings for 10–15 minutes following application, the subsequent decrease in pain is dramatic.

Synthetic Dressings

In recent years, several types of barrier dressings have been developed from synthetic materials such as plastic film, which seals the wound like pigskin. Although these agents will not usually adhere to the wounds as do biological dressings, not become vascularized or form fibrin bonds as do homografts, they can or will effectively seal the wound. This decreases pain and prevents dehydration. Lack of adherence to the wound seems to be their biggest advantage.

Opsite (Smith & Nephew of Welwyn Garden) (22), a transparent plastic film dressing, is most effective when applied over small, clean, relatively dry, superficial wounds which are free of eschar and necrotic tissue. It has the added advantage of eliminating the need for daily wound care and dressing changes, especially important for infants and small children. An additional advantage is that it is waterproof thereby preventing contamination of wounds from urine and feces in burns of the perineum. This transparent plastic film has an adhesive back. It is cut to fit the wound, overlapping the wound edges by approximately one-half inch onto the undamaged skin to prevent leakage. The backing is then removed and the film applied to the wound much as one would apply contact paper to a counter top.

Another of the newly developed synthetic dressings is Hydron (Abbott Laboratories, Chicago, IL), a mixture of polyhydroxyethylmethacrylate monomer powder and polyethylene glycol (16, 36, 38). The mixture is the consistency of thick syrup and can be applied to the wound by "painting" with a tongue blade or gloved finger. It is then allowed to dry for 20 or 30 minutes until it sets. Since it will soften and slough when wet, it is not used on weeping wounds or parts of the body subject to moisture. Another disadvantage of this type of dressing is that it tends to become incorporated into any bandage applied over it. It is relatively expensive, more difficult to apply, sometimes difficult to remove, and other less expensive dressings tend to work as well.

Dressings used extensively on inpatients and often applicable for outpatients are wet-to-wet and wet-to-dry four × four gauze sponge dressings. Wet-to-wet soaks are seldom indicated in outpatient care except to protect small areas of exposed bone or tendon. It is difficult to keep the dressings moist, without causing maceration of surrounding tissue. Thus, they are more easily utilized only on inpatients.

Wet-to-dry dressings, however, can be helpful with small outpatient wounds that show signs of local infection, remain excessively moist or purulent, or that require additional débridement beyond the hydrotherapy and wound care treatment. Several layers of mesh are soaked with a solution such as sterile saline or triple antibiotic solution and bandaged onto the wound. The dressing is allowed to dry completely. It is then removed, the area is washed, and another wet dressing is applied. This can be done two to four times daily.

BANDAGES

Bandages are generally applied over topical agents, biological or barrier-type dressings. However, in some instances, the open method is utilized, whereby no bandages are applied. This is a simple method of treatment, is well-suited for the hospital environment, and is advantageous for areas as the face and perineum. It is not generally recommended for outpatients as the wound must be protected during transportation to and from the hospital, during work, school, and leisure activities. It is often a messy treatment if topical agents are used and the agents may stain bed clothes and furniture. Infants and small children are difficult to manage as outpatients by the open method. In selective cases, it can be effective in the outpatient setting with the cooperative and intelligent patient who is in control of his activities and home environment; the patient remains unclothed as much as possible or necessary, and must wash and apply the topical agents two to three times daily. The most practical and easily controlled method for outpatients is the closed method, utilizing light bandages.

Bulky occlusive bandages have little place in an effective outpatient treatment program; however, they may be used as a temporary measure to immobilize grafts, or early in the acute phase, to help decrease swelling of hands or feet that cannot be controlled with elevation. Generally, a light dressing will hold the topical agent or biological dressing, in place, protect the wound from the environment, and provide coverage for a self-conscious patient.

One to three layers of mesh are sufficient to hold the topical agent in contact with the wound. A single layer is sufficient over pigskin when it is moist; if the pigskin is dry and adherent, a single layer of a nonadherent dressing (Adaptic, Johnson & Johnson Products, Inc., New Brunswick, NJ) is indicated. If bandages are indicated over synthetic dressings, a mesh layer is sufficient over the plastic film.

A light layer of conforming gauze bandage (Kling, Johnson & Johnson) is usually applied over the mesh or nonadherent dressing to hold the entire bandage in place. In small children and on hard to wrap areas such as the axilla, an expandable net dressing (Surgifix, FRA Surgifix, Inc., Elmsford, NY) is helpful (29). Bandages should be applied in a manner that does not restrict movement. In the hand, fingers should be wrapped individually using a layer of gauze (Fig. 7.9) and the smallest size net bandaging (12). This facilitates functional use of the hand.

Outpatients should also be instructed in the application of elastic bandages to the upper extremities if swelling occurs, although early elevation and avoidance of dependent positioning are best. Lower extremity burns require elastic bandage support during healing to decrease pain and swelling, and to offer circulatory support (29).

Skin Care

As healing occurs, skin care and scar control become major concerns. Skin problems are related to the fragility of the new epithelium and its decreased natural lubrication and suppleness. Blister formation, splitting of the skin, and post-healing trauma are problems common in the recovering burn (Fig. 7.10). Patients who initially heal with little scarring and full range of motion may develop loss of joint motion as the skin thickens and hypertrophic scarring develops (7).

CLEANSING OF HEALED WOUNDS

Submersion therapy in a tank or whirlpool should continue only until the wounds can be managed with local wound care. Prolonged submersion hydrotherapy has a drying effect on the skin, eventually causing cracking and breakdown of healed areas with resultant decrease in range of motion (5). The use of astringents and strong antiseptic soaps at this time should

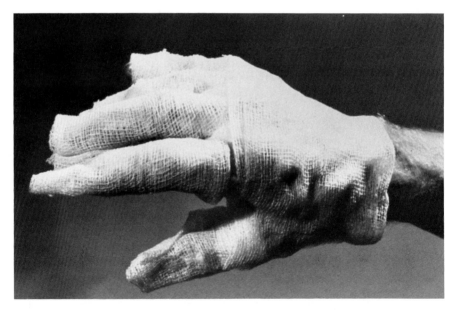

Figure 7.9. Fingers are wrapped separately to facilitate functional use of hand.

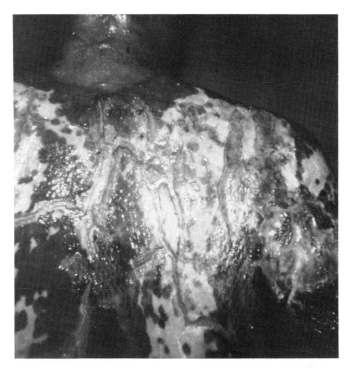

Figure 7.10. Splitting and breakdown of skin after healing.

be avoided. Mild soaps without dyes or perfumes can be effectively used. The cleaning program is now designed to allow for removal of oil and debris without further drying or injury to the healing skin.

A basin or sink can be used for small open areas and the tank or whirlpool used with a spray system when necessary for larger or multiple scattered wounds. Patients should be instructed to shower instead of soaking in a tub, and to limit baths and showers to only the time necessary to wash and rinse thoroughly.

POST-HEALING BLISTERING

Blistering of the healed skin can be disheartening to the patient (Fig. 7.11). He should be informed that this is possible and sometimes a common, recurrent problem during convalescence. The severity and extent varies greatly from patient to patient. As healing progresses, blistering will become less frequent, but may last six months or more. Care should be taken by the patient to keep the skin clean and lubricated, and to avoid friction and trauma to healed areas as much as possible.

Small blisters can be drained with a sterile needle, and flattened with a dressing. These areas will usually dry, crust, and heal without further problems.

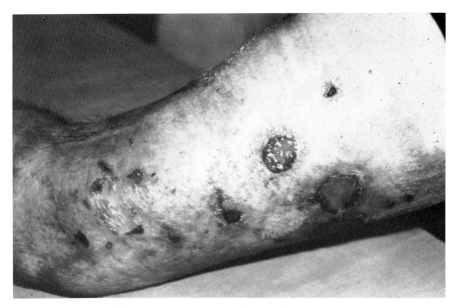

Figure 7.11. Blistering of skin after healing.

Large blisters may require removal of the bullae, leaving open areas that need conservative treatment. Crusts that form over small open areas should be left alone as long as the areas are dry and clean. Repeated removal of scabs at this point can be traumatizing to the skin and prolong healing. Gentle daily washing should be sufficient. Crusts that drain or become purulent, however, should be removed.

ALLERGIC REACTIONS

Occasionally patients will develop allergic reactions with areas of skin breakdown over healed burns. Oral medications can be the cause but the reaction is more commonly a contact dermatitis. It is often very difficult to determine the irritating agent. All soaps, lotions, and topical agents used in the area of the reaction should be discontinued for two to four days. Gentle washing with water and covering the area with a dry dressing will often alleviate the problem. The patient should understand that there will be increased discomfort during this period as the skin will become dry, itch, and be painful with movement. Once the irritated area is under control, the soaps and lubricants can be reintroduced, one at a time, often without further problems. Areas that remain moist and weeping generally respond to Domeboro (Miles Pharmaceuticals, West Haven, CT) soaks for 20–30 minutes two to three times a day.

CONVALESCENT PHASE DRESSINGS

For the wounds seen in the convalescent phase of burn care, a dry mesh dressing is usually sufficient. However, if the area is large and a dry dressing would be uncomfortable, wounds may be dressed with a nonadherent type dressing or with a topical agent such as a neomycin. If the dry mesh dressing is indicated on larger areas, the pain and pulling sensation associated with removal can be lessened by applying multiple small patches to the wound instead of one large layer of gauze.

For a limited number of small wounds, further bandaging over the patches is not necessary unless they are in an area where clothing will rub (Fig. 7.12). On exposed areas of the body they will either stay in place until moistened for removal, or become dry and fall from the wound. Larger open wounds or areas with multiple small wounds can be covered with a conforming gauze bandage. Small areas of overgranulated tissue not controlled with fine mesh patches can be treated by cautery with silver nitrate sticks.

LUBRICATION

In healed burned skin, there is a lack of lubrication and pliability. Dryness and decreased elasticity contribute to skin problems such as cracking and skin breakdown, and can lead to a rapid loss of motion. Lubrication of the healed areas will help alleviate some of these problems. All healed areas should be kept lubricated with a mild nonirritating agent such as cocoa butter, aloe vera cream, Vaseline Intensive Care Lotion (Warner-Lambert Co., Morris Plains, NJ),Lubriderm (Chesebrough-Ponds Inc, Greenwich, CT), etc. Patients respond differently to various agents, and several may be tried before finding the one that gives the patient the most relief from itching and dryness.

Lubricants can be applied as often as necessary throughout the day to keep the patient comfortable and the skin supple. They should be applied lightly and rubbed gently up to and around all open areas. Care should be taken to avoid leaving a greasy residue on the skin or allowing a "build up" of oils to remain on these areas, as this can lead to the formation of pimples and whiteheads. A heavy layer of oil or grease will make the patient more uncomfortable, feel hotter, and itch more.

MASSAGE

Massage of scar tissue aids in maintaining or increasing its pliability (Fig. 7.13). Gentle massage should be started as healing occurs with care to avoid friction to superficial layers that could cause blistering. A light stroking motion when applying lubricants is easily tolerated when beginning massage techniques. After the skin becomes less fragile and blisters are no longer present, deep massage to the subcutaneous tissue is begun. Massage will

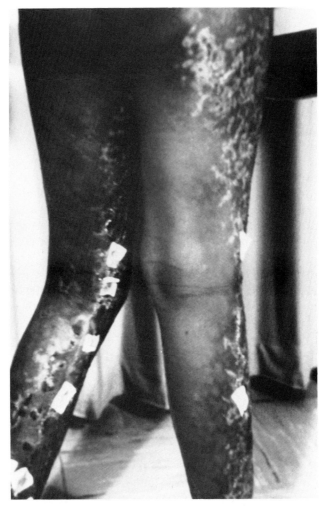

Figure 7.12. Fine mesh patches on small open areas.

not only increase pliability but will also aid in decreasing sensitivity of the healing skin and scar tissue.

DESENSITIZATION

A program of desensitization should begin in the acute phase when open wounds are still present. Patients who are treated in nonaggressive settings where the wound and healing skin are rarely touched have more problems with scar pain and hypersensitive skin. A program of daily wound care, dressing changes, activities of daily living, and early mobilization of wounds promote less sensitive skin when healing occurs (Fig. 7.14). Of more limited

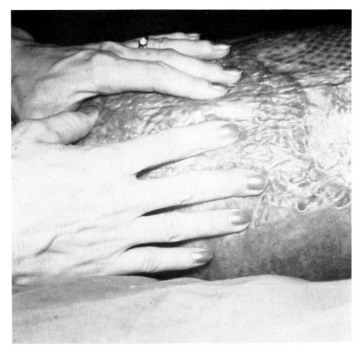

Figure 7.13. Massage of scar tissue.

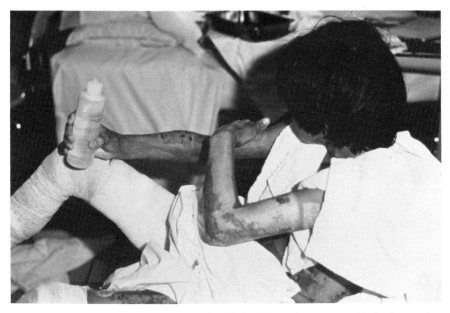

Figure 7.14. Early patient participation for lubrication and massage aids in decreasing hypersensitive and painful scars.

use, ultrasound and transcutaneous nerve stimulation are sometimes helpful in the convalescent phase for control of persistent skin hypersensitivity and scar pain.

Graduated gradient pressure has been shown to promote desensitization and to increase the skin's tolerance to the shear force encountered with the application of commercial pressure garments (6). As healing occurs, gentle pressure can be applied early with an elastic bandage, elastic stockinette, or hand-made elastic garments. These can be applied over bandages before healing is complete as long as friction or shear force is not exerted on the wound bed or newly healed skin. As skin becomes less fragile and the patient's tolerance increases, additional pressure may be applied using double layers of elastic or increasing the tension of the elastic wrap. This should prepare the skin for the fitting of the commercial pressure garments.

PROBLEM AREAS

Skin Discoloration

It is erroneous that the application of oils and other agents will aid in returning the skin to its natural preburn condition. Quality lotions and oils may be used, but anything exotic, especially those recommended by "friends" should be investigated thoroughly and physician advice sought before their use. The color of the skin changes gradually over a period of several months (Fig. 7.15) As long as the skin has a red discoloration, it is

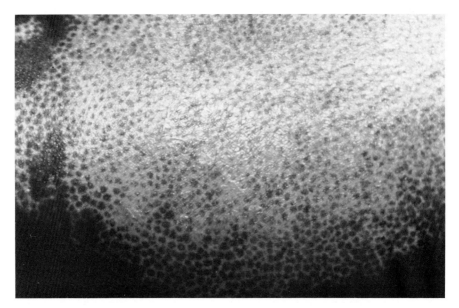

Figure 7.15. Pigment returning in healed burn; dryness and flaking remain a problem.

subject to blistering, breakdown, hypertrophic scarring, and contracture formation. As the redness decreases, so should the other skin problems.

In addition, the intensity of the color may change from day to day, ranging from pale pink to deep purple. These changes are influenced by the temperature, the level of activity of the patient, whether or not the part was dependent for prolonged periods, and the wearing of the pressure garments. Even though any one of these factors may tend to cause skin to become purple, it is usually a temporary condition. Severe discoloration is an indication to the patient that pressure garments should be continued or that dependent positioning should be limited or avoided.

Pruritis

Pruritis is a continuing and universal problem for the recovering burn patient and no permanent solution is available. Medications such as antihistamines are generally prescribed, but are of limited value.

Lightly applied lubrication to dry or scaly areas will provide some relief, as will cool towels and cool showers. On a long-term basis, the wearing of pressure garments is as effective as any other method for controlling itching. Patients should be instructed to stay in cool areas as much as possible, especially during the hot summer months, and to avoid scratching or continual rubbing of the areas as this will severely irritate the skin.

Exposure to Sunlight

As long as skin discoloration is present, the patient should avoid direct sunlight to healed areas, as a sunburn can occur easily. Patients are usually advised to avoid sunlight for six months following healing, and then to proceed with extreme caution. Applying sunscreens, covering healed areas with clothing, and planning outdoor activities in the early mornings and in the evenings will allow the patient to resume outdoor activities on a gradual basis. In time it may be possible to tan the healed skin and achieve color blending of the burned and nonburned areas, but this should not be done for at least a year after healing and then only with short, numerous exposures.

Heat and Cold Tolerance

Large partial-thickness burns with heavy scar tissue and large full-thickness burns adversely affect the patient's tolerance to extremes in temperature on a temporary or permanent basis. Patients with such intolerance are warned to avoid prolonged exposure to heat or cold. They are also warned against vigorous outdoor activities in summer or winter until reactions and tolerances are determined.

Cosmetics

Once wounds are healed and the skin is past the fragile blistering stage, patients (male, female, and children) should be encouraged to explore the possibilities of cosmetics to cover the scarred areas. Scarring presents several problems when choosing cosmetics. There is little or no natural skin lubrication; there may be only a few or distorted pores, and the skin textures and color may vary considerably. Traumatized skin requires gentle cleansing, moisturizing, and environmental protection. Assistance from a professional cosmetologist and/or make-up artist may be necessary. There are specialized lines of cosmetics commercially available for the express purpose of covering or minimizing scarring. Most large department stores carry these lines, and have someone trained in their use and to act as a consultant.

Burn patients are beset with many problems in wound healing and skin care. With early initiation of proper techiques of care, and attention to the minute details of care, problems can be minimized with good functional and cosmetic results.

REFERENCES

1. Arturson G: Pathophysiology of the burn wound. *Ann Chirurg Gynecol* 69:178–190, 1980.
2. D'Aiuto ML: Progress in burn management: Retrospective look. *Conn Med* 45:695–698, 1981.
3. Gotshall RA: Sodium depletion related to hydrotherapy for burn injury. *JAMA* 203:182–184, 1968.
4. Hartford CE: The bequests of Moncrief and Moyer: An appraisal of topical therapy of burns—1981 American Burn Association presidential address. *J Trauma* 21:827–834, 1981.
5. Head M, Helm P: Paraffin and sustained stretching in the treatment of burn contractures. *Burns* 4:136–139, 1977.
6. Helm P, Head MD, Pullium G, et al: Burn rehabilitation—A team approach. *Surg Clin North Am* 58:1263–1278, 1978.
7. Helm PA, Kevorkian CG, Luschbaugh M, et al: Burn injury: Rehabilitation management in 1982. *Arch Phys Med Rehabil* 63:6–16, 1982.
8. Herzog SR: The role of the physical therapist in burn management. (From Duke University Medical Center, Durham, NC).
9. Jurkiewicz MJ, Hill HL: Open wounds of the scalp: An account of methods of repair. *J Trauma* 21:769–889, 1981.
10. Koepke GJ: The role of physical medicine in the treatment of burns. *Surg Clin North Am* 50:1385–1399, 1970.
11. Krier D, Mani MM: Thermal injuries—Assessment and treatment for outpatient care. *Kansas Med Soc* 80:550–553, 1979.
12. Labandter H, Kaplan I, Shavitt C: Burns of the dorsum of the hand: Conservative treatment with intensive physiotherapy versus tangential excision and grafting. *Br J Plast Surg* 29:352–354, 1976.
13. Levenson SM, Gruber DK, Gruber C, et al: Chemical debridement of burns: Mercaptans. *J Trauma* 21:632–644, 1981.
14. Lindberg RB: Agents used for topical degerming of the burn wound. *Rec Antisepsis Tech—Burn Wound Mgmt* 3–11, 1974.
15. Luterman A: Topical chemotherapy and burn wound care. *Ann Chirurg Gynecol* 69:210–212, 1980.
16. MacMillan BG: Closing the burn wound. *Surg Clin North Am* 58:1205–1231, 1978.
17. MacMillan BG: Local care and infection in burns. *J Trauma* 5:292–305, 1965.
18. Miller SF: Outpatient management of minor burns. *Am Fam Phys* 16:167–172, 1977.
19. Monafo WW: *The Treatment of Burns: Principles and Practice.* St. Louis, Warren H. Green, Inc., 1971.

20. Monafo WW, Ayvazian VH: Topical therapy. *Surg Clin North Am* 58:1157–1171, 1978.
21. Mullick F: Hexachlorophene toxicity—Human experience at the Armed Forces Institute of Pathology. *Pediatrics* 51 Part II:395–399, 1973.
22. Neal DE, Whalley PC, Flowers MW, et al: The effects of an adherent polyurethane film and conventional absorbent dressing in patients with small partial thickness burns. *Br J Clin Prac* 35:354–357, 1981.
23. Niederhuber SS, Stribley RF, Koepke GH: Reduction of skin bacterial load with use of the therapeutic whirlpool. *Phys Ther* 55:482–486, 1975.
24. Ollstein RN, McDonald C: Topical and systemic antimicrobial agents in burns. *Ann Plast Surg* 5:386–392, 1980.
25. Peacock EE Jr, Van Winkel W Jr: *Surgery and Biology of Wound Repair*. Philadelphia, W. B. Saunders Company, 1970.
26. Peacock EE Jr, Van Winkle W Jr: *Wound Repair*. Philadelphia, W.B. Saunders Company, 1976.
27. Pruitt BA Jr: The burn patient: Initial care. *Curr Prob Surg* 16:4–95, 1979.
28. Salisbury RE, Carnes R, McCarthy LR: Comparison of the bacterial clearing effects of different biologic dressings on granulating wounds following thermal injury. *Plast Reconstruc Surg* 66:695–698, 1980.
29. Schuck JM: Outpatient management of the burned patient. *Surg Clin North Am* 58:1107–1117, 1978.
30. Shuck LW, Shuck JM: The outpatient burn. *Curr Con Trauma Care* 5:15–21, 1982.
31. Schumann L, Gaston S: Commonsense guide to topical burn therapy. *Nursing* 9:34–39, 1979.
32. Simonetti A, Miller R, Gristina J: Efficacy of povidone-iodine in the disinfection of whirlpool baths and hubbard tanks. *Phys Ther* 52:1277–1282, 1972.
33. Smith R, Blasi D, Dayton SL, et al: Effects of sodium hypochlorite on the microbial flora of burns and normal skin. *J Trauma* 14:938–944, 1974.
34. Steve L, Goodhart P, Alexander J: Hydrotherapy burn treatment: Use of choramine-t against resistant microorganisms *Arch Phys Med Rehabil* 50:301–303, 1979.
35. Stone LL, Dalton HP, Haynes BW: Bacterial debridement of the burn eschar: The in vivo activity of selected organisms. *J Surg Res* 29:83–92, 1980.
36. Tavis MJ, et al: Current status of skin substitutes. *Surg Clin North Am* 58:1233–1248, 1978.
37. Turner AG, Higgins MM, Craddock JG: Disinfection of immersion tanks (hubbard) in a hospital burn unit. *Arch Environ Health* 28:101–103, 1974.
38. Warren RJ, Snelling CRT: Clinical evaluation of the Hydron burn dressing. *Plast Reconstr Surg* 66:361–368, 1980.
39. Wolf DL, Capozzi A, Pennisi VR: Evaluation of biological dressings. *Ann Plast Surg* 5:186–190, 1980.

ADDITIONAL READINGS

1. Abraham EA, McMaster WC, Krigger M, et al: Whirlpool therapy for treatment of soft tissue wounds complicating extremity fractures. *J Trauma* 14:222–226, 1974.
2. Ariyan S, Enriquez R, Krizek TJ: Wound contraction and fibrocontractive disorders. *Arch Surg* 113:1034–1046, 1978.
3. Artz CR, Moncrief JA, Pruitt BA: *Burns: A Team Approach*. Philadelphia, W. B. Saunders Company, 1979.
4. Asch MJ, Curreri WP, Pruitt BA: Thermal injury involving bone: Report of 32 cases. *J Trauma* 12:135–139, 1972.
5. Bhasker SN, Cutright DE, Hunsuck EE, et al: Pulsating water jet devices in debridement of combat wounds. *Milit Med* March: 264–266, 1971.
6. Bowser BH, Caldwell FT, Cone JB, et al: A prospective analysis of silver sulfadiazine with

and without cerium nitrate as a topical agent in the treatment of severely burned children. *J Trauma* 21:558–563, 1981.

7. Brown PW: The fate of exposed bone. *Am J Surg* 137:464–469, 1979.

8. Edlich RF, et al: *Fundamentals of Wound Management in Surgery: Technical Factors in Wound Management*. Chirurgecom, Inc., 1977.

9. Glover DM: Necrosis of skull and long bones resulting from deep burns, with evidence of regeneration. *Am J Surg* 95:679–683, 1958.

10. Grower MF, Bhaskar SH, Horan MJ, et al: Effect of water lavage on removal of tissue fragments from crush wounds. *Oral Surg* 33:1031–1036, 1972.

11. Hamit HF, Moser E, Walker J: The use of nylon net in the management of skin grafts applied to burn wounds. *Surg Gynecol Obstet* 143:809–810, 1976.

12. Hunter JM, Schneider LH, Mackin EJ, et al: *Rehabilitation of the Hand*. St. Louis, C.V. Mosby Company, 1979.

13. Lushbaugh M, Hunt JL, Sato RM, et al: Thermal injury: Outpatient care of minor burns. A slide-tape presentation developed by the Texas Regional Burn Care System, Dallas, TX, 1979.

14. Lushbaugh M, et al: Thermal injury: Antimicrobial therapy. A slide-tape presentation developed by the Texas Regional Burn Care System, Dallas, TX, 1979.

15. Matthews RN, Bennett JP, Faulk WP: Wound healing using amniotic membranes. *Br J Plast Surg* 32:76–78, 1981.

16. McComb H, Annear DI: A bath-bed for burn management. *Plast Reconstr Surg* 102–104, 1975.

17. Medical News; Encouraging news on temporary covering for burn wounds. *JAMA* 244:2493–2495, 1980.

18. Noe JM, Kalish S: The problem of adherence in dressed wounds. *Surg Gynecol Obstet* 147:185–188, 1978.

19. Park GB: Burn wound coverings—A review. *Biomat Med Dev Art Org* 6:1–35, 1978.

20. Schwope AD, Wise DL, Sell KW, et al: Evaluation of wound covering materials. *J Biomed Mat Res Dev* 11:489–502, 1977.

21. Teh BT: Why do skin grafts fail? *Plast Reconstr Surg* 63:323–332, 1979.

22. Wright Et, Haase KH: Keloids and ultrasound. *Arch Phys Med Rehabil* 52:280–281, 1971.

8

Management of Hypertrophic Scarring

ELIZABETH A. RIVERS

Introduction

The major emphasis of this chapter is the management of scars following thermal injury. Hypertrophic and keloid tissue is defined, the problems unique to hypertrophic scars are outlined, and early factors that influence wound healing and scar formation are discussed. The management is presented in an illustrated format describing the application of pressure to hypertrophic scars organized according to anatomic areas. In addition, detailed scar treatments for the face and neck are included. Treatment of the hand is mentioned, but will be discussed in greater detail in Chapter 9.

Description of Hypertrophic Scars

Historic records include descriptions of a wide variety of scar overgrowths. Considerable effort was made initially to differentiate hypertrophic scars from keloids (22, 23, 42).

Hypertrophic scars bulge directly above the original wound (Fig. 8.1) and hypotrophic scars (Fig. 8.2) appear indented below the level of the surrounding tissue surface (22, 23, 36, 42). Keloids (Fig. 8.3) are defined as massive, noncancerous lesions that extend beyond the boundaries of the original wound and frequently recur after excision. Recently, electron microscopy and detailed analysis of wound composition have given researchers more complete understanding of normal wound healing (9, 26, 27, 36, 42, 47, 49). By 1977, Ketchem (23) called the hypertrophic scar a "morbid variant" of the keloid. Peacock et al. (42) stated that "keloids seem to differ from severe hypertrophic scarring only in the amount of scar production." For the purpose of clarity in this chapter, the term "hypertrophic scar" will be used to describe all overgrowth of connective tissue.

Hypertrophic scars are predominantly fibrous tumors that usually develop within a year after trauma (15). They appear as firm, variably pruritic or tender growths near a site of injury, often a burn (15). The epidermis over

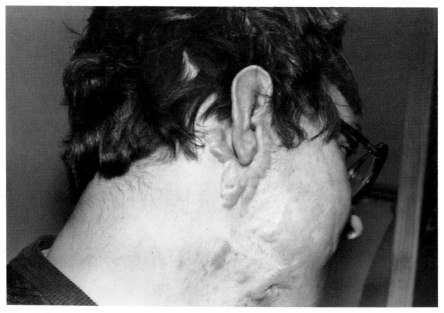

Figure 8.1. Hypertrophic scar of loose tissue surrounding ear is shown four months after healing of partial-thickness burn.

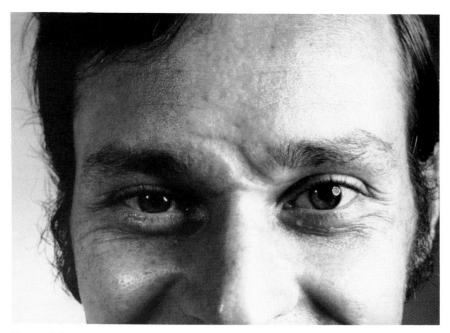

Figure 8.2. Hypotrophic scar is shown one year following healing of partial-thickness tar burn.

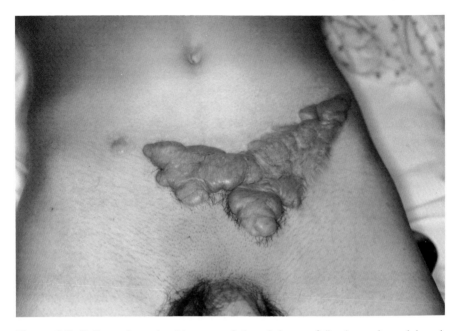

Figure 8.3. Bulbous hypertrophic scar of the abdomen following a burn injury is shown. (Photo courtesy of Alan Shons, M.D., SPRMC.)

such a scar is usually thinned. Kischer and Shetlar (25) stated that "hardness and rigidity are characteristics of all scars on the surface of the body. In the case of hypertrophic scar they contribute in large measure to the grotesque and bizarre appearance of the scar." Feller (15) described the scar formation process as "intense erythema followed by a raised lesion." The patient reports paresthesia and dysesthesia. The most prominent symptom is pruritis. The lesion continues to increase in thickness and becomes firm, dark red, and almost cartilaginous in consistency. The final color, size, hardness, and tenderness of the scar varies. Usually the scar is noticed in the first weeks after healing, but it may appear at any time until the collagen is mature and light colored (14, 22, 36). The time of onset, duration, and time of involution varies (15).

A familial predilection for hypertrophic scar formation has been noted (36). Hypertrophic scars develop more often in black people (23) and in people with dark pigmentation (22). They seem to occur most frequently in patients between 10 and 30 years of age, although they are seen at every age (36). No consistent differences in the incidence between males and females have been noted. These scars seem to enlarge during pregnancy and puberty and to resolve after menopause (23, 25). After several years of normal scar-tissue remodeling, the scars become greatly reduced in thickness and also are more supple to the touch.

Early Factors Influencing Scar Resolution

Early in wound healing, certain factors influence the final scar formation. The presence of bacteria in the burn wound increases the inflammatory process (2, 22). The synthesis and deposition of collagen are thought to be increased in response to macrophages that are stimulated by bacteria or toxins (22). Abnormally high fibroplasia is noted if tension is increased on the wound margins when they are surgically closed (17, 22). This is observed especially in wounds that cross the relaxed skin tension lines described by Borges and Alexander (5) and by MacMillan and Lang (31). Suture materials used for skin grafts may cause inflammation and, therefore, increase scar formation. Crushing or irritating the wound and surrounding tissues during operative procedures also increases the likelihood of hypertrophic scarring (22). Some topical antibiotics such as Sulfamylon (mafenide) increase hypervascularity in the healing wound.

Wound repair is inhibited by poor microvascular circulation. Transportation of oxygen and glucose to the cell must be adequate for normal wound healing (22). Steroid hormone excesses also decrease healing. Systemic corticosteroids can be so high that wound healing is totally absent (22).

Factors that can improve wound healing, improve its quality and reduce scar tissue are thorough wound care to minimize infection (42), meticulous and delicate care of the burn wound during surgical procedures (35), and early skin grafting (2, 5, 7, 14). Adequate nutrition and early pressure and splinting speed healing (22).

The Challenge of Hypertrophic Scar Control

Hypertrophic scar formation after thermal injury is a challenge to the entire burn treatment team (2, 21). To achieve optimal long-term outcome, early scar control is crucial and should begin as soon as wound healing commences (22). Scar control frequently must be re-evaluated for effectiveness. It is essential that conservative control continue until the healed tissue appears flat, soft, and supple, and light pink, white or brown (32, 35). Often the total process takes more time than either the physician or the patient anticipated. Some hypertrophic scars remain active as long as four years. Most scars resolve in 12–18 months.

In some primitive cultures near the equator hypertrophic scars are considered beautiful embellishments or body jewelry (Fig. 8.4). Scars are valued as a status symbol. However, burn victims in technologically advanced civilizations do not share this attitude toward scars. Raised bumps of tissue are offensive defects, often inviting stares and ridicule. Overgrown scars and physical deviations, such as scar contractures, seem to arouse upsetting feelings reflexly in observers and victims. Often a person who is scarred or appears unusual is avoided, and being shunned confirms the victim's opinion that he is ugly. In cultures that exaggerate the importance of a flawless,

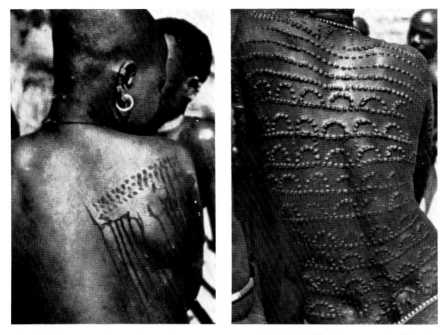

Figure 8.4. Hypertrophic scar being produced on Africans. (Photo courtesy of Appleton-Century-Crofts from *Fundamentals of Wound Management in Surgery.*)

youthful-appearing skin, thin, flat, light-colored scars are preferred. However, this is the final outcome of natural wound healing for few people—mainly fair skinned, blonde, blue-eyed caucasions (23). Wound healing with no effort to control collagen overgrowth or to assist the degenerative phase of remodeling frequently results in an unnecessarily strong scar that is bulky and aesthetically displeasing (22, 23). "Optimal scarring" as defined by Ketchum (23) is "the least amount of scar tissue produced by the wound that is compatible with normal function." The burn team, especially the Physical Medicine and Rehabilitation component, undertakes to influence the healing process so that the appearance of the final scar will be acceptable.

EXPECTATIONS AND GOALS OF THE PATIENT

Many burn patients expect to return to their former activities and employment with no loss of function and with no change in income level. They may anticipate a final appearance and self-identity unchanged from that before the injury. They believe their healed skin will be tough and pliable, will protect them from heat and cold, and will have normal sensation without pain, itching, burning, or stinging. Burn victims expect to regain their strength, dexterity, and coordination quickly. They believe hospital dismissal is the beginning of a future uncomplicated by surgical reconstructions or hospital admissions for rehabilitation. These goals are rarely achieved by a seriously burned person. Hypertrophic scars that contract thwart the patient's efforts to achieve smooth supple skin. The patient and family need frequent, kind, resolute explanations to overcome their naive optimism. Hopefully such explanations will prevent their becoming depressed, bewildered, and unable to continue the rigorous therapy program.

COMPLICATIONS UNIQUE TO HYPERTROPHIC SCARS

Permanent musculoskeletal alterations may result from hypertrophic scar growth and contraction, especially at flexion creases. Decreased chest expansion and postural flexibility, accompanied by limited joint motion, often give the burned person an obvious "robotlike" gait. Another serious complication of collagen overgrowth is the unsightly distortion of facial features and hand contours. Contracture of the collagen adds to disfigurement such as by pulling nose, eyelids, mouth and ears out of alignment (Fig. 8.5). Pain, burning, and itching of the scar often interfere with the patient's ability to concentrate or sleep. Habitual scratching of the scar may invite social ridicule. Excoriations may result in open areas that are painful, that increase the risk of infection, and which may cause further scarring. Carcinomas

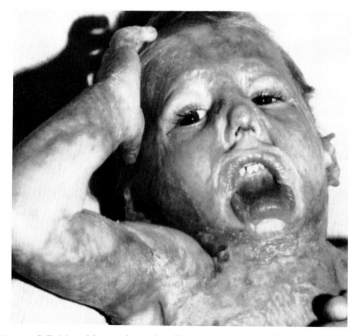

Figure 8.5. Lip, chin, neck, and axillary contractures distort appearance.

may develop at chronically open scar sites of 10 or more years (38), but this problem can be avoided by appropriate surgical intervention. Reconstructive operations to remove scars interrupt work, are accompanied by renewed pain and fear, and may require prolonged rehabilitation. Surgical procedures for scar removal do not guarantee a successful outcome and each procedure has its own inherent risks.

These complications present a unique composite of factors that interfere with rehabilitation. With exasperating tenacity, the myofibroblasts remain active in the scar 24 hours a day until an unknown factor causes their regression, usually some 9–18 months after injury. An acceptable functional and cosmetic outcome can be more assured if the injured tissue has been kept flat and supple. Ths is accomplished by the patient and burn staff demonstrating more tenacity than the burn scar itself.

Treatments Available to Decrease Hypertrophic Scar Formation

For years, scar control was largely a matter of luck. In recent years, the following treatments have been tried for minimizing hypertrophic scars: surgery, radiation (33), cryotherapy (29), intralesional steroids (8), laser therapy (1), topical vitamins E (12) and A (11), oral vitamins A C, (3), and E (12), cytotoxic or immunosuppressive drugs such as methotrexate (39), topical corticosteroids (49), external pressure (40), and any combination of these. Table 8.1 lists the advantages and disadvantages of several possible treatments. Only external pressure will be dealt with in this chapter.

The use of external pressure for scar control has been widely used and well accepted by numerous burn centers for successful treatment of hypertrophic scars (4, 16, 31, 34, 40). It has the distinct advantage of minimal side-effects. Overcompression may cause tissue breakdown or impaired nerve function; however, with proper supervision this will not occur.

EXTERNAL PRESSURE

Scar resolution can be accelerated by application of external pressure approximating capillary pressure over the healing body surface (Fig. 8.6). Usually the patient must wear a custom-made elastic stocking and a total-contact splint (4); sometimes traction is necessary at night (28). Typically, patients view use of these compression applicances as an annoyance. Assuring compliance for the recalcitrant patient requires an inordinate amount of support, reassurance, and commitment by the professional staff. Family and community must be recruited to encourage the burned person. It is crucial that the burn team not succumb to insistence by the patient or family to discontinue scar controls. Follow-up appointments are critical even after initial scar activity appears to be diminishing. The scar may re-form so insidiously that it will not be noticed early enough to respond to resumption of pressure. The final result will then be less than optimal. Therefore, follow-up clinics must be extended for a year or more and must

Table 8.1.
Scar Prevention Methods for Burns

Method	Advantages	Disadvantages
Early surgical excision with split-thickness sheet or unexpanded mesh grafts	Nearly always flat, supple and cosmetically acceptable Decreases pain Shortens hospitalization	Skilled surgeon needed Blood loss limits procedure to 20% of body surface area
Surgical excision of already formed scar		Regrowth of scar larger than original in 1–5 years
Radiation	Simple Painless	Possibly carcinogenic
Corticosteroids	Topical: Simple and painless to apply	Not consistently effective Side-effects of systemic absorption severe
	Intralesional: Shortens time to scar maturity	Painful Local overdose may result in skin atrophy pigment changes and telangiectasia Systemic absorption causes Cushing-like symptoms
External pressure	Accelerates collagen tissue breakdown bringing the scar to maturity earlier Accurate support to healing tissues can be provided from initial injury until the scar is mature Properly applied external pressure cannot cause any permanent tissue damage Controlling scar from day of injury also prevents contracture, increases patient comfort, decreases itching and reduces edema	Pressure must be applied continuously for 9–36 months Patient and family must take active responsibility to assure success Jobst garments, face masks, and orthoses are expensive Experienced therapists with considerable skill and imagination needed It is possible for elastic wraps to be applied as serial tourniquets and result in tissue loss

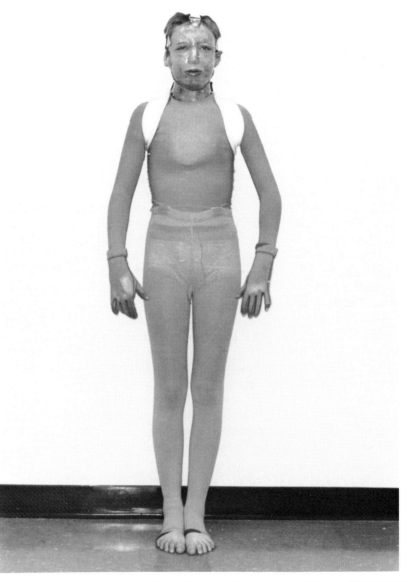

Figure 8.6. External pressure to body from elastic garments (Jobst or Bioconcepts), transparent face mask, transparent neck orthosis; extra pressure to intradigital web spaces with lambs wool packing and thumb web otoform K or elastomer inserts, chest elastomer insert, and figure of eight clavicle strap overlay are shown. Total-contact axillary splint is worn on right arm under clavicle strap at night.

include psychological support for the patient and family as well as supervision of wound healing and pressure control devices.

Hunt (22), Larson et al. (28) and others (22, 34) state that application of firm pressure (10–30 mm Hg) and of external traction, if needed, to all injured tissue 23 hours a day will decrease hypertrophic scarring. According to Moncrief (35) "pressure must be exerted constantly for twelve to eighteen months during the period of collagen remodeling and maturation."

When first applied, the pressure devices decrease edema by enhancing lymphatic and venous return. When less protein-rich fluid is available for the inflammatory process, fibroblastic activity will be reduced. It is postulated that external pressure reduces the bulk of hypertrophic scars by enhancing collagen lysis and retarding synthesis through diminished circulation in the tissues and cell hypoxia (22, 24–28).

Bulky rigid scars rarely develop after injuries that do not involve the reticular dermis or that heal spontaneously in two to three weeks (22). Also, raised hard scars rarely form after injuries in which all pigment and color changes resolve in two months (22, 40). These patients, however, must be observed for up to 12 months so that pressure can be initiated if hypertrophic tissue is noted. Prophylactic external pressure should be applied to all other burned areas from the time of injury until skin maturation.

The objective of using elastic garments and splints is to apply perpendicular pressure, approximating capillary pressure, to all injured tissues while allowing full active motion of all body parts. No pressure device is ideal. In addition, the exact pressure under these devices probably cannot be accurately determined (41). Achievement of effective scar control, while maintaining the skin coverage, full sensory function, and free body movement, requires considerable imagination, trial and error, and skill on the part of the therapist, the patient, the family, and the physician. A sense of humor as well as determination and perseverance are valuable qualities in this challenging pursuit.

Prescription and use of orthotic devices should be under the supervision of a physician who is knowledgable in burn wound care, tissue healing, and rehabilitation medicine and who realizes the limitations and timing of plastic reconstructive surgery. The orthoses should be comfortable, durable, easy to apply, and cosmetic. Ease of fabrication decreases the cost of the device and the time required to fit the patient. Precautions to be observed in the use of orthoses include avoiding excessive or insufficient tissue compression, preventing nerve compression, and preventing skin irritations or infections.

Noncompliance is a difficult problem. This may result from difficulty in donning the garment or device, from pain while wearing the appliance, from inadequate understanding of the scar healing process, and from psychological problems and lack of emotional support. Patient and family compliance may be improved by increasing patient control in appropriate related decisions, clear explanations of the action of pressure, and a behavior modification program. Earnest concern and enthusiasm by the burn team also is helpful, especially if combined with realistic descriptions of scar build-up if treatment is not consistent.

Total-contact splints of low temperature thermoplastic often give dramatic results in a short time. These orthoses have several advantages over open or three point splints. When secured with elastic wraps or Tubigrip, they provide firm pressure to the scar. The plastic keeps underlying tissue warm and prevents the evaporation of perspiration. This moisturizes the scar tissue making it more supple. In addition, the patient pulls away from the plastic, to control the amount of pain during motion; therefore, the patient is often more cooperative. Improvement in scar configuration often can be observed after two to eight hours of pressure.

Scar tissue can be modified by static total-contact pressure appliances or by dynamic orthoses that apply stretching forces by means of rubber bands or springs (Fig. 8.7). Dynamic splints work best when the patient is relaxed. Care must be taken to assure that the stretching force does not lead to breakdown of the skin surface due to ischemia or tearing of the underlying tissue. The traction attachments must be wide enough for adequate distribution of pressure, and the orthosis must be properly constructed and fitted to the patient. The stretching force is most effective if it is gentle and

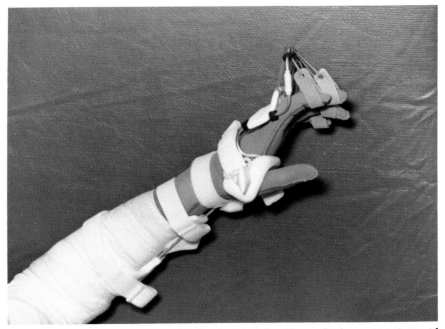

Figure 8.7. Dynamic rubber band splint for stretchng finger flexion contractures of palmar burn is shown; it also strengthens finger flexion if desired.

applied for prolonged periods. Safe and successful use of dynamic orthoses often depends on the patient's cooperation. The risks of tissue damage and increased scarring must be considered carefully when these devices are prescribed.

General Application Techniques and Principles

Burn victims benefit from well-established and accepted techniques of tissue compression. Initially, pressure bandages prevent or decrease edema by supporting the severely damaged vascular system. Tissue support not only prevents or limits edema but it decreases pain when extremities are dependent, such as a burned lower extremity during ambulation. Tissue support at this time also prevents skin graft hemorrhage in the dependent part from increased intravascular pressure. Later, edema control decreases scar formation by preventing protein rich fluid from becoming a matrix for the formation of unnecessary scar tissue. During the final stages of healing, tissue compression decreases pruritus. Rigid, total-contact tissue compression helps prevent the connective tissue of an immature hyperemic scar tissue from contracting, thereby helping to prevent joint contractures.

Timing of pressure application to the burn varies widely throughout the country. Elastic bandage supports are routinely used on legs during ambulation from admission through hospital discharge for most burn victims. Outpatients are routinely treated with edema control bandaging at some centers. Other centers do not use elastic supports for edema and/or scar control. In general, if the wound heals spontaneously in two to three weeks with no pigment changes, pressure for scar control is unnecessary. These burns are rarely deep enough into the reticular dermis to cause hypertrophic scar development.

The use of tissue compression after skin grafting varies widely from center to center. Elastic wraps, casts, cotton stent dressings, elastomer with prosthetic foam dressings, total-contact splints, tubular and commercial elastic garments have all been used as postoperative dressings of both grafts and donors. Few studies comparing the results of graft or donor healing with or without pressure have been published.

When hypertrophic scars are red, raised, hard, and painful, tissue compression is nearly universally used to control the scar and to improve patient comfort. This pressure is applied 23 of 24 hours a day until all the redness fades and the scars remain flat for at least three days after removal of the pressure. This end point occurs roughly about 18 months after injury, but the time is extremely variable.

If the tissue becomes red or hard at a later time, pressure should be resumed 23 hours a day.

In some cases, inactive, contracted connective tissue can be kept elongated by use of a total contact night splint. However, if the tissue is active, pressure must be continuous, 23 or 24 hours a day, because the myofibro-blasts are active during the entire 24 hours a day!

No pressure device is ideal, and all healed or grafted skin has differing durability; therefore, a graded variety of materials must be used to achieve tissue compression without causing tissue breakdown. Shearing, a common factor in skin breakdown, must be avoided.

As the skin and connective tissue tolerate, pressure and subsequent tissue compression can be increased. The staff and patient can monitor the effect of each type of pressure device and change to the most effective technique as early as possible. Initially a soft, conforming type of gauze and a nylon stocking under the elastic wrap may be needed to protect fragile tissue. Distal-to-proximal elastic wraps are usually the first compression used. The elastic bandages may be unwrapped over joints to allow range of motion exercises, and then reapplied. After elastic wraps are tolerated well, the patient may progress to tubular elastic support. Occasionally, this will provide adequate compression for the entire treatment course. This is most often true for cylindrical-shaped body parts. Custom made elastic garments may be needed to provide compression to difficult areas such as finger webs and axillae. The garment must be frequently revised until optimal fit is obtained.

To achieve total-contact pressure to contoured body parts, it is necessary to add inserts or overlays. Adhesive foam, nonadhesive foam, elastomer silicone and/or prosthetic foam, orthopedic felt, isoprene and other low temperature plastics as well as high temperature plastics, or Otoform K silicone can be used as inserts or as an overlay and can be elastic wrapped or strapped over a tubular elastic or elastic garment. The insert must be beveled to provide equal pressure and to avoid tenting of the pressure device at the insert's edge.

Table 8.2 lists the name, source, characteristics, and uses of various orthotic materials for burn scar compression.

Techniques for Application of External Pressure by Body Area

HEAD AND FACE

Methods of applying pressure to the newly burned, edematous head include elastic wraps over the forehead and around the chin or the use of elasticized tubular bandage material to secure gauze strips. Usually the swelling resolves rapidly after the third day, but may be evident until the 10th day. At this time, more individualized and costly pressure devices may be initiated. A custom-fitted elasticized hood can be made with openings for eyes, nose, mouth, and ears, if desired (Fig. 8.8). If only the mandibular area is involved, an elastic custom-made chin strap can provide total contact pressure. Elastic wraps, tubular bandages, and custom-fitted elastic garments provide excellent total-contact pressure to any body surface that is

Table 8.2.
Orthotic Materials Used for Burn Scar Control

Name (Source)	Characteristics	Uses
Compression wraps Elastic wraps 2-inch, 3-inch, 4-inch, 6-inch, ½ length, double length (Any medical company)	Effective compression; proper width conforms well to irregular body parts; easy to vary tension; rubber deteriorates on exposure to oils Nylon bandages cut into fragile tissue; laundering is time consuming	Gradient pressure wrap; most pressure at distal point with support to most proximal point Spiral or figure of eight wrap to any body part
Elset (Tubiton House, Medlock Street, Oldham 011 3HS, England)	Very soft, flexible elastic fabric; conforms for stump wraps and finger wraps	Early compression when little tension is tolerated
Tubular products Elastic net Tubigauze (Scholl Hospital Products Division, 213 W. Schiller St., Chicago, IL)	Open mesh net; conforms to regular body parts; cuts into tissue if no interface is present, due to swelling around fibers in mesh	Secure gauze bandages; may slightly reduce swelling; allows individual bandaging of fingers
Tubigrip elastic bandage (Tubiton House) Compressogrip (Fred Sammons, Box 32, Brookfield, IL 60513)	Rib weave stockinette covered with latex rubber yarns introduced into the fabric in continuous lengths; shaped support bandage available for arms and legs; friction to tissue diminished if applied from applicator; Tubigrip: 34% rubber and 67% cotton and is therefore more effective to maintain compression because rubber is elastic; Lycra or Spandex products change in compression after 30-minute stretch due to viscoplasticity of synthetic fibers; laundering is easier than elastic wraps; fabric may roll at proximal edge and cause decubiti	Compression of any cylindrical body part, particularly effective in applications involving knee or elbow because bandage does not gather in joint space One to three layers may be used to achieve adequate pressure; several sizes may be combined for cone-shaped body parts
Commercially produced individual garments	Gradient pressure lycra garments individually fit-	Head and face—hood neck—turtleneck, soft

Table 8.2—*Continued*

Name (Source)	Characteristics	Uses
Jobskin garments (Jobst, Box 653, Toledo, OH 43694)	ted to specific body measurements Jobskin elastic pressure covers are engineered to apply physiologically correct counterpressure to newly formed scar tissue	collar Chest and arms—vest with sleeves Legs—stocking torso and legs—2-leg stocking with panty
Elastic garments (Bioconcepts, 7324 N. 71st St., Scottsdale, AZ 85253)	Bioconcepts garments are also individually fitted to specific measurements	Any combination of areas can be compressed with these garments Concave areas need inserts or overlay for extra pressure
Pre-sized garments, Tubigloves (Tubiton House); Jobst pre-sized standard glove; Isotoner gloves (Aris, 417 5th Ave., New York, NY 10016); Tubigarments (Tubiton House)	Costly; deteriorate from exposure to oils, detergent or heat; fabric synthetic and viscoplasticity causes compression to relax after 30 minutes Presized garments may be used to toughen tissue for final individual garment; frequently fit is less than ideal	
Insert or overlay materials (preformed) Adhesive backed foams Reston (3M) Spenco padding (Spenco Med Products, Inc., P.O. Box 8113 Waco, TX 76710) poly cushion (Fred Sammons) Vigilon (C.R. Bard, Inc., Berkeley Hts., NJ 07922)	Soft padding may be stuck to garment, patient's shoe, etc; may cause excessive sweating May macerate tissue due to moisture collection; may collect bacteria if patient's hygiene is not meticulous Cut with scissors Prolonged drying time if laundered	Inserts or overlay to increase pressure on scars; especially effective if beveled for concave areas such as breast and buttock cleavage Protection at irritated skin creases Finger web spreaders
Open cell foam Alimed (Alimed, 172 W. Newton, Boston, MA 02118) cushion foam backpacker's mattress		

Table 8.2—*Continued*

Name (Source)	Characteristics	Uses
Tubifoam and arthro-pads LMB finger pressure wraps (LMB, Hand Rehab Products, Inc., P.O. Box 1181, San Luis Obispo, CA 92406)		
Closed cell polyethylene sheets aliplast plastazote	Resilient Light weight Flexible Fairly durable Cut with scissors Can be heated and molded to patient	Shoe inserts, support for neck foam collars Temporary "wraparound" knee extension splint
Orthopedic felt, ¼-inch, ½-inch (Any medical company)	Polyester felt can be washed and dried Cut with tin snips or felt shears Does not usually cause sweating; can sew to garments or secure with pocket	Beveled inserts or over-lays
Insert Materials (liquid with catalyst) Otoform K (WFR Aqua-plast Corp., P.O. Box 215, Ramsey, NJ 07446)	Silicone type material cures in 5 minutes with catalyst Viscous enough to setup without running to edges Moderately flexible when setup	Beveled inserts especially effective in thumb webs
Silicone Medical elasto-mer 382 (Dow Corn-ing Corp., Medical Products, Midland, MI 48640)	Liquid silicone sets up with stannous octoate cata-lyst; may cause exces-sive sweating Odor controlled somewhat by boiling elastomer Conforms to all irregulari-ties	Postoperative dressing over interface for skin grafting (½ elastomer-½ prosthetic foam)
Prosthetic foam Q7-4290 (Dow Corning)	Expands seven times when mixed with cata-lyst Forms open cell foam Odor may be offensive Conforms perfectly to scar	Positioning splint espe-cially for hands of chil-dren Hand web expanders Insert or overlay adhered to tee-shirt or tubular elastic

Table 8.2—*Continued*

Name (Source)	Characteristics	Uses
Strapping material Velfoam Beta pile Duravel (LMB) Polyester wicking (Fred Sammons)	Soft nap; easy to secure with Velcro	Splint strapping Finger web spreaders Beveled insert or overlay for scars
Low temperature plastic K-splint (Sammons) Polyform (Rolyan, P.O. Box 555, N93-W14475 Whittaker Wax, Menomonee Falls, WI 53051)	Plastic material Easily removable. Secure with elastic wrap, tubular elastic or straps Bonds with heat. Washable Hard, smooth surface at room temperature. Cut with scissors at 70° (140°F). Shape conforms perfectly to patient and to raised scars May need silicone or sponge insert to keep pressure on raised area. If perforated, may retain bacteria. Scars may grow into perforation if no interface is used. Swelling of tissue at perforations may cause itching	Draping plastic Insert or overlay to prevent or stretch contractures Static or dynamic splinting materials
Orthoplast isoprene (Johnson & Johnson Products, Inc., Chicago, IL)	Synthetic rubber, smooth, relatively stable surfaces at room temperature. Cut with scissors and mold at 60°C (130°F) Does not conform exactly to scar. Must be stretched with some pressure to conform. Bonds with surface clean and heat. Washable. Easily removable	Used as above Usually does not require insert for scar compression because plastic does not conform accurately to scar
Casting Materials splints rolls	Variety of plaster widths and setup times; becomes warm during	Total-contact splint which must be removed with cast cutter

Table 8.2—*Continued*

Name (Source)	Characteristics	Uses
	setup Can be fit for total contact pressure to scars; must be applied over interface, e.g., webril	Impression material for positive cast of neck

High temperature plastics
  Cellulose acetate butyrate (Eastman Kodak) Uvex
  Polycarbonate
  "Lexan"
  "Tufak" (Any plastic company)
  Thermovac-clear or Suralyn (U.S. Manufacturing, 180 No. San Gabriel Blvd., P.O. Box 5030, Pasadena, CA 91107)
  Tenite Butyrate
  Aquaplast-clear (WFR Company)
	Stable to 350°; must be cut warm or cut with saw or moto-tool
	Must be vacuum formed or shaped by hand over plaster cast of body part
	Tissue can be observed through splint
	Tissue must be observed for contact dermatitis
	Washable
	Easily removable
	
	Polycarbonate bubbles if not dehydrated at 250°F for 6 hours
		Transparent face and neck orthosis
		Inserts or overlays in circumscribed scar areas
		Individual splints to compress areas needing more pressure than circumferential elastic can provide without impairing circulation or nerve function

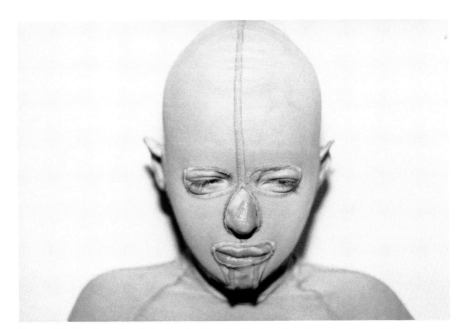

Figure 8.8. Custom-fitted elastic stocking for the head and face is shown (Bioconcepts or Jobst). Elastomer or otoform K inserts or plastic overlay is needed for contours.

barrel-shaped and where the pressure can, therefore, be exerted perpendicular to the scar. However, these garments tent over body contours and folds, encouraging the scar to fill these areas. An insert of adhesive foam (16), silicone foam sponge, felt, isoprene (7, 28), or elastomer (30) around the nose and lips will prevent this result when secured by a custom-made facial compression hood. A low temperature isoprene splint also can be fitted to the face and secured with elastic straps (43).

All of these appliances have the disadvantage of being opaque. Pressure that blanches the hyperemic tissue cannot be evaluated continuously. A transparent face mask, fitted from an accurate plaster mold of the head (Figs. 8.9–8.12), allows the patient and the rehabilitation team to check the blanched tissue and to monitor the orthotic fit (45, 48). The disadvantage of this compression device is the time and experience needed in fitting the splint.

If the patient has an eyelid burn, and a transparent night mask is used, it should be domed to provide corneal humidity and protection (Fig. 8.13). The dome should be used during the day if the patient is unable to blink, either because of cerebral function or because of loss of eyelid tissue. A child should be fitted with two additional transparent masks if the total face is badly injured. A night mask should be domed for burned eyelids and fitted with a microstomia correction device (Fig. 8.13). A feeding mask

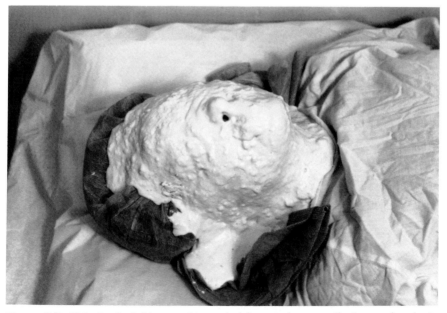

Figure 8.9. Alginate dental impression material poured over patient records minute details of facial scars. It is reinforced with plaster strips to take the negative facial impression.

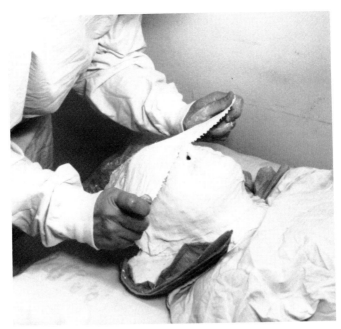

Figure 8.10. Plaster strips reinforce the negative impression material to allow removal without distortion.

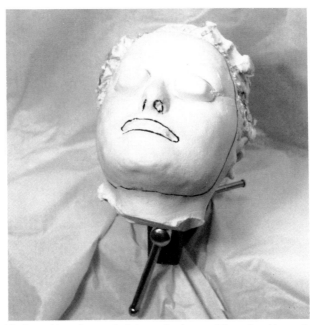

Figure 8.11. A positive plaster facial cast is shown. The raised hypertrophic scars are removed and the entire plaster mold sanded smooth with sanding cloth (Durite). This mold includes humidity domes for night use if the patient cannot blink.

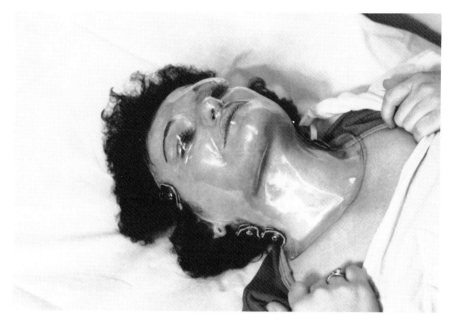

Figure 8.12. One-piece night neck and face mask with humidity domes is shown. The 400 degree transparent plastic is conformed to the plaster mold, trimmed and fitted to the patient. Elastic straps apply pressure to blanch the hyperemic scar. Areas needing additional pressure are revised by spot heating with a heat gun. This night splint covers neck and face. Usually the neck splint is applied separately, over the face mask.

should be fitted to put pressure on cheeks, forehead, and nose, but should allow breathing through both mouth and nose for bottle feeding if necessary. The eyes should be left open so the child can spend at least four hours a day developing normal binocular vision. Plastic, although transparent, can change visual acuity, and some children who have worn the domed day mask for several months have had difficulty adjusting to spatial relationships when the mask was removed, especially if they had not had many periods of unobstructed vision. The eye openings are made in the feeding mask because an adult will be present to prevent injury to the cornea when it is unprotected. Often it is easier for parents to remove one mask, dry the skin, encourage exercising of the mouth, face, and eyes, and then apply a new mask. When the mask is taken off for meals and exercise, replacing it is often delayed because of other demands on the adult. This prolongs the final scar resolution.

If a burned adult does not need a microstomia correction device at night, the day mask can be fitted if necessary with a removable, transparent adhesive plastic dome to humidify the cornea at night. This treatment may reduce the need for tarsorrhaphy. Meticulous hygiene is vital and the tissue and mask must be cleaned and reapplied frequently if the area around the

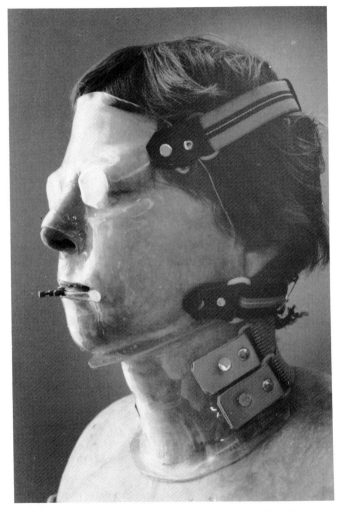

Figure 8.13. Modification of transparent splints is shown. A night mask domed for corneal humidification and fitted with Iowa City Microstomia Prevention Device in place. Nostril catheters would be added if the nasal passage became occluded by development of hypertrophic scars.

eye is draining. The night dome has the advantage of protecting the eye while allowing enough vision for independent care.

NOSTRIL

The cone-shaped connection of a silicone catheter can be cut 1 mm long and placed in the nostril to keep it patent and to minimize hypertrophic scarring (Fig. 8.14). Some patients prefer to wear this device four to eight hours during the day, removing it at night. Massage and stretching of the tissues with an obturator are also necessary to control the scar and contracture around the nostril.

MOUTH

Widely varied devices for prevention and correction of microstomia have been described (20). All devices can be applied with any of the facial conformers (Fig. 8.13) or elastic hoods (Fig. 8.8). Wearing the orthosis all night is usually adequate to preserve the horizontal lip opening. Massage plus vertical stretching of the lips and jaws must be done four times a day to avoid scar contractures. Even if surface pressure is used compulsively, the lips will contract until resistance is met. Circular distance of the obicularis muscle can be maintained with 5-minute hourly stretching during

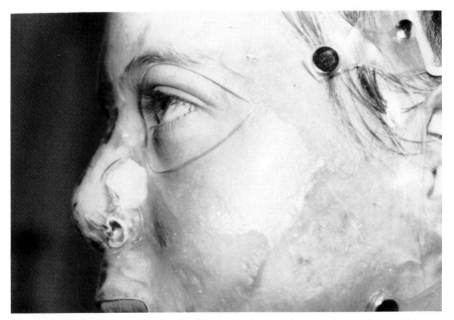

Figure 8.14. Catheter or mediastinal tubing cut 1-mm long and worn in nostril keeps airway patent under transparent orthosis. Silicone insert temporarily adds pressure on nostril wall. Separate, clear, nostril and nose compression splint may be worn under transparent face mask.

waking hours. The facial compression device must be replaced after stretching exercises.

Facial injuries that are obviously full-thickness or that do not heal in two weeks must be grafted. Usually split-thickness sheet or unexpanded mesh grafts are used. These are applied in symmetrical "cosmetic" units along the lines of relaxed skin tension (5). If skeletal halo traction (Fig. 8.15) is not utilized for immobilization an accurate elastomeric moulage under an elastic hood may be used to stent the graft (30) (Fig. 8.16). The moulage and hood are left in place for five days and then removed daily for skin care, exercise, and washing of the elastomer and hood. To decrease shearing forces on the grafts, the patient should not chew during the first three days after grafting. Use of the hood and elastomer is continued until an accurate transparent day splint is fitted. Some centers use this method of compression, remolding the elastomer as needed until the facial scars mature. Transparent splinting can similarly be used. With meticulous care, open areas will heal under any type of splint (Figs. 8.17–8.19).

A pad of elastomer or other material may be needed behind the ear to preserve the contours and to maintain the erectness of the pinna. A special

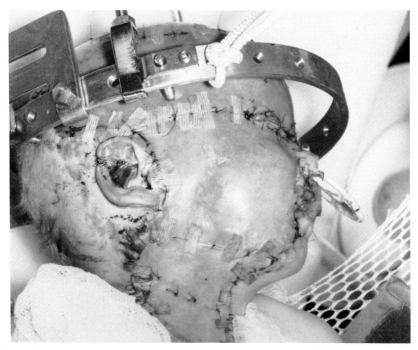

Figure 8.15. Halo traction immobilization for open graft and donor care if healing of entire head is needed. Note tarsorrhaphies to prevent eyelid contractures and protect corneas.

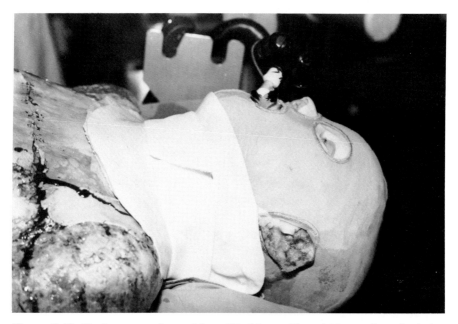

Figure 8.16. Elastomer moulage of face fitted to positive plaster cast made during grafting can be secured over grafts with Bioconcepts hood. Graft may be observed daily for serum collections if desired but stent pressure is maintained for five days. Elastomer silicone dressing over neck grafts is secured by K-splint overlay.

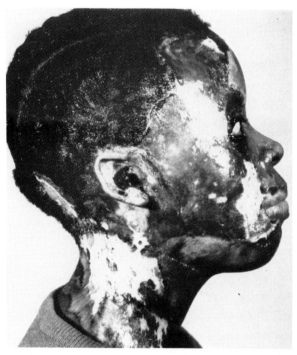

Figure 8.17. Open healing granulation tissue following nitric acid burn in mastoid area, neck, lip-cheek fold, and on forehead is shown.

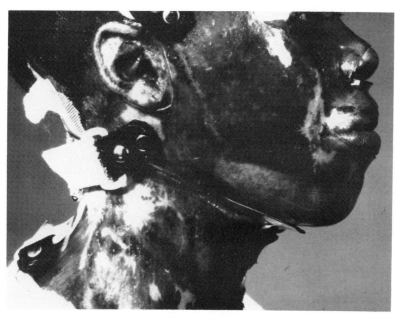

Figure 8.18. Transparent splinting 23 hours dally over open areas is shown; it is removed hourly for five-minute cleaning of skin and splint.

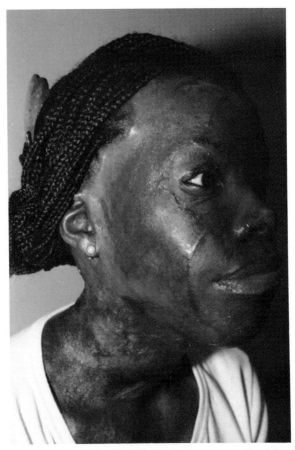

Figure 8.19. Healed tissue shown two years after injury.

earring (6) can be fitted for the ear lobe to control scars. A transparent clip can be fitted for patients who do not wear earrings.

After reconstructive "Z" plasties, grafting, or dermabrasion, the same orthoses can be used and will be needed to control hypertrophic scarring. Since bacteria are rarely present in the wound after these operations, the likelihood of inflammation is reduced. Therefore, external pressure can be discontinued earlier because the scar will mature faster. Properly supervised prophylactic pressure cannot injure the healing tissue and often it will prevent recurrences of hypertrophic scars. The total time required for use of pressure is prolonged if the scar is already raised when pressure is instituted.

NECK

In 1961, Cronin (10) first described a horsehide, felt, and Silastic splint that kept the grafted neck wrinkle free and soft. Later, early grafting and constant foam splinting to prevent flexion contracture and hypertrophic scarring of the neck were suggested (50). Willis (51) pioneered the use of total contact splinting with easily fabricated isoprene. Feldman and MacMillan (13) reported a declining need for neck reconstruction in children, and related this to the use of total contact orthoses of polyvinyl chloride.

Gentle pressure can be applied to the edematous neck by a cervical collar of foam or a gauze covered perineal pad. In the opinion of some burn teams, a custom-fitted foam orthosis provides adequate pressure for the entire healing process (Fig. 8.20).

In addition to using pressure, the patient must exercise the neck in all directions to prevent muscle weakness and contractures of soft tissues. Another technique to maintain tissue length and to stretch the scar tissue is to hyperextend the neck over a short mattress or wedge (Fig. 8.20). The head of the bed must be elevated on shock blocks eight inches or more to avoid possible cerebral edema and headaches.

Immediately after grafting, proper pressure to the healing tissue and immobilization of the neck can be obtained by using an elastomer, a prosthetic foam elastomer-elastic wrap stent, or a cotton stent with or without a rigid support (Fig. 8.21). Two weeks after the graft, a rigid, total contact transparent neck orthosis can be fitted (46). This assures accurate pressure to the neck, which can be assessed continuously by the patient and the burn team. The rigid splint can be fitted to stretch the tissue from the

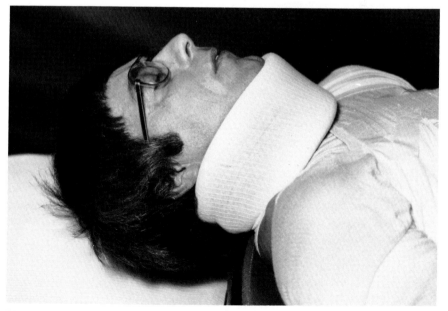

Figure 8.20. Foam neck orthosis is less irritating to denuded areas early after injury. Wedge or double mattress assists neck stretch to maintain scar tissue length.

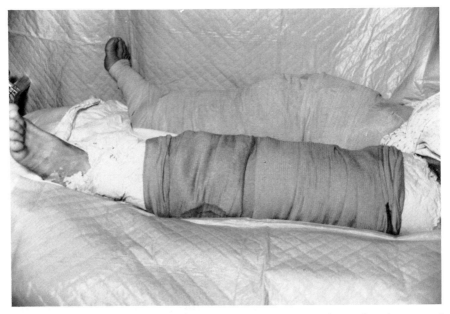

Figure 8.21. Prosthetic foam with elastomer elastic wrapped over leg donors and circumferential graft shown which stents the graft, immobilizes the leg, provides perfect total-contact tissue support, distributes pressure, and allows drainage. It replaces tibial and calcaneal pin in circumferential leg grafts.

clavicles to the mandible. Care must be taken to avoid impingement of the neck splint on the deltoid muscle if shoulder stretching also is required. A night splint that depresses the shoulder and laterally bends the neck can be attempted. However, use of this splint for more than four hours daily requires an unusually motivated patient. The neck splint should be made to extend beyond the chin shelf of the face mask if the two are to be worn simultaneously. The patient can then rotate the head slightly without pinching the tissue at the seam.

A four-post neck orthosis has been recommended but it does not provide a total-contact pressure. With this splint, the chin will be held parallel to the floor, but the scar in the open neck area will still thicken. A turtle neck added to the elastic support garment or an elastic covered sponge has also been suggested. These devices, however, do not conform to the contours of the neck as well as temperature molded plastics, and therefore they allow greater scar build-up.

AXILLA

Control of hypertrophic scar about the very mobile shoulder joint is very difficult. Although initially somewhat painful, a commercially available, soft, figure of eight clavicular strap (Fig. 8.6), worn over the burn dressings for 23 hours a day, can prevent hypertrophic scarring and contractures of the anterior and posterior axillary folds.

A wide variety of open immobilizing axillary splints for graftings have been described (see Fig. 5.25). A small patient can be immobilized in a prosthetic foam elastomer-elastic wrap total-contact stent dressing (Fig. 8.22). It is removed after five days.

Once skin coverage has been achieved, the axilla remains one of the most difficult areas for preservation of skin integrity while at the same time controlling scars and contractures. In the axillary area, a figure of eight elastic wrap using foam crescents can provide pressure to the arm pit and prevent irritation from motion (28). This wrap and the commercial clavicular strap are difficult for the adult to use when skin is still easily abraded. Occasionally, excessive breakdown of the skin makes it necessary to remove elastic garments or elastic wraps for shoulder exercise. In these cases, each exercise period should be restricted to 30 minutes.

For small children, a splint at 160 degrees of forward flexion (Fig. 8.23) has been used for 20–24 hours daily for as long as four months while active deltoid strength develops. Thereafter, the splint is used only at night and during naps. In patients thus treated, complications were not noted and shoulder reconstructions were not needed.

Elastic garments fit poorly in the axillary area. Refitting and revising

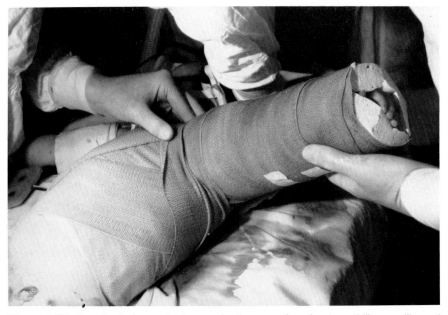

Figure 8.22. Prosthetic foam-elastomer elastic wrap dressing immobilizes axilla and stents graft. Arm will be supported in foam airplane to slightly forward rotate axilla.

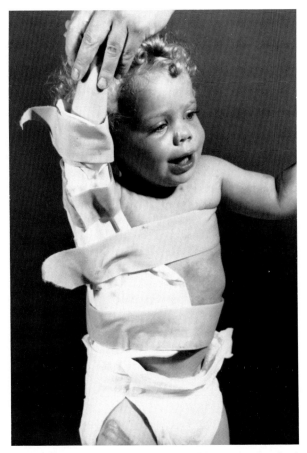

Figure 8.23. Total-contact axillary splint was worn 20 hours a day for four months by this child. Splint was worn over Jobst custom body suit.

these garments to obtain optimal contact with the axillary tissue is important. It must be remembered that the scar will build up until the pressure of the garment exceeds the force of the contracting hypertrophic scar. Night splints (Fig. 8.23) added over the elastic garments and secured with elastic wraps or Velcro straps are helpful, but inconvenience, pain, and perspiration may cause the patient to discontinue the use of these orthoses.

ARMS AND LEGS

Scar control of these cylindrical structures has been relatively successful. Early elastic wraps or Tubigrip bandages provide adequate compression. Later, when the healed tissue will tolerate the shearing force of donning custom-fitted elastic garments, such garments will provide excellent scar control. Complications may be noted at the antecubital space, the olecranon, the posterior popliteal space, and the medial and lateral malleoli. Frequently, motion of the elbow, knee, or ankle will cause hypertrophic scars in these areas to become denuded by shearing against the elastic support. Some adaptation must then be made to allow frequent exercise without tissue breakdown. Occasionally, use of elastic garments must be discontinued temporarily and Tubigrip or elastic wraps must be resumed. A nylon interface, a felt pad or a foam pad, or any combination of these may be adequate to protect the skin. If zippers are inserted in the elastic garment, they should be discontinued as soon as possible because the zipper does not provide uniform pressure. Unwrapping of the knee or elbow permits stretching of the joints at the extremes of motion. Exercise of this type should last only 30 minutes and the support should then be immediately replaced. A patient who develops severe blistering or venous stasis of a newly grafted area may need to curtail walking and follow a strictly graded exercise program with the leg dependent. The goal of this program would be normal walking with intact tissue and use of pressure garments 23 hours a day.

Ropelike hypertrophic scars, often seen at the medial and lateral borders of the antecubital and popliteal spaces, frequently need the additional pressure of a total contact isoprene splint or a draped K-splint wrapped over the elastic garment at the flexion creases during rest and sleep. Hypertrophic scarring over the flexion crease of the hip is extremely difficult to control, especially in children still wearing diapers. Elastomeric inserts are waterproof, but it is difficult to prevent them from slipping and blistering the tissue of an active child. Lying prone for several hours during rest periods and sleep will increase the pressure on anterior hip scars and decreases the thickness of the scar. An extra bikini-type panty can be worn under the regular tights to prevent tenting at the hip during sitting.

Grafted areas often mature months before partial-thickness, spontaneously healed areas. Additional pressure to second degree burn scars can be applied with elastomeric inserts, felt, open-cell sponge, folded fabric, fabric-covered sponge, or custom-fitted transparent plastic strips. These devices can be applied under the custom-fitted garment or, if the insert tents the garment in a burned area, the device can be wrapped with elastic bandages over the garment.

Many authors advocate three-point positioning splints for extension of elbow and knees. Such splints apply pressure only in the three areas of contact. When a healing wound intervenes, it is helpful to provide pressure the full distance of the injury by means of a thermoplastic splint.

HANDS

Only general principles of scar control for the hand are mentioned in this chapter. Hand burns are dealt with in greater detail in Chapter 9. Deep partial-thickness burns of the hands which heal slowly over four to six weeks usually have considerable overgrowth of granulation tissue and subsequently scar tissue which does not become tough, durable, and free of pain for many months. After successful early excision and grafting of the hand with complete removal of nonviable tissue and 100% take of the graft healing is much more satisfactory and less hypertrophic scarring develops (2, 14). Full active range of motion can usually be achieved one week after the grafting unless the burn destroyed tendons or nerves. Elastic-wrap support, Isotoner gloves, Tubigrip gloves, Jobst (Fig. 8.24), or BioConcepts gloves may be needed while the healing tissue matures, but the healing after early excision is rarely prolonged.

All hand burns initially require elevation to control edema. Severe burns may require a night splint. The night splint should place the wrist in some extension (15–30 degrees), the metacarpophalangeal joints in 70 degrees of flexion and the interphalangeal joints extended and the thumb rotated into opposition. This splint can be used for immobilization after grafting if the burn is not circumferential. If single fingers are involved in hypertrophic

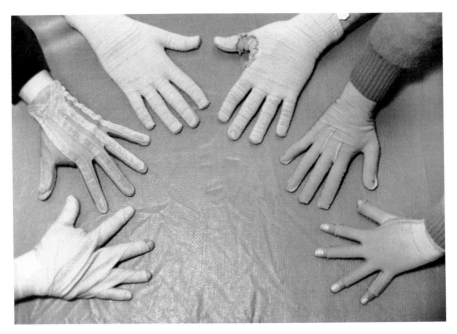

Figure 8.24. Compression devices which are available for hand support. Applied in graded program as tissue will tolerate shearing force of donning support. Left to right: (1) elastic figure of eight "boxer" wrap of hand; (all finger webs separated by lambs wool and thumb webs stretched by otoform K day spacers); (2) Isotoner slightly elastic glove; (3) Tubigrip glove; (4) Tubigrip glove with expanded thumb web; (5) Jobst presized glove; (6) Jobst custom elastic glove with slant back at finger webs.

scarring and contracture, individual gutter splinting is most effective and may be used in combination with static or dynamic hand and wrist splints.

If closed dressings are being used immediately after grafting, a prosthetic foam elastomer-elastic wrap can provide appropriate uniform pressure and positioning. From the third to the fifth day the foam is removed and gentle active motion is resumed. Elevation is continued until edema is resolved. Graded total-contact pressure to the hand can be applied as the grafts tolerate, initially by spiral Elset or elastic bandage wrapping, progressing to figure of eight wrapping, then to commercial gloves, and finally by custom-fitted elastic gloves with slant-back web spaces if these are needed (Fig. 8.24). Inserts for the interdigital web spaces, and especially for the first web space, may be needed to prevent limitation of motion in these areas. Lambs wool makes a very effective, disposable insert. Elastomer has been well accepted by patients who need thumb-web spreaders. These can be applied over or under the elastic glove and should allow full use of the hands.

Numerous dynamic splints using rubber-band or spring traction are available to stretch hand contractures. However, these splints are less successful in hypertrophic scar control than other methods and may cause discomfort and tissue breakdown.

Serial plaster casting can be used successfully in the recalcitrant patient who refuses to wear pressure devices. The hand can be serially casted into a position of function. The cast should be removed once or twice daily for exercise and skin care. If the hand is stiff in both flexion and extension, the serial casting can be done in flexion alternating with extension. This treatment requires very careful supervision and a skilled therapist. After approximately one week of serial casting the tissue will become flatter, softer, and more supple. Additionally improved range of motion can be accomplished.

FEET

Hypertrophic scars are seldom seen on the soles of the feet where the skin is thick and tethered to an aponeurosis. Wearing shoes and walking apply considerable pressure to the bottom of the foot, controlling the scar process. Soon after the burn, foam boots or sandals may be used, making ambulation more comfortable (Figs. 8.25 and 8.26). Cutouts in shoe inserts result in increased swelling into these openings and therefore increased tissue breakdown. Differing densities of insert materials covered by a smooth foam insole may aid in pain-free ambulation and avoid edema to insole cutouts.

Following grafting the foot may be immobilized with prosthetic foam elastomer-elastic wrap stent dressing or by skeletal traction. Dorsal foot scars and contractures are a problem (37), especially for children. These

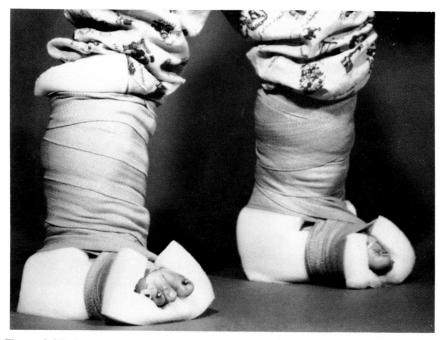

Figure 8.25. Sponge rubber "boots" for early ambulation are shown. They are worn over elastic wrap and wrapped in place with second elastic wrap. Note rivets glued to toes for night traction in dynamic metatarsal flexion splint.

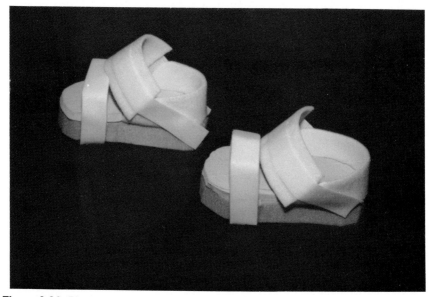

Figure 8.26. Plastazote and Velcro shoes are shown for ambulation of a child burned on sole of foot.

may result in hyperextension of the metatarsophalangeal joints. A posterior ankle-foot orthosis that ends at the metatarsophalangeal joint fitted with an anterior splint to provide plantar flexion of the toes can help to prevent scar contracture. This splint can be lined with sheepskin to decrease shearing on newly healed tissue. It is worn at all times except when the patient is walking. When the tissue is stable, after grafting, fleecelined high-top double-depth tennis shoes can be worn (Fig. 8.27). If the toes are becoming hyperextended, an insert will be needed to flex the metatarsophalangeal joints. Ultimately, the patient can wear regular toe lacing orthopaedic shoes. A double-depth insert allows plantar flexion of the toes when used with a felt-padded tongue. The shoes are often needed day and night to reduce scarring and contractures. It may be necessary to put a steel shank in the shoes to prevent curling of the toe of the shoe which would exaggerate the contracture (Fig. 8.28). Custom-fitted elastic garments can be made with soft, closed toes to improve total contact. They can also be fitted with a soft lining at the heel. Toes should be separated with lambs wool. An elastic "foot-mitten" with a divider for the big toe can be fitted but this frequently causes discomfort. Often padding will be needed under

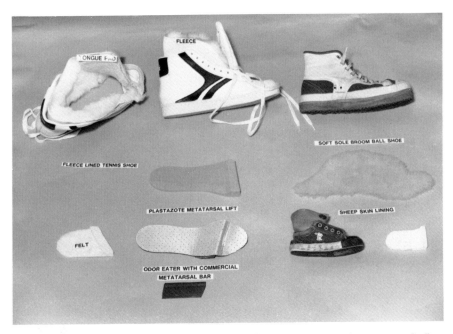

Figure 8.27. Sheepskin-lined tennis shoes apply extra pressure to scars and allow ambulation without shearing away grafts. Metatarsal bar may be of foam or felt. Tongue of toe lacer shoe may be padded with fleece or felt to compress dorsum of foot. Two pair of shoes are lined, one for day wear and one for night wear. Toe may curl because steel shank cannot be used.

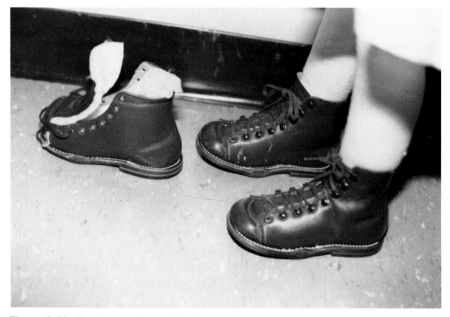

Figure 8.28. Toe lacer orthopaedic shoes with sole insert ending at metatarsals, steel shank, metatarsal bar and felt padded tongue are worn during the day. A bivalved cast, splint, or adapted tennis shoe may be worn in bed.

the stocking on the dorsal aspect of the hindfoot to prevent tissue breakdown.

GENITALIA

Controlling hypertrophic scars in the genital area is nearly impossible. For the female, perineal pads in several thicknesses, secured with an elastic girdle or custom-made bikini-type elastic garment may be helpful. Using a banana-type bicycle seat both for exercise and rest periods can increase pressure to the genital area. Gymnastic exercises are needed if hypertrophic scars are contracting.

Hypertrophic scarring can deviate the penis from midline, interfering with the urine stream and causing painful erections. The penis may be folded over a cylinder-shaped foam in the opposite direction of the scar. If a tight bikini-type short is worn over this, pressure can be applied to diminish the scar. A cylindrical elastic tube also can be fitted for the penis, but few patients are willing to wear this device, unless scarring is significant or incapacitating.

TRUNK

Elastic wraps and custom-fitted elastic garments control trunk scars quite well. The breast cleavage, the interscapular area, and the buttock creases

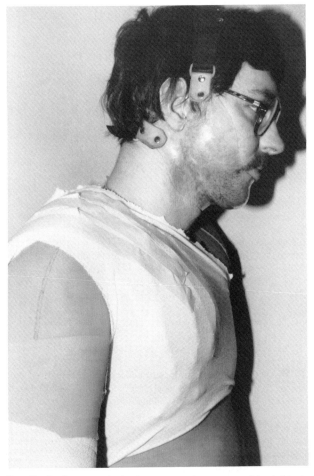

Figure 8.29. Prosthetic foam and elastomer overlay secured to tubigrip tube, worn over Jobst in chest area to apply additional pressure in concave areas.

are exceptions. Inserts of elastomer or similar material are needed for scar control in these areas (Fig. 8.29). These inserts can be secured or sewed to Tubigrip or to an undershirt (19). This also helps keep children from removing the inserts (19). Inserts must be washed frequently since they may cause increased perspiration of the uninjured tissue.

Summary

The challenge of controlling hypertrophic scarring is being met with a wide variety of modalities. Each burn center has different scar treatment protocols, but the general principle is the application of pressure through the use of inexpensive and non-damaging materials. There is yet no method that will allow safe, complete control of scarring. However, external pressure has dramatically decreased disfigurement and the need for reconstruction for the burn victim.

REFERENCES

1. Apfelberg DB, Maser MR, Lash H: Extended clinical use the argon laser for cutaneous lesions. *Arch Dermatol* 115:719–721, 1979.
2. Artz CP, Moncrief JA, Pruitt BA: *Burns: A Team Approach.* Philadelphia, W.B. Saunders Company, 1979.
3. Barnes MJ: Function of ascorbic acid in collagen metabolism. *Ann NY Acad Sci* 258:264–277, 1975.
4. Bartlett RH, Wingerson E, Simonton S, et al: Rehabilitation following burn injury. *Surg Clin North Am* 58:1249–1262, 1978.
5. Borges AF, Alexander JE: Relaxed skin tension lines, Z-plasties on scars, and fusiform excision of lesions. *Br J Plast Surg* 15:242–254, 1962.
6. Brent B: The role of pressure therapy in management of earlobe keloids: Preliminary report of a controlled study. *Ann Plast Surg* 1:579–581, 1978.
7. Buchan NG: Experience with thermoplastic splints in the post-burn hand. *Br J Plast Surg* 28:193–297, 1975.
8. Callen JP: Intralesional corticosteroids. *J Am Acad Dermatol* 4:149–151, 1981.
9. Cohen IK, McCoy BJ, Mohanakumar T, et al: Immunoglobulin, complement, and histocompatibility antigen studies in keloid patients. *Plast Reconstr Surg* 63:689–695, 1979.
10. Cronin TD: Excision of scar contracture of the neck. In Feller I, Grabb WC: *Reconstruction and Rehabilitation of the Burned Patient.* Ann Arbor, MI, National Institute for Burn Medicine, 1979.
11. DeLimpens J: The local treatment of hypertrophic scars and keloids with topical retinoic acid. *Br J Dermatol* 103:319–323, 1980.
12. Ederton MT, Hanrahan EM, Davis WB: Use of vitamin E in the treatment of keloids. *Plast Reconstr Surg* 85:224–233, 1951.
13. Feldman AE, MacMillan BG: Burn injury in children: Declining need for reconstructive surgery as related to use of neck orthoses. *Arch Phys Med Rehabil* 61:441–449, 1980.
14. Feller I, Grabb WC: *Reconstruction and Rehabilitation of the Burned Patient.* Ann Arbor, MI, National Institute for Burn Medicine, 1979.
15. Feller I: Hypertrophic scarring and keloid: Shaving and overgrafting. In Feller I, Grabb WC: *Reconstruction and Rehabilitation of the Burned Patient.* Ann Arbor, MI, National Institute for Burn Medicine, 1979.
16. Fujimori R, Hiramoto M, Ofuji S: Sponge fixation method for treatment of early scars. *Plast Reconstr Surg* 42:322–327, 1968.
17. Furnas DW, Fischer GW: The Z-plasty: Biomechanics and mathematics. *Br J Plast Surg* 24:144–160, 1971.
18. Grigsby L: An approach for applying additional pressure material and maintaining its position under pressure vests in the treatment of pediatric burn patients. American Burn Association, Burn Rehabilitation Special Interest Group, 1981, Abstract 1.
19. Guin JD: Complications of topical hydrocortisone. *J Am Acad Dermatol* 4:417–422, 1981.
20. Hartford CE, Kealey GP, Lavelle WE, et al: An appliance to prevent and treat microstomia from burns. *J Trauma* 15:356–360, 1975.
21. Helm PA, Head MD, Pullium G, et al: Burn rehabilitation—A team approach. *Surg Clin North Am* 58:1263–1278, 1978.
22. Hunt TK: *Fundamentals of Wound Management in Surgery, Wound Healing: Disorders of Repair.* South Plainfield, NJ, Chirurgecom, Inc., 1976.
23. Ketchum LD: Hypertrophic scars and keloids. *Clin Plast Surg* 4:301–310, 1977.
24. Kischer CW, Bunce H, Shetlar MR: Mast cell analyses in hypertrophic scars, hypertrophic scars treated with pressure and mature scars. *J Invest Dermatol* 70:355–357, 1978.
25. Kischer CW, Shetlar MD: Collagen and mucopolysaccharides in the hypertrophic scar. *Connect Tissue Res* 2:205–213, 1974.
26. Kischer CW, Shetlar MR: Microvasculature in hypertrophic scars and the effects of

pressure. *J Trauma* 19:757–764, 1979.

27. Kischer CW, Shetlar MR, Shetlar CL: Alteration of hypertrophic scars induced by mechanical pressure. *Arch Dermatol* 111:60–64, 1975.

28. Larson DL, Abston S, Dobrkovsky M, et al: The prevention and correction of burn scar contracture and hypertrophy. Shriners Burn Institute, Galveston, TX, University of Texas Medical Branch, 1973.

29. Lubritz RE: Cryosurgery of benign lesions. *Cutis* 16:426–432, 1975.

30. MacDonald LD, Covery MH, Marvin J, et al: The risk to graft when elastomere/thermoplastic pressure devices are applied immediately after grafting the head and neck. American Burn Association Thirteenth Annual Meeting, 1981, Abstract 73.

31. MacMillin BG, Lang D: Nursing care in the operating room. *Burns: A Team Approach.* Philadelphia, W.B. Saunders Company, 1979.

32. Making the least of burn scars. *Emerg Med* 4:24–45, 1972.

33. Malaker K, Ellis F, Paine CH: Keloid scars: A new method of treatment combining surgery with interstitial radiotherapy. *Clin Radiol* 27:179–183, 1976.

34. Mani MM, Robinson DW, Masters FW, et al: Burn update—Management of scars and contractures. *J Kans Med Soc* 79:118–120, 1978.

35. Moncrief JA: Grafting. In Artz CP, Moncrief JA, Pruitt BA: *Burns—A Team Approach.* Philadelphia, W.B. Saunders Company, 1979.

36. Murray JC, Pollack SV, Pinnel SR: Keloids: A review. *J Am Acad Dermatol* 4:461–470, 1981.

37. Nothdurft D, Pullium G, Bruster J: Management of feet and ankle burns: Orthotic management of pre-existing deformity and protocol for prevention of deformity. *Burns* 5:221–226, 1978.

38. Novick M, Gard DA, Hardy SB, et al: Burn scar carcinoma: a review and analysis of 46 cases. *J Trauma* 17:809–817, 1977.

39. Onwukwe MF: Treating keloids by surgery and methotrexate. *Arch Dermatol* 116:158, 1980.

40. Parks DH, Larson DL, de la Houssaye AJ: Hypertrophic scarring: Pressure dressings. *Reconstruction of the Burned Patient.* Ann Arbor, MI, National Institute for Burn Medicine, 1979.

41. Patterson RP, Fisher SV: The accuracy of electrical transducers for the measurement of pressure applied to the skin. *IEEE Trans Biomed Eng* 26:450–456, 1979.

42. Peacock EJ, Madden JW, Trier WC: Biologic basis for the treatment of keloids and hypertrophic scars. *South Med J* 63:755–760, 1970.

43. Petersen P: A conformer for the reduction of facial burn contractures: A preliminary report. *Am J Occup Ther* 31:101–104, 1977.

44. Peterkofsy B: The effect of ascorbic acid on collagen polypeptide synthesis and proline hydroxylation during the growth of cultured fibroblasts. *Arch Biochem Biophys* 152:318–328, 1972.

45. Rivers EA, Strate RG, Solem LD: The transparent face mask. *Am J Occup Ther* 33:108–113, 1979.

46. Rivers EA, Walbruch BJ, Collin TL, et al: The superiority of the transparent neck splint in the management of hypertrophic scars and neck contractures. Proceedings of the Twelfth Annual Meeting of the American Burn Association, 1980, Abstract 35.

47. Ryan GB, Cliff WJ, Gabbiani G, et al: Myofibroblasts in human granulation tissue. *Hum Pathol* 5:55–67, 1974.

48. Shons AR, Rivers EA, Solem LD: A rigid transparent face mask for control of scar hypertrophy. *Ann Plast Surg* 6:245–248, 1981.

49. Soyka P, Zellweger GA: Bethamethasone in the treatment of hypertrophic scars. *Helv Chir Acta* 47:137–140, 1980.

50. Tanzer RC: Burn contracture of the neck. *Plast Reconstr Surg* 33:207–212, 1964.

51. Willis B: The use of Orthoplast isoprene in the treatment of the acutely burned child. *Am J Occup Ther* 23:57–61, 1969.

9

Hand Management

ROGER E. SALISBURY

The phrase, rehabilitation of the burned hand, has practically become a cliché, synonymous with motherhood, baseball, and apple pie. It is fashionable to express concern for the hand, and yet the definition of rehabilitation is extremely variable to those in health care. Daily whirlpool and squeezing a ball do not constitute hand rehabilitation. Returning to work or school expeditiously is always the desirable end result, but how to reach this goal is confusing. Interestingly, a recent survey (5) conducted by the Committee on Organization and Delivery of Burn Care for the American Burn Association revealed that too often the healed burn patient goes back to his community and never benefits from the considerable rehabilitation potential of the center's staff. The purpose of this chapter is to identify common burned hand problems, (often resulting from inadequate rehabilitation efforts) and to discuss how to avoid problems and treat optimally.

Probably the greatest impediment to good rehabilitation for the working man or woman is lack of a team effort initially. Specifically, the patient should be seen and evaluated during his first week in the hospital by the rehabilitation team consisting of the physician, occupational therapist, physical therapist, vocational rehabilitation counselor, and social worker. Most often it is possible to determine (a) if the patient will survive, (b) if the hand function will be significantly compromised, (c) about how long the patient will be in the hospital and out of work, and (d) whether or not the patient will be able to return to his/her old job. Armed with this information, the team can communicate with the employer and involve him/her in some of the decision-making process. In fairness to all, the employer should be informed if he/she will need to hire a replacement in the patient's old job. It may happen that the patient regains 80% of function, but is unable to perform his/her previous job. In the present climate of a shrinking job market, it is very possible that such a patient with reasonable hand function will find himself unemployed. This unfortunate situation reflects a failure of the system, not of the patient. It is important to determine early if job retraining and schooling are necessary and then get the process started, saving many months of "down" time. Of course, there are some cases in which the patient will have to try his/her previous occupation to determine if he/she can still do it.

Of real concern is a lack of a hand rehabilitation team in many hospitals. Most of the patients treated at burn centers come from great distances. To minimize family disruption and expense, they often are referred back to their local physician and hospital. Unfortunately these hospitals often do not have health care professionals experienced with treating and rehabilitating hand burns. The ability to correct a contracture, "to flip a flap" or skin graft is not the essence of treatment. The key is to be able to ask the right questions of the patient and plan a sequence of procedures (if necessary, several years ahead) to restore function in concert with the efforts of the other members of the team. To formulate a rehabilitation program one must ask:

(1) Is the dominant hand involved?
(2) What is the age of the patient?
(3) What are the economic past and future, including job history?
(4) What were any associated injuries?
(5) Are there any medical diseases?

Controversies surrounding choice of early treatment are not really hard to resolve. Enzymes vs. early excision and grafting vs. topical chemotherapy all have their advocates. Simply, each can yield an excellent result and rapid rehabilitation if the patients are chosen carefully. For instance, superficial and intermediate partial-thickness burns will do well regardless of choice of treatment. Charred hands will do poorly with all forms of treatment. It is the deep partial-thickness or full-thickness injury that sparks controversy. In these injuries, Dr. Gant (4) has shown that early use of enzymes followed by grafting gives excellent function. Drs. Robson (2) and Salisbury (6) in two prospective studies found no difference in the functional results of early excision and grafting vs. topical chemotherapy and late grating. There is no single perfect treatment to the exclusion of all others. Rather a good aggressive team can get excellent results with different treatment modalities. With each treatment, a well-organized splinting and exercise program for many months is a cornerstone to success. Incorrect application of any of the three treatment modalities gives a poor result and the technique a "bad name." For instance, this hand (Fig. 9.1) is seven weeks after injury, managed by topical chemotherapy. The hand is chronically edematous from disuse. It is obvious that skin grafting is long overdue. It is rare that any wound treated with chemotherapeutic agents, débridement, and grafting should go beyond four weeks without being healed. If so, a different treatment should be employed, excision and grafting. A vigorous exercise and splinting program might have prevented this edema formation. It must be noted that a chronically edematous hand can also result from poor technique in excision and grafting, if one inadvertently removes the dorsal veins. Not using a large enough skin graft after early excision can

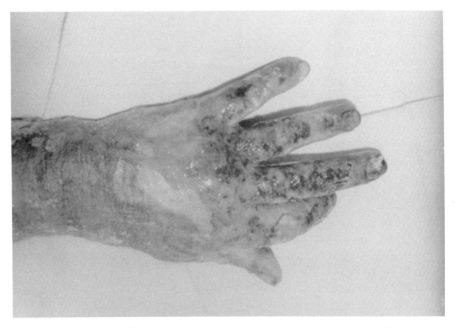

Figure 9.1. A chronically edematous hand was inappropriately treated for seven weeks with topical chemotherapy.

also result in dorsal shortening and extension contractures (Fig. 9.2). Nevertheless, the proper splinting during and after surgery might have prevented the hyperextended metacarpophalangeal (MP) joints and first web space adduction contracture. To hasten rehabilitation, the early treatment choices might be as follows:

(1) Superficial or intermediate burn: use topical chemotherapy and active exercise until healing. Splint only if necessary because of noncompliance with the exercise program.

(2) Deep second degree, third degree burns: if the total body burn is small and the hand burns are the reason for hospitalization, then excision and grafting will shorten morbidity and hospitalization. If the total body burn is large, treat with chemotherapy, exercise and splinting, skin graft if necessary. The limited donor site is best meshed and used over large areas to save the patient's life.

(3) Deeper burns (fourth degree): topical chemotherapy and graft when granulated. Expectations are guarded for these hands regardless of treatment.

Volar hand burns are rarely excised because they usually heal. Unlike the dorsum, there is no dissection plane and excision is very bloody and difficult. Deep volar burns (Fig. 9.3) must be splinted in the antideformity position (Fig. 9.4) with the wrist and fingers in extension, or narrowing of the palm

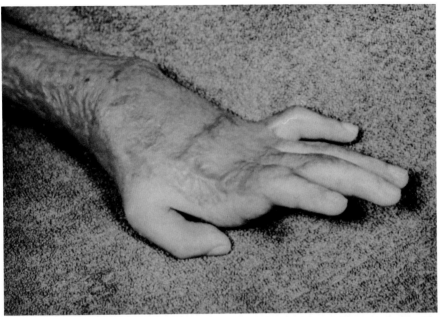

Figure 9.2. Placement of too small a skin graft on the dorsum and fingers resulted in extensor contracture.

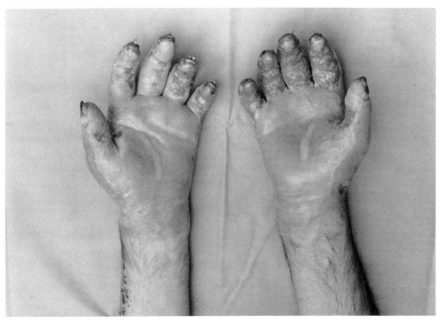

Figure 9.3. Deep burn of palm and fingers results in narrowing of the palm and flexion contractures.

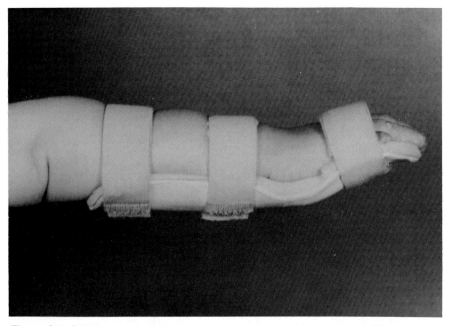

Figure 9.4. Splinting a volar burn with the wrist and fingers extended will help prevent flexion contractures.

and finger contractures will result. Managing an established contracture, (Fig. 9.5) can be very difficult. One might start with serial splinting. As with other contractures, if diagnosed and treated early, the process may be arrested and reversed. For an established contracture, surgical release must be done. Although this is not an atlas and technique is not to be stressed, one must be aware that the surgeon is actually retarding rehabilitation if he does the release incompletely. It is inappropriate to depend on the therapist to finish the surgery as therapy cannot overcome a mature thick scar.

Dorsal hooding, web space contractures, and frank syndactyly can interfere with both dexterity and power. Yet all can be easily prevented by early surgery and splinting. Web space contractures and syndactyly usually result from not grafting burned fingers and allowing them to heal by scarring. Dorsal hooding often results from poor placement of lines of tension of grafts. Suture lines should not go horizontally across web spaces. Padding the spaces with foam and then wearing a glove will apply pressure, retaining their integrity.

The first web space (Fig. 9.6) adduction contracture is particularly debilitating and usually results from lack of early aggressive splinting. In the position of comfort for the patient, the thumb is held in adduction resulting in shortening of skin and soft tissue of the web space as well as the adductor

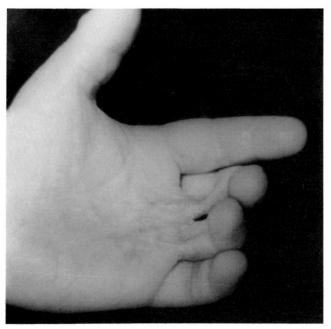

Figure 9.5. A mature contracture that usually will require release by surgery.

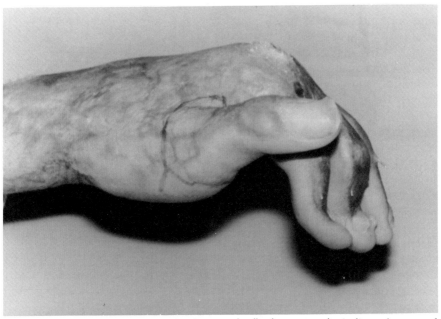

Figure 9.6. A first web space contracture markedly decreases dexterity and power of the hand.

muscle. Early splinting with a C bar (Fig. 9.7A), followed by dynamic traction (Fig. 9.7B) will prevent this problem. Once the contracture has developed, several surgical techniques have been employed for correction. Incision and grafting is usually successful as long as one extends the incision dorsally and volarly for completeness. A particular hazard of cutting through the web anteriorly is the possibility of injuring the digital nerve on the radial aspect of the index finger. A Z plasty is usually inadequate if the flaps themselves consist of scar. Finally, if the adductor is tight, one must partially incise its insertion to allow for complete mobilization.

Tendon complications include disruption and adhesions. Because the dorsal skin is thinner than the volar, and the tendons more superficial, they are more frequently damaged than flexors. In Figure 9.8, the very deep injury has resulted in several tendon complications. The patient is attempting to extend his fingers but the dorsum was badly burned, normal fat replaced with scar and the extensors adherent. No normal extension was possible. The hoods had been destroyed over the proximal interphalangeal (PIP) joint and the lateral bands slipped below the axis of the joint creating a boutonniere deformity. The choices of repair of this type of injury are not as plentiful as in the unburned but traumatized hand. For instance, tenolysis is rarely effective as the extensor is usually encased in scar over great distances, rather than having several discrete adhesions. Attempted extensor tenolysis can result in skin devascularization and subsequent slough. The indications for a flap to restore normal soft tissue are rare because adhesions often extend distally along the course of the fingers. Movement would not occur unless soft tissue was restored to the fingers, followed by tenolysis.

Although multiple operations and splints are available for the boutonniere deformity, many cannot be used in the healed burn hand. For instance, splints are rarely useful because the healed dorsal skin cannot tolerate pressure (without developing ulceration) and all boutonniere splints depend on pressure of some kind. Dorsal dislocation of the PIP joint with severe skin shortening and ulceration makes tendon reconstruction highly unlikely as one is attempting reconstruction through a scar field. In these instances, it is best to shorten the bone ends and do an arthrodesis in 30 degrees of flexion. For the occasional finger in which the dorsal skin is of good quality, a tendon reconstruction such is that proposed by Elliot (3) has been successful in our experience.

The most difficult tendon rehabilitation problem is also the least commonly diagnosed correctly. Intrinsic muscle tightness secondary to ischemia results in limited phalangeal flexion. Early post-burn edema in circumferential injuries, if severe enough, can destroy the blood supply of the intrinsics, severely hampering small muscle function. This problem is easily missed and stiffness attributed to other reasons, but a positive Bunnel test

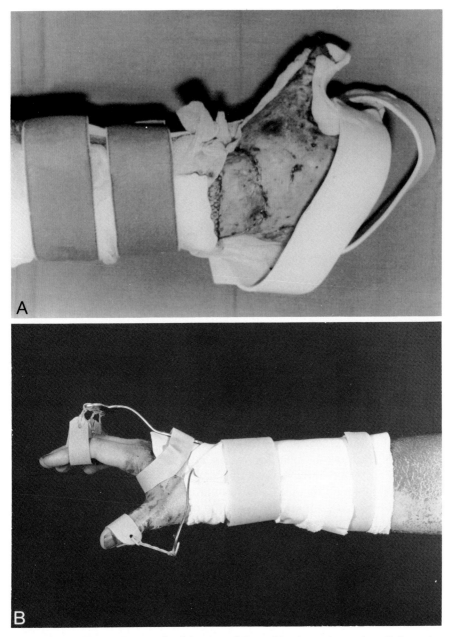

Figure 9.7. A. The early use of a C bar was followed by dynamic traction. B. It retains the integrity of the first web space.

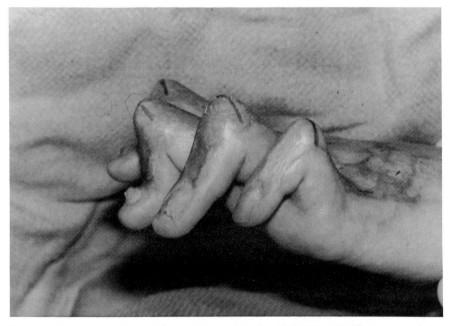

Figure 9.8. A deep dorsal injury was caused by extensor adhesions as well as disruption over the PIP joints.

is diagnostic. Therapy will rarely improve this problem, and a Littler procedure is indicated. It is extremely important for therapist and surgeon to keep this diagnosis in mind whenever examining a stiff hand or one will waste his time, and the other do incorrect surgery.

Joint injuries may be open or closed and affect one or more fingers. Severe dislocation (Fig. 9.9) involving only a little finger (with multiple tissue injury) may be best treated by amputation. The multiple procedures required for rehabilitating a relatively unimportant finger would actually retard rehabilitation when one considers time lost from work or activity.

The most common MP joint problem is shortening (Fig. 9.8) in a neutral or extended position. Flexion of the MP joints is severely retarded and the arch is flattened. This is a totally preventable problem arising usually because the patient has not been splinted correctly or has had no active exercise program. The hand should be splinted nightly with MP joints in 80 degrees of flexion, the interphalangeal joints in 15 degrees of flexion, and the wrist in neutral. If the patient will not or cannot exercise his hand during the day, day splinting will have to be started. Poor MP flexion markedly reduces power grasp or pinch. The reader is referred to the excellent papers by Raymond Curtis (1), discussing the stiff MP and PIP joints. Limitation of flexion of the MP joints may be due to:

(1) skin shortening;

(2) adhesions between extensor and skin;

(3) thickened dorsal capsule;

(4) contracted collateral ligaments in the shortened, neutral, or extended position.

If the patient has 75 degrees of flexion, continued therapy efforts are warranted as future gains are probable. However, if the fingers are fixed in extension or less than 65 degrees of flexion possible, surgery is indicated. This surgery is done through individual dorsal longitudinal incisions. If a single transverse incision was attempted, then as the fingers flexed at operation, a large defect would be created requiring grafting over the exposed joints.

The reasons for limited flexion of the interphalangeal joints are multiple. Hyperflexion often occurs due to destruction of the extensor slip as previously mentioned. Reasons for difficulty flexing include:

(1) scar contraction of the skin over the dorsum;

(2) contracted long extensor;

(3) contracted interosseus;

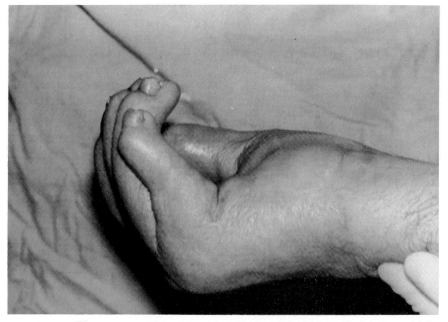

Figure 9.9. Severe dislocation of the little finger with tendon, soft tissue, and joint damage may be best treated by amputation if the rest of the hand is normal.

(4) retinacular ligament adherent to the lateral capsular ligament;

(5) contracted collateral ligaments;

(6) volar capsular ligament adherent to the proximal phalanx;

(7) flexor tendon adherent to the sheath.

The surgeon and the therapist must be aware that in the burned hand multiple causes may be contributing to a decrease in motion and preoperatively the diagnosis is not always apparent. Unfortunately, a common complication of dorsal burns is that more than one set of joints becomes damaged. For example (Fig. 9.8), the MP joints are fixed in neutral and the PIP joints are severely dislocated. To shorten rehabilitation, it is best to reconstruct both sets of joints during the same operative procedure. MP joint capsulectomies combined with PIP fusions will increase motion and stability and hasten recovery.

Open joints are extremely painful and the therapist's attempts stymied to increase range of motion in the rest of the hand. Injudicious activity can also increase the amount of damage. Stabilization and healing should occur before activity is restarted. One can reconstruct by the following techniques:

(1) Move a local or distant flap.

(2) Rongeur the bone to bleeding marrow and pin in a functional position, grafting when granulations form. A pseudoarthrosis results.

(3) Shorten the bone, arthrodese the joint, and close the wound primarily.

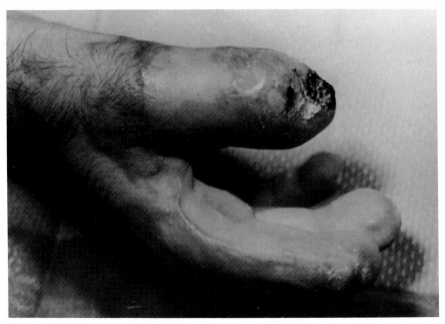

Figure 9.10. Exposed distal phalanx with edema and inflammation of thumb strongly suggests osteomyelitis.

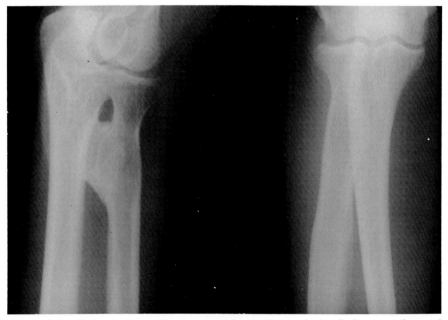

Figure 9.11. Heterotopic ossification involving radius and ulna limits pronation and supination.

Procedures 2 and 3 will give stability and should decrease pain, whereas procedure 1 will only result in a closed wound.

Bony complications can surely prolong rehabilitation if not attended to promptly. An exposed (Fig. 9.10) blackened distal phalanx, edematous thumb that is painful, strongly suggests osteomyelitis. When bone is exposed and has been burned, there may be no surrounding inflammation and x-ray may be read as osteomyelitis when in reality changes are secondary to thermal injury. If the marrow has been destroyed, there may be bacterial contamination, but the underlying process is tissue death secondary to burning, and extirpation of the involved phalanges should be performed. Exposed, viable, but infected bone with surrounding inflammation might best be treated with excision if it was just one phalanx. If more than one was involved, one might consider a trial course of intravenous antibiotics. For wounds with intact skin, osteomyelitis may occur from a previously placed traction wire and a course of intravenous antibiotics should be instituted.

Heterotopic ossification (Fig. 9.11) remains an enigma both in etiology and treatment. It usually affects the elbow region or the distal radius and ulna. The first indication of trouble is a decreased range of motion after the patient has been doing well. No drug or treatment modality has been found to alter its occurrence. Appropriate therapy remains a question mark. Some suggest a nuclear scan of the area to determine the level of osteoblastic activity. If high, surgery should be postponed. Some suggest surgical extirpation of the involved bone and irradiation, but regardless of the treatment there is no guarantee against recurrence.

Loss of part or all of the extremity represents a significant challenge to the patient and whole burn team. Unfortunately, amputation of part or all of the hand is a common occurrence following severe thermal or electrical injury. To hasten rehabilitation, a major question is whether reconstructive surgery or a prosthesis is indicated. A person with an amputation through the metacarpals without a useful thumb metacarpal or through the wrist would do best with a prosthesis. Considering the time involved in multiple surgical procedures, intervals for therapy and treatment of other injuries, more rapid rehabilitation will result with a prosthesis. No prosthesis, however, has sensation and if there is palmar sensory bearing tissue, and something to grasp with, reconstruction is preferable.

The surgeon must:
(1) preserve the palm for stability in grasping;
(2) retain all length of whatever is left;
(3) provide a working cleft between thumb and remaining tissue;
(4) build two poles for pinch and grasp.

To accomplish these goals one might have to resect the metacarpal, deepen the first web space by incision and grafting, or Z plasty, pollicize the index finger, do tendon grafts and transfers, repair or graft digital nerves. For instance, the baby in Figure 9.12 would be best helped by resecting the index metacarpal to widen the first web space and improve grasp.

When reconstruction has not been successful or has been refused by the patient, a partial prosthesis might be helpful. For a partial prosthesis to be successful one must have:
(1) good skin coverage;
(2) sensation of the mobile part of the stump;
(3) at least one movable digit for prehension against a prosthesis;
(4) adequate stump length;
(5) good range of motion of the wrist.

In developing a temporary prosthesis, the patient and the therapist must work together and consideration be given to the patient's age, life style, general physical condition, job, and motivation.

Sometimes rehabilitation following partial or total amputation is limited because of hypersensitivity. A hypersensitive stump can make the patient afraid to use the good portion of the hand. A well-organized therapy program can overcome this problem, through percussion, massage, graded pressure activity, and handling materials of different texture. A graded activity program can often desensitize the area and allow normal activity.

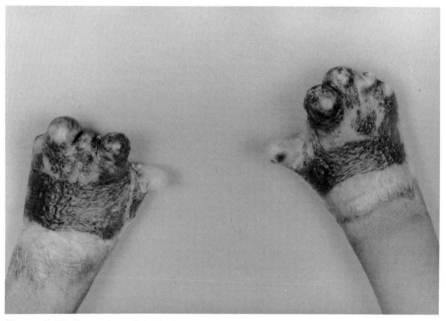

Figure 9.12. Resection of the index metacarpal would widen the first web space and improve grasp.

Although this discussion is primarily about the hand, it would be remiss to forget that it is attached to the rest of the upper extremity. The commonest burn problems are contractures of the axilla and the elbow. If these are identified early, serial splinting may reverse the problem. If not, a K wire through the radius and continuous traction can often straighten the contracture in several days. A splint must be applied immediately to maintain the correction and worn for 6–12 months. It is obvious that maintaining the axilla in an abducted position most of the day will limit functional activity and certain aspects of rehabilitation. To allow the arm to remain in the adducted position, however, will surely result in a severe axillary contracture which will markedly reduce dexterity and power. Likewise, the elbow flexion contracture may well impede pronation and supination. If splinting is unsuccessful, incision and grafting is usually necessary for correction. It is rare to find isolated bands that can be released by local flaps. Surrounding tissue is usually compromised, making flaps risky. The amount of contracted missing tissue is often underestimated (Fig. 9.13A and B) and when the bands are incised, released, and full correction made, the defect is often startling. In releasing severe axillary and elbow contractures it is frequently necessary to incise unburned but contracted tissue. The mature chronic contracture also involves underlying soft tissue, fascia,

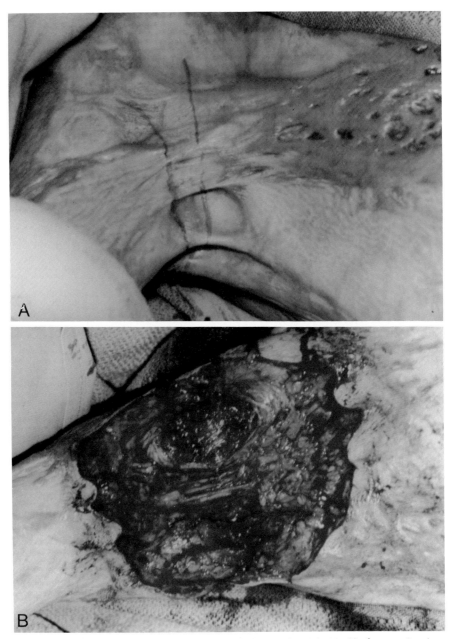

Figure 9.13. A and B. The true tissue deficit is often underestimated before contracture release. A Z-plasty would not have solved this problem.

and muscle that have shortened. Therefore, incision and gradual release by cutting all fibrotic structures is necessary until the desired result is achieved. It is inappropriate, however, to cut the latissimus dorsi or biceps completely and totally lose the function of these muscles and a compromise must be made. One must be very aware of the anatomical changes that are possible with severe contractures and look for an abnormal position of the median nerve and brachial artery at the elbow and even the brachial plexus in the

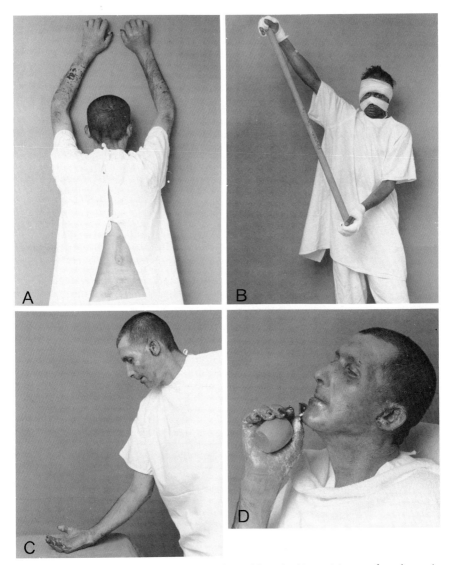

Figure 9.14. A–D. Excellent therapy can be achieved with a minimum of equipment.

axillary release. A true disaster for the patient and rehabilitation team is a brachial plexus traction injury that can occur as a chronically adducted axilla is released, abducted and fully externally rotated.

While other chapters are devoted to physical and occupational therapy, it is important to emphasize that the efforts of these professionals not only help decrease the need for surgery, but improve postoperative results. Enthusiastic therapists in smaller hospitals with less equipment and facilities should be encouraged to greater creativity, not dismayed by their budgets. Much of burned upper extremity therapy can be done with a minimum of equipment if the patient is cooperative. For instance, every hospital has walls and wall climbing exercises (Fig. 9.14A) are superb for stretching the axilla. A simple broom handle (Fig. 9.14B) is an excellent device to force the elbow into neutral. Leaning on a table (Fig. 9.14C) will force the stiff wrist into flexion or extension. Adaptive devices that allow shaving (Fig. 9.14D), eating, and the activities of daily living are often designed by interested patients at no cost. Ingenuity and enthusiasm invariably overcome budget shortages. Getting the patient involved both in active exercise and designing helpful pieces of equipment lifts everyone's spirits.

In summary, there are complications of the burned upper extremity that result from the magnitude of the injury, in spite of our best therapeutic efforts, and other preventable iatrogenic ones. After a logical assessment of the extremity in terms of the involved tissue, one can anticipate and prevent many of these problems. Involving a full rehabilitation team will shorten back to work "lag" time, whether it be in an old or new job. With the input of the entire team, one can determine if the plan should concentrate on attempting to achieve power, dexterity, or both. Perhaps it will be best for the patient to concentrate efforts on correction of deformities of other parts. Although the ability to release a contracture or to restore range of motion measurements is significant, true rehabilitation entails so many considerations such as age, profession, dominance of hand, employment history, and associated diseases that one realizes the hand is merely a small part of a very complicated story, but a very important part.

REFERENCES

1. Curtis RM: Capsulectomy of the interphalangeal joints of the fingers. *J Bone Joint Surg* 36A:1219–1232, 1954.
2. Edstrom L, Robson MC, Macchiaverna JR: Management of deep partial thickness dorsal hand burns. *Orthop Rev* 8:27–33, 1979.
3. Elliot RA: Boutonniere deformity. In: *Symposium on Surgery of the Hand*. St. Louis, C.V. Mosby, 1971, pp. 42–57.
4. Gant T: The use of proteolytic enzymes for burns of the hand. San Antonio, American Burn Association Pres., 1980.
5. May SR: Report of the Subcommittee on Rehabilitation Manpower in Burn Treatment Facilities. Boston, American Burn Association, 1982.
6. Salisbury RE, Wright P: Evaluation of early excision of dorsal burns of the hand. *Plast Reconstr Surg* 69:670–675, 1982.

10

Neuromuscular Considerations

PHALA A. HELM

Introduction

Neurological problems in burn injured patients can be the result of diverse etiologies. Many are preventable. It is important to understand how various neurological deficits occur so precautions can be taken for prevention. Early recognition and intervention for treatment of a deficit can prevent permanent musculoskeletal deformities and additional complications because of impaired function. Careful repeated neurological assessments are necessary even though these patients are difficult to evaluate because of their multiple concurrent problems. Predisposing factors make some patients more susceptible to neurological trauma; the aged are more prone to develop compression neuropathies because their peripheral nerves do not tolerate pressure well and older patients are less mobile (6). Alcoholics and diabetics are also prone to neurological complications because of diseased nerves. Problems commonly seen include peripheral neuropathies, localized stretch or compression neuropathies, intramuscular injection injuries, and electrically induced neurological sequelae.

Peripheral Neuropathy

Peripheral neuropathy is the most common neurological disorder seen in the burned patient. It usually occurs in patients with burns greater than 20% total body surface area. An exception to this is the electrical burn patient who can develop a peripheral neuropathy with a lesser percent burn.

Peripheral nerves may be damaged by a variety of disorders including infections and postinfectious conditions, nutritional deficiencies, metabolic abnormalities, toxic conditions, and drugs. Some neuropathies may cause damage primarily to motor fibers or primarily to sensory fibers while other neuropathies affect both motor and sensory fibers. A symmetrical polyneuropathy with findings manifest in the distal portion of the extremities is seen in both toxic and metabolic neuropathies. Initially, sensory symptoms predominate (2).

The burn patient with a peripheral neuropathy generally presents with symmetrical distal weakness of both upper and lower extremities with or without sensory symptoms. In severe cases, though rare, there may be marked muscle atrophy and weakness, causing "foot drop" and "intrinsic minus" hands. Most conditions improve with time although the patient may complain of lack of endurance and easy fatigability for months or even years after burn. The incidence ranges from 15% determined in a study by Henderson et al. (5) to 29% as determined by Helm et al. (4). The etiology of this condition is uncertain; however, metabolic complications and neurotoxic drugs have been implicated.

Localized Stretch or Compression Neuropathies

In addition to peripheral neuropathy, the patient is subject to localized nerve compression or stretch injury. Unfortunately both a peripheral neuropathy and localized nerve injury can occur simultaneously and cause severe debilitation. Commonly affected nerves are the peroneal, ulnar, and the brachial plexus. Other nerves can be involved but less frequently. The various causes of peripheral nerve injury include improper positioning both in bed and in the operating suite, tourniquet injury, ischemia, and tight bulky dressings.

IMPROPER POSITIONING

Following burn injury, patients are reluctant to change positions because of pain involved with movement. The least painful position is assumed; this is normally a position that keeps the burned tissue on a slack or, in many cases, a flexed posture. A "frog leg" position (Fig. 10.1) (hip flexion, abduction, external rotation; knee flexion; foot plantar flexed and inverted) is often assumed by patients with tender medial thigh and perineal burns, patients who are exceptionally tall, those who keep urinals between their legs because of hand burns, or it is the position of comfort. Prolonged positioning in this manner can cause a stretch injury to the peroneal nerve, resulting in complete paralysis with a foot drop, or varying degrees of weakness of muscles of the anterolateral compartments. The nerve is vulnerable to injury as it courses around the fibular head where it makes contact with the bone over a distance of four to five centimeters. It is covered only by skin and superficial fascia, making it readily compressible and it has limited longitudinal mobility of approximately one-half centimeter, increasing its susceptibility to stretch injury. Another cause of injury to the peroneal nerve because of improper positioning is compression of the nerve at the fibular head as seen in prolonged side lying. Preventive measures are positioning knees in extension, feet in dorsiflexion, and rotating side-lying positions at least every two hours.

A typical position seen in patients with upper extremity burns is with the arms resting on pillows with the elbows flexed and pronated. A similar

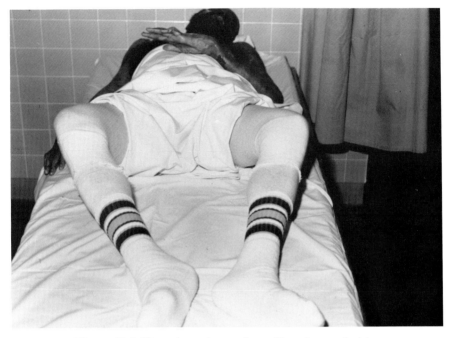

Figure 10.1. The peroneal nerve is positioned on a stretch.

position is seen when the patient is prone. Lengthy static positions of this type can cause injury to the ulnar nerve in the cubital tunnel. According to Wadsworth and Williams (10), the ulnar nerve in the cubital tunnel is at risk of compression when the elbow is flexed at 90 degrees because of internal pressure exerted by the arcuate ligament. The arcuate ligament forms the roof of the tunnel and is slack in elbow extension (Fig. 10.2) but taut with 90 degrees of elbow flexion (Fig. 10.3). He also notes that when the elbow is pronated the cubital tunnel makes contact with a surface whereas with supination the cubital tunnel is lifted from a surface (10) (Fig. 10.4). Thus, the ulnar nerve can receive external compression from lengthy pronated positioning, and receive both internal and external compression with 90 degrees elbow flexion and pronation. Because of the topography of the ulnar nerve in the cubital tunnel, compression of the nerve spares the fibers to the flexor digitorum profundus and flexor carpi ulnaris and damages the sensory fibers to the hand and motor fibers to the intrinsics. Weakness of ulnar intrinsics causes a claw hand deformity. Obviously preventive positioning is recommended.

Another "position of concern" is shoulder positioning supine, prone, and side-lying. Proper positioning of the shoulder is critical to prevent injury to the brachial plexus. A common prone position is with the shoulder in external rotation, abducted to 90 degrees or greater, and the elbows flexed.

ELBOW IN EXTENSION

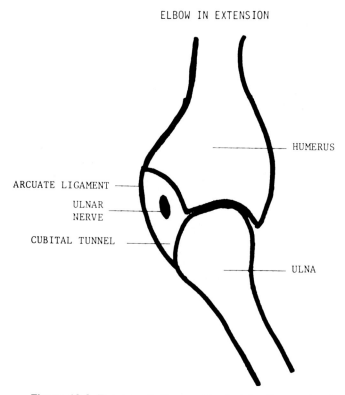

Figure 10.2. The arcuate ligament is slack in elbow extension.

ELBOW IN FLEXION

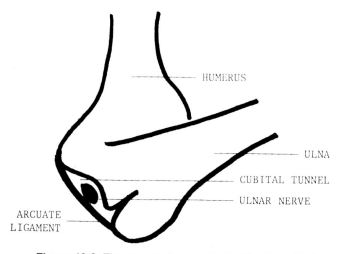

Figure 10.3. The arcuate ligament is taut in elbow flexion.

SUPINATION   PRONATION

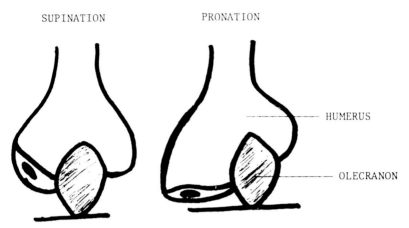

HUMERUS

OLECRANON

Figure 10.4. The cubital tunnel in elbow supination and pronation is shown.

Burn patients frequently must maintain prone positions after grafting for days to weeks, depending on the number of procedures required. Following this type of positioning, weakness of one or both upper extremities may be seen (3).

One possible mechanism of injury, described by Dhuner, is compression of the brachial plexus between the first rib and the clavicle during certain movements of the shoulder (3). When the arm is abducted 90 degrees or more and externally rotated, the clavicle approximates the first rib. Jackson and Keats (7) studied similar positioning of the shoulder in 15 fresh cadavers. They found stretching of the plexus with shoulder abduction, external rotation and posterior shoulder displacement, but minimal or no compression between the clavicle and first rib. They also noted that stretch on the plexus can be alleviated with 15 centimeters of horizontal adduction of the arms. In prone positioning, this can be accomplished with pillows under the chest.

Injury to the plexus can also occur in the lateral decubitus position when the upper arm hangs across the chest and off the bed. In most cases of injury, weakness is primarily of the proximal muscles of the extremity and good return of function is expected.

Awareness of the effects of improper positioning is probably most crucial in the operating suite. The problem is accentuated by the patient's unconsciousness and relaxed muscle tone.

TOURNIQUET INJURY

Compression neuropathies can occur during surgery from prolonged application of an elastic tourniquet to create a bloodless field. With the advent of the pneumatic tourniquet nerve injuries have been less frequent. However, not all surgeons use the pneumatic tourniquet and in spite of its use, nerve injuries can occur. The tourniquet can be harmful in two ways (1): by direct pressure on the structure beneath, as peripheral nerves, and by congestion and ischemic injury to tissues distal to the tourniquet. Pressure of the cuff and tourniquet time can be critical, especially in those with low tolerance as in patients with advanced vascular disease and patients with old scarring and thus, poor blood supply. Pressures of 270–300 mm Hg for adults and 250 mm Hg for children are suggested for one hour's duration with a 10-minute release period before reapplication (1).

TIGHT BULKY DRESSINGS

Another cause of localized nerve injury from direct pressure over the nerve is the application of tight bulky dressings after grafting. The nerve most commonly compressed is the peroneal at the fibular head. A window in the dressing, or a loose dressing in this area, is recommended for prevention.

Intramuscular Injection Injuries

Failure to rotate intramuscular injections can cause muscle and small nerve fiber damage. The damage is due to (1) chemotoxicity of the drug, (2) pressure from the volume injected, (3) physical trauma from the needle, and (4) inflammatory reaction (8). The deltoid is frequently involved and is usually the one on the nonburned side or the side most accessible. Patients complain of pain in the shoulder, and present with deltoid weakness and limitation of shoulder motion. Patients and nursing personnel should be aware of the importance of rotating injections.

Electrically Induced Neurological Sequelae

A variety of neurological complications and sequelae produced by electricity have been reported in the literature; yet there has been little or no progress in determining the pathophysiology of the effect of electricity on the nervous system. A few of the complications reported are temporary paralysis of an extremity, cerebellar dysfunction, paraplegia and quadriplegia, localized nerve damage in areas of tissue injury, and mononeuritis of various nerves. In our experience the most common complications have been central nervous system damage manifest as either paraparesis or quadriparesis with spasticity, peripheral nerve damage close to entrance or exit wounds, and radiculopathies.

Weakness with spasticity can occur within the first one to two weeks after burn or be delayed up to one year; some authors report a delay as long as two years. In some cases the paresis and spasticity have been transient, in some permanent without progression, while others have shown marked improvement with minimal residual deficits. Silversides' review of the pathological changes that occur includes hemorrhage into the grey matter of the spinal cord, wide separation of pia and arachnoid, patchy focal myelin degeneration and chromatolysis in the pyramidal, medullary, Purkinje and anterior horn cells (9).

Peripheral nerve damage can easily occur in the electrically injured by the passage of current through the nerve. The median and ulnar nerves have been noted to be frequently involved. This can result from an entrance wound at the wrist or in close proximity. Depending upon where entrance and exit wounds are, peripheral nerves in the area may be injured. Pathologically, ballooning of the myelin sheath and axon fragmentation may occur in the nerve anywhere along its trunk (9). The nerve injured may be permanently damaged or may recover completely.

Radiculopathies seen in patients with electrotrauma commonly occur in the cervical region. The mechanism of injury is thought to be root compression secondary to the intense tetanic muscular contraction and the opisthotonos position caused by the severe contraction of muscles. The patient is predisposed to radiculopathic problems if he has pre-existing cervical spine pathology.

Summary

Neurological problems in the burn patient are not uncommon, and a significant number of the conditions are preventable. Treatment of patients with deficits should be instituted immediately to prevent further complications and prolonging the rehabilitation phase.

REFERENCES

1. Bruner JM: Safety factors in the use of the pneumatic tourniquet for hemostasis in surgery of the hand. *J Bone Joint Surg* 33A:221–224, 1951
2. Collins WF, Burns RO, Johns TR, et al: Common neuromuscular disorders and injuries to the peripheral and cranial nerves and spinal cord. *Arch Neurol* 36:771–781, 1979.
3. Dhuner KG: Nerve injuries following operations: a survey of cases occurring during a six-year period. *Anesthesiology* 11:289–293, 1950.
4. Helm PA, Johnson ER, Carlton AM: Peripheral neurological problems in the acute burn patient. *Burns* 3:123–125, 1977.
5. Henderson B, Koepke GH, Feller I: Peripheral polyneuropathy among patients with burns. *Arch Phys Med Rehabil* 52:149–151, 1971.
6. Hope T: Pinpointing entrapment neuropathies in the elderly. *Geriatrics* 35:79–89, 1980.
7. Jackson L, Keats AS: Mechanism of brachial plexus palsy following anesthesia. *Anesthesiology* 26:190–194, 1965.
8. Johnson EW, Braddom R, Watson R: Electromyographic abnormalities after intramuscular injections. *Arch Phys Med Rehabil* 52:250–252, 1971.
9. Silversides J: The neurological sequelae of electrical injury. *Can Med Assoc J* 91:195–204, 1964.
10. Wadsworth TG, Williams JR: Cubital tunnel external compression syndrome. *Br Med J* 1:662–666, 1973.

11

Musculoskeletal Considerations

GEORGE VARGHESE

Bone and Joint Changes

Bone and joint changes are by no means rare following burn injury and are reported to occur in about two to five percent of severely burned patients (7, 15).

Structural abnormalities following burn can be categorized as follows (6, 16):

(1) Internal changes in bone: osteoporosis, bone necrosis, bone growth disorders, periosteal new bone formation.
(2) Periarticular changes: Heterotopic ossification, calcific tendinitis.
(3) Joint changes: Septic arthritis, joint dislocation, and ankylosis.
(4) Changes secondary to soft tissue contracture: Scoliosis, kyphosis, joint contractures.
(5) Amputation.
(6) Miscellaneous: Arthritis, shoulder-hand syndrome, pre-existing conditions.

INTERNAL CHANGES IN BONE

Osteoporosis

Shiele et al. (21) reported osteoporosis in 36% of severely burned patients. In addition to prolonged immobilization, other factors may play a role in the development of osteoporosis. Hyperemia which often follows burns may cause decalcification. Increased adrenocortical activity following burns may influence the metabolic shift which subsequently results in bony demineralization (14, 15). Reflex sympathetic dystrophy and contractures can cause localized osteoporosis (8).

Early mobilization of the patient can minimize osteoporotic changes. Active range of motion exercises, tilt table, and ambulation should be started as soon as possible.

Bone Necrosis

Deep thermal injury can occasionally cause necrosis of the periostem and cortex of a superficially located bone, such as the tibia. The skull and olecranon process of the ulna are other common sites (2). Usually bone necrosis results in sequestration of the avascular portion. It is difficult to graft this area because the sequestrum will not accept a graft. Removal of the sequestrum and drilling the bone to stimulate the growth of granulation tissue will provide a surface for subsequent skin grafting (8).

Bone Growth Disorders

Growth disturbances can occur in children following burns. If the burn damages the epiphyseal cartilage, bone growth can be retarded. If damage occurs in a part of the epiphysis, then growth continues in the remainder, resulting in angulation of the bone and joint (12).

Periosteal New Bone Formation

Periosteal new bone formation has been reported especially in the hand, and is usually seen in areas of local inflammation or infection (7, 21).

PERIARTICULAR CHANGES

Heterotopic Ossification

Heterotopic ossification is defined as new bone formation in tissues that normally do not ossify. Such ossification has been reported in burn patients as well as in certain neurological conditions such as spinal cord injury, head injury, and poliomyelitis. In a prospective study of 70 patients with upper extremity burns, Schiele et al. (21) reported the incidence of heterotopic ossification as 23% (16/70). Six of the patients required surgical resection of the bone because of functional limitations. In another prospective study, Munster et al. (18) reported an incidence of heterotopic ossification in burn patients as 13.6%. Both Schiele et al. and Munster et al. reported a high incidence of spontaneous resolution of the bony mass. This might explain why retrospective studies (7–9, 15) reported only two to three percent incidence of heterotopic ossification in severely burned limbs. No definite etiological factors have been established. Superimposed trauma or repeated minor trauma, resulting in local hemorrhage have often been suspected as predisposing factors (13). Overzealous joint manipulation (19), immobilization, local factors as infection, circulatory stasis, and tissue hypoxia may also play a role in the pathomechanism. High protein intake resulting in alteration of calcium transport by the kidneys has also been implicated (5, 10). It is known that heterotopic ossification can occur in severely burned patients even though the burn does not involve the bone or joint. Generally periarticular changes are seen in the area of a deep burn although they have been reported away from the burn site (7, 8, 18, 21). The elbow joint is by far the most common joint involved (Fig. 11.1) followed by shoulder, hip, and knee joints.

The onset of heterotopic ossification may be from 3 to 12 weeks following injury (7, 13, 15). The usual signs and symptoms of heterotopic ossification such as pain, redness, and swelling may not be easily appreciated in burn patients. Pain and loss of motion precede the x-ray changes of new bone formation (18, 19, 21). Sudden loss of range of motion in a previously mobile joint is usually the first warning sign (1, 19). The initial x-ray change is a fluffy-looking bony mass which later becomes a more defined bony mass. Serum calcium and phosphorus are normal (15). Alkaline phosphatase is sometimes elevated. This differs from heterotopic ossification following neurological injury such as spinal cord injury and head injury where there is a signficant elevation of alkaline phosphatase (11). A bone scan can be helpful in making the diagnosis and is usually positive before the x-ray changes.

Spontaneous resolution of the bony mass can occur especially in children (11–13). Management consists of the following:

(1) Active assistance to active range of motion; forceful stretching should be avoided.

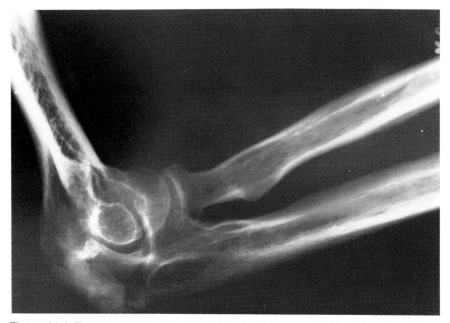

Figure 11.1. The patient had deep second degree burn around the elbow. The patient developed heterotopic ossification in the posterior aspect of elbow resulting in complete loss of range of motion. The patient underwent surgical resection with good results.

(2) Alternate resting splints for maximal flexion and extension.

(3) Surgical excision of heterotopic ossification is controversial. Some of the earliest reports do not recommend excision because of the recurrence of an even worse bony mass (4, 9, 15). Many of the recent reports, however, recommend excision. Several authors have reported significant improvement in joint range of motion following surgical excision (6, 11–13, 17). Surgery should be delayed at least until the skin lesions are completely healed (7, 14). According to some authors, although there is recurrence, it is much less than what it was before excision. Active range of motion and splinting in alternate positions should be carried out after surgical excision (11).

(4) Etidronate disodium may be of value in preventing recurrence of heterotopic ossification. It has been reported useful in preventing heterotopic ossification following spinal cord injuries. Further studies need to be conducted regarding the value of this drug.

Calcific Tendinitis

Evans and Smith (8) have reported calcific tendinitis following burn injury. This can occur in both children and adults and can result in severe pain and limitation of movement. The shoulder joint is a common site. Superimposed trauma could be a factor in the development of tendinitis. Treatment consists of active assistive and active range of motion exercises, combined with deep heating modalities (ultrasound) and anti-inflammatory agents.

Steroid injection may be indicated when other treatment modalities fail.

JOINT CHANGES

Septic Arthritis

Wound infection can cause transient bacteremia or septicemia in burn patients and the subsequent problem of septic arthritis (7). Often it is difficult to diagnose septic arthritis because of burn wound pain and swelling which can mask the signs and symptoms. When the diagnosis is suspected, treatment consists of vigorous antibiotic therapy and splinting of the involved joint in an antideformity position. Septic arthritis can result in not only degenerative arthritis but also joint dislocation and ankylosis.

Joint Dislocation and Ankylosis

An acute dislocation as a part of the original trauma should be reduced without regard to the burn (7, 8). Fracture dislocation can often occur in electrical injuries as a result of a fall or strong muscle contraction during the accident (7, 13). Dislocation can also be provoked by faulty positioning during the acute stage or can be a result of scar tissue contracture. Evans et al. (7) reported an incidence of dislocation as one percent in all hospitalized patients. Destruction of a joint with eventual ankylosis has been reported in children (8). The onset of bone changes may be up to several months following injury. There is progressive destruction of articular surfaces resulting in new bone formation and subsequent ankylosis (8, 21). The most common joints involved are the hips, ankles, and elbows. Arthrodesis can also occur in the small joints of the hand as a result of deep thermal necrosis.

CHANGES SECONDARY TO SOFT TISSUE CONTRACTURES

Scoliosis

Scoliosis can occur in children with asymmetrical trunk burns (7, 17) (Fig. 11.2). Scar tissue contractures can result in scoliosis with the concavity toward the side of the contracture. Knee and hip flexion contractures can cause a leg length discrepancy, later leading to scoliosis. Frequent follow-up visits for scoliosis evaluation are necessary in children with asymmetrical trunk, shoulder, and hip girdle burns. Trunk mobilization should be started early to prevent scoliotic deformities.

Kyphosis

When a burn involves the anterior shoulders, neck, and trunk, a kyphotic posture may develop. Scar tissue can cause a flexion contracture of the neck

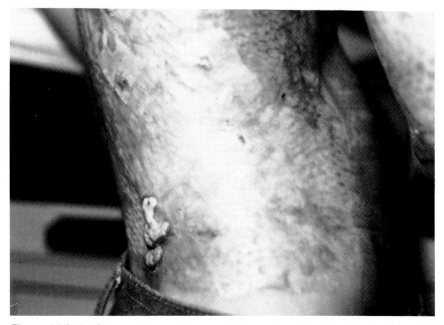

Figure 11.2. A 10-year-old boy with second degree burn involving the trunk on right side is shown. He developed scoliosis with concavity toward the side of scar.

and rounding of the shoulders. The scars from the neck, shoulders, and abdomen often converge along the midsternum and the pull of the scar tissue can cause this kyphotic posture (3, 20). Pressure garments used to minimize the scar are frequently ineffective and may even create additional posture problems. Unfortunately the topography of the anterior chest wall make it difficult to get a proper fitting (3). The uneven surfaces of the anterior chest reduces effectiveness of pressure garments and inserts need to be applied under the garment to assure even pressure. A cervical collar can help prevent the flexion deformity of the neck. Postural exercises emphasizing horizontal abduction and protraction of the shoulders should be carried out. Using a roll between the shoulder blades will be helpful in acute phase positioning. In cases which do not respond to the above procedures, a polyurethene total-contact body jacket has proven successful (3). If conservative treatment is not successful, excision and surgical release of the scar may be indicated.

Joint Contractures

Contractures are the most common sequelae of burn injury and have been discussed extensively elsewhere in the book.

AMPUTATION

Tissue destruction can result in amputation following burn injury particularly following electrical injury. Management of this problem is discussed in another chapter.

MISCELLANEOUS

Arthritis

Osteoarthritis of the hip joint as well as seropositive arthritis have been reported following burn injuries (1, 22)

Shoulder-Hand Syndrome

Burn injuries involving the hands can result in reflex sympathetic dystrophy. The precipitating factor is thought to be excessive sensory stimulation from the burn producing sympathetic overactivity. Patients usually present with a swollen hand, smooth shiny skin, and pain in the shoulder, wrist, and hand. The elbow joint may be pain free, if not burned. Management of reflex sympathetic dystrophy includes active assistive and active range of motion, splinting, and use of anti-inflammatory agents.

Pre-existing conditions

Some patients, especially the elderly, have preinjury osteoarthritic conditions. Immobilization in bed can result in exacerbation of these conditions particularly those with lumbar and cervical problems. Subsequent mobilization can also result in significant increased pain that prolongs the rehabilitation phase. Application of heat and oral analgesics are indicated to help relieve the painful conditions.

Summary

Bone and joint changes are often overlooked in the management of burn patients. Physicians and therapists should be aware of such changes and patients should be frequently evaluated to minimize potential deformities.

REFERENCES

1. Alarcon-Segovia D, Reyes PA: Transient seropositive arthritis after thermal injury. *Lancet* 1:1019, 1972.
2. Asch MJ, Curreri PW, Pruitt BA Jr: Thermal injury involving bone. Report of 32 cases. *J Trauma* 12:135–139, 1972.
3. Becker BE: Hypertrophic burn scarring: Control of chest deformities with a new device. *Arch Phys Med Rehab* 61:187–189, 1980.
4. Boyd BM Jr, Roberts WM, Miller GR: Periarticular ossification following burns. *South Med J* 52:1048–1051, 1959.
5. Dusansky AN, Maylan JA, Linkswiler H, et al: Calciuretic response to protein loading in burn patients. *Burns* 6:198–201, 1979.
6. Evans EB: Orthopedic measures in the treatment of severe burns. *J Bone Joint Surg* 48-A:643–669, 1966.
7. Evans EB, Larson DL, Yates S: Preservation and restoration of joint function in patients with severe burns. *JAMA* 204:91–96, 1968.
8. Evans EB, Smith JR: Bone and joint changes following burns. A roentgenographic study—preliminary report. *J Bone Joint Surg* 41A:785–799, 1959.
9. Griswold ML Jr: Extra-articular bone formation as a burn complication. *Plast Reconstr Surg* 32:544–548, 1963.
10. Heslop JH: Heterotopic periarticular ossification in burns. *Burns* 8:436–438, 1982.
11. Hoffer MM, Brody G, Ferlic F: Excision of heterotopic ossification about elbows in patients with thermal injury. *J Trauma* 18:667–670, 1978.
12. Jackson DM: Destructive burns. Some orthopaedic complications. *Burns* 7:105–122, 1980.
13. Jay MS, Saphyakhajon P, Scott R, et al: Bone and joint changes following burn injury. *Clin Pediatr* 20:734–736, 1981.
14. Kolar J, Babicky A, Bibr B, et al: Systemic effects of burns on bone mineral metabolism. *Acta Chirurg Plast* 13:133–140, 1971.
15. Kolar J, Vrabec R: Periarticular soft tissue changes as a late consequence of burns. *J Bone Joint Surg* 41A:103–111, 1959.
16. Kubacek V, Fait M, Poul J: A case of heterotopic ossification in the hip joint area following skin burn. *Acta Chirurg Plast* 19:209–214, 1977.
17. Mani M: Periarticular ossification: A burn complication. Unpublished personal manuscript, 1982, pp. 1–5.
18. Munster AM, Bruck HM, Johns LA, et al: Heterotopic ossification following burn: A prospective study. *J Trauma* 12:1071–1074, 1972.
19. Pruitt BA Jr: Complications of thermal injury. *Clin Plast Surg* 1:667–691, 1974.
20. Quinby WC Jr: Restrictive effects of thoracic burns in children. *J Trauma* 12:646–655, 1972.
21. Schiele HP, Hubbard RB, Buick HM: Radiographic changes in burns of the upper extremity. *Diagnostic Radiol* 104:13–17, 1972.
22. Taylor K: Hip joint arthritis presenting 20 years after an extensive childhood burn. *Br J Plast Surg* 27:330–331, 1974.

12

Electrical Injuries

JOHN L. HUNT

Introduction

Although acute electrical injuries constitute a small portion of most burn unit admissions, they nonetheless represent one of the most devastating types of thermal injuries encountered by a physician. Their overall incidence ranges between 5 and 10% of patients admitted to hospitals treating thermal injuries and their average total body surface area burn is about 15% (6). This latter percentage is quite deceiving as electrical injuries notoriously involve underlying muscle. Unfortunately, the appearance of the cutaneous injury often gives no indication as to whether underlying muscle is damaged, and if so, to what extent and therefore, an electrical burn is described as an "iceberg"-type injury. Most victims with serious injuries are in the 20- to 30-year age range and are often injuried while on the job, such as high tension linemen or construction workers. Another major population segment suffers electrical injury in nonwork-related activities such as installing of home TV and CB antennae, and recreation-related injuries. These accidents are most often preventable and are caused by carelessness and/or lack of common sense. Electrical injuries cause significant monetary loss in patient income, and represent significant dollar loss for compensation of injuries, medical expenses, rehabilitation costs, and legal claims. Prolonged post-injury physical, occupational, and psychological rehabilitation are often necessary. Of all types of burn injury, the greatest number of amputations occur in patients with electrical burns, and consequently, many individuals are unable to return to their previous occupation, and some, due to their limited education and narrow vocational skills, are unable to return to any type of work.

Pathophysiology

Electrical injuries are no more than a heat-related injury. Tissue temperatures generated at the time of the electrical accident can exceed 4000° C in lightening strike victims. An explanation of electrophysics is essential for understanding both the pathophysiology of the injury and its clinical ramifications. In an electrical circuit, three components are essential for current to flow. These are voltage, amperage, and resistance, and are expressed by the equation, $V = I \times R$, Ohm's law. In most clinical circumstances, the approximate voltage is known but resistance and amperage are unknown. In an experimental acute electrical injury animal model with a known voltage, amperage and resistance can be measured (3). At the onset of the electrical shock, amperage remains low, then rises very rapidly, "peaks," and falls to zero as arcing between the electrical contact and the skin surface occurs (Fig. 12.1). If voltage remains constant and amperage rises, resistance must decrease, otherwise current would not flow. Measurement of tissue temperature reveals it is highest directly underneath and adjacent to the contact site, i.e., entrance and exit wounds. The further away the tissue is from the contact site, the less the current density and, therefore, the less heat generated. Electrical energy is converted to heat energy as expressed by Jule's law: power or heat equals amperage squared times resistance ($P = I^2 \times R$). In all clinical circumstances the higher the voltage, the greater the amperage and, therefore, the greater the amount of heat generated. It is readily apparent that amperage is of greater importance in causing tissue destruction than voltage.

In most electrical accidents, the point(s) where the electrical current enters and leaves the body are easily identified. These skin sites generally represent the deepest areas of cutaneous injury. Initially, the skin acts as a resistant organ and current does not flow well. Because the skin of the palm and sole is very thick and cornified, initial electrical flow is impeded even more than in areas with thinner skin such as on the forearm and calf. Once

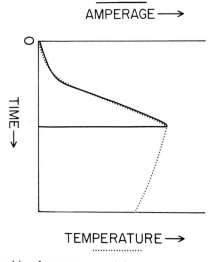

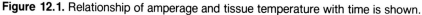

Figure 12.1. Relationship of amperage and tissue temperature with time is shown.

sufficient heat is generated at the skin surface, tissue volitalization and breakdown occur and current breaks through the skin and flows into the deeper regions of the body. Various tissues have different resistance to current flow and in order of increasing resistance, they are: nerve, blood vessel, muscle, skin, lung, tendon, cartilage, and bone. For all practical purposes, although theoretically the various tissue resistances do affect current flow, once skin resistance is overcome, individual tissue resistance with the exception of bone, is unimportant. Because bone has a high resistance, current tends to flow at its surface and, therefore, the temperature is greatest at the periosteum. This is relevant for two reasons. First, muscle damage is often most extensive adjacent to bone. In fact, superficial muscles may grossly appear minimally injured, yet the deeper muscles next to the bone may be nonviable. Second, the periosteum and a portion of the outer cortex may be nonviable. With the exception of small bones such as a phalanx in a finger or toe, through and through irreversible bone damage is unusual. The volume of a finger is so small that dissipation of the heat is minimal and, therefore, tissue damage maximal. Because heat apparently is dissipated by the rapid flow of blood, vascular thrombosis does not occur with the exception of small vessels or in vessels directly under or adjacent to contact sites.

Deep tissue destruction is always greatest in areas of the body with small volume such as a finger, toe, wrist, or ankle. Because of the small volume of a digit, there is often total destruction of tendons, nerves, and bone. In body areas of large volume such as the chest or abdomen, current is diffused so rapidly that very little heat is generated internally. Therefore, it is unusual to have damage to internal organs unless they are directly under a major contact site.

Electrical injuries can be divided arbitrarily into low voltage, no greater than 500–1000 volts, and high voltage, those greater than 1000 volts. Most home accidents involve 60-cycle current and either 110 or 220 volts. These injuries are associated with very little cutaneous and rarely any deep muscle damage. A common low voltage injury occurs when a child bites on an electrical cord and sustains a burn at the commissure of the lips. Low voltage accidents are most apt to be associated with cardiac standstill or rhythm irregularities of a transient nature. High voltage electrical accidents are most often work-related and involve 7600 volts. This is the common voltage carried in high tension lines 15–20 feet above road surfaces in urban areas. Obviously higher voltages, greater than 100,000 volts, can be encountered by persons working for power companies on cross-country lines. High voltage accidents are also associated with a high incidence of cardiorespiratory arrest. Generally speaking, the greater the voltage, the greater the associated amperage and consequently the greater the likelihood of deep muscle damage.

Initial Resuscitation—Scene of Accident

It is imperative that anyone associated with or treating an injured patient must be sure the victim is not still in contact with the electrical source, otherwise the rescuer may become a victim. Under most clinical circumstances, the victim does not remain in contact with the electrical source for more than a few seconds. Cardiorespiratory arrest must be treated by the prompt institution of cardipulmonary resuscitation (CPR). If CPR must be administered to an injured person hanging from a high tension line or a utility pole, five quick breaths by mouth to mouth resuscitation are administered followed by promptly bringing the victim to the ground. It is not unusual for patients to fall from heights such as high tension lines or be thrown against or away from and into some nearby object, thereby potentially sustaining blunt trauma. Because associated trauma may coexist with an electrical injury, the rescue personnel must exercise extreme care when moving and transporting the victim. They must be acutely aware of potential spinal cord injuries and institute appropriate backboard immobilization. At the scene of the accident the patient may be confused or in a dazed mental state and will often be unable to remember the details of the accident. It is imperative that a quick assessment of neurological function be made. All fractures and dislocations must be splinted. If the patient is to be transported from one medical facility to another or if paramedical personnel in the field determine that longer than 20 minutes will elapse between the time of pick up and transportation to a hospital facility, an intravenous line should be inserted through unburned skin.

Emergency Room Care

Assessment of the patient's airway, breathing, and circulation (ABCs) should be carried out. The patient may present in a very clear and lucid state or may be confused, disoriented, combative, and even unconcious. All clothing is removed and a rapid physical assessment to identify any associated injuries such as open and/or bleeding wounds, fractures, and bony dislocations is performed. If an intra-abdominal injury is suspected in an unconscious person, peritoneal lavage is performed. Auscultation of the chest should be performed in all patients. A large-bore intravenous catheter is inserted into a vein and secured in place. Placement of a subclavian line is contraindicated because of the potential iatrogenic complications that might result, the most common being a pneumothorax. The large percentage of unburned skin in these patients affords ample opportunity to identify a suitable vein for cannulation. A urine specimen is obtained. A portwine or blood color is indicative of chromogens, myoglobin, or hemoglobin, and signifies the presence of underlying damaged muscle. A 12-lead electrocardiogram is obtained to assess the presence of myocardial injury and/or cardiac arrhythmia. A nasogastric tube is inserted into the stomach to prevent gastric distension otherwise aspiration of gastric contents might occur and result in bronchopneumonia. A burn diagram utilizing the "Rule of 9s" is made of all cutaneous injuries. If possible, areas of second degree and third degree burn are specifically noted and entrance and exit points are identified. A complete neurological examination is performed and documented in the medical record. This has both prognostic and potential medical legal importance. Notation is made of the presence or absence of arterial pulses in all extremities. Contact wounds about the face, neck, and shoulder may be associated with rapid soft tissue swelling and acute upper airway obstruction. This potential catastrophic event can be anticipated and "prophylactic" intubation, preferably with a nasotracheal tube performed.

Not all patients with acute electrical burns need to be admitted to the hospital, but the following patients should be considered for admission: high voltage accidents, a cutaneous burn of greater than 15% total body surface areas (TBSA), history of loss of consciousness, cardiorespiratory arrest, the presence of an associated injury, cardiac arrhythmia, chromagens in the urine, suspected or obvious deep muscle damage.

Types of Wounds

It is not unusual for some patients who are injured fatally to have no evidence of a cutaneous burn. On the other hand, most patients do have demonstrable entrance and exit sites. Entrance sites are commonly noted about the upper extremities or upper torso while exit sites commonly occur on the lower extremities about the feet and ankles. These wounds are most often third degree, appear dry or charred, and vary in color from gray to black. Because of local tissue volitilization secondary to the extreme heat generated by the passage of the current, the wounds are often contracted, appear concave, and may have a cracked surface. Exit sites are often larger than entrance sites and clinically appear as a "blowout"-type wound because the electrical current collects under the skin and literally bursts through to the surface to exit the body. Not only the skin and subcutaneous fat, but often underlying fascia, muscle, bone, or joint may be destroyed at the contact site. The electrical current may arc between the palm and the wrist between the forearm or arm and axilla. This produces the physical finding of two adjacent or "kissing" wounds with intervening unburned skin. Rings and wrist watches make ideal electrical conductors and are frequent entrance sites.

Some patients may exhibit cutaneous "splatter" marks. These are small partial- or full-thickness punctate skin burns caused by current arching or splattering from the electrical contact point to the skin. Underlying muscle is generally not injured. Minor skin lesions can include petechial hemorrhages and welt marks. Lastly, electrical burns can be a purely cutaneous injury with no underlying muscle damage. In this circumstance, contact sites are not present and, therefore, no current has passed through the person's body. The victim's burn was caused by the clothes igniting.

Resuscitation

As with any thermal injury, early and aggressive fluid resuscitation is mandatory. Extravasation of fluid into areas of cutaneous burn and underlying muscle results in a significant intravascular fluid deficit the first 24 hours after injury. Ringer's lactate is used for the resuscitation fluid. The minimal amount of fluid required in the first 24 hours is based on the percentage of cutaneous burn and body weight (4 cc/kg/% TBSA burn). If underlying muscle is damaged, an indeterminant amount of additional intravenous fluid will be necessary to adequately resuscitate the patient. Unfortunately there is no way to predict this volume of fluid, therefore, the adequacy of volume replacement is determined by closely monitoring the patient's mental status, blood pressure, pulse, and urine output during resuscitation. A urine output of 50–70 cc per hour is sufficient. At the end of the first 24 hours after burn, the serum pH should be normal. Metabolic acidosis signifies hypovolemia with inadequate tissue perfusion and the need for further volume replacement.

Colloid is unnecessary during the first 24 hours of resuscitation. It offers no advantage as a resuscitation fluid over Ringer's lactate and is far more expensive. Unlike a pure cutaneous burn, a significant plasma volume deficit does not occur in an acute electrical injury with a cutaneous injury of less than 15%–20% TBSA. If the accompanying cutaneous injury is greater than 20%, a plasma deficit, which can be hemodynamically significant, occurs regardless of the amount of electrolyte-containing fluid administered (1). The plasma volume deficit at the end of the first 24 hours can be measured either with I^{131} tagged albumin or estimated at one-half cc of colloid/kg/% burn. The plasma deficit is replaced with purefied protein fraction (PPF) or Plasmanate[R] because of its near zero incidence of hepatitis risk. It is given over a two- to four-hour period. Beginning with the second 24 hours after burn only five percent dextrose and water is administered to replace both evaporative losses and maintenance fluid. The serum sodium is maintained between 130–135 mEq/L.

If gross chromagens, myoglobin, or hemoglobin are present in the urine, then the intravenous fluid is administered at a rate sufficient to maintain a urine output of between 100–150 cc per hour until all gross pigment clears. After the urine clears, the intravenous fluid is administered at a rate sufficient to maintain a urine output of 40–50 cc per hour. In order to obtain an initial rapid diuresis, 12.5 grams of mannitol is given intravenously at the onset of resuscitation. By doing this, a urinary diuresis is established earlier than if only intravenous Ringer's lactate is given. In some instances it would require one to four liters of Ringer's lactate to initiate a significant urinary diuresis. In addition, one to two ampules of seven and one-half percent sodium bicarbonate are added to every 1000 cc of Ringer's lactate to alkalinize the urine. This lessens the chances of pigment precipitation in the renal tubules and decreases the risk of acute renal failure. Urine output is monitored hourly and once alkaline urine is established, sodium bicarbonate is given on an as necessary basis in order to maintain continued alkalinization. Significant hyperkalemia occurs secondary to both injured skin and muscle, therefore potassium is not administered during the first 24 hours after injury.

Continuous cardiac monitoring is mandatory for the following patients: those who sustained a cardiorespiratory arrest; those who have or had any cardiac arrhythmias; and if the current passed through the chest. Monitoring is continued for a minimum of 24 hours. In addition a technetium^{99m} stannous pyrophosphate myocardial muscle scan is obtained 24 hours after injury to rule out myocardial damage. Abnormalities of cardiac rate and rhythm are not treated unless the patient becomes hemodynamically unstable, i.e., develops hypotension. Cardiac arrhythmias generally spontaneously revert to normal sinus rhythm within 24–48 hours of injury.

Muscle Injury—Diagnosis and Treatment

It is often very difficult early after injury to say with medical certainty whether or not there is underlying muscle damage. Unfortunately, the physical examination early after injury, with the exception of the cutaneous burn, is often unremarkable. Patients who have sustained high voltage electrical injuries, those with extensive tissue loss at entrance and exit wounds, or if chromagens are in the urine, must be suspected of having underlying muscle damage. Initial absence of palpable pulses or no arterial flow as detected by Doppler ultrasound indicates arterial thrombosis and obvious underlying muscle damage. This characteristically occurs in extremities that are "mummified" (Fig. 12.2). Absence of arterial pulses that were once palpable or decreased arterial flow as detected by the Doppler flow meter indicates increasing subfascial edema. Progressive accumulation of subfascial edema causes muscle compartment pressure to increase, initially it exceeds lymphatic, then venous, and finally arterial pressure and if unrelieved, results in tissue ischemia and necrosis. Numbness and tingling, the earliest clinical symptoms of tissue ischemia, precede loss of pulses or dampened arterial flow as detected by the Doppler flow meter. Unfortunately soft tissue edema, pain or tenderness to palpation may be related to an overlying or adjacent burn and not clinical signs or physical findings indicative of underlying nonviable muscle. Muscle that has a "woody" induration to palpation is generally not viable. Muscle paralysis is a very late sign of ischemia and is usually associated with muscle necrosis.

X-rays of contact sites taken immediately after an injury may either reveal nothing or show air in the soft tissue. The air has entered through

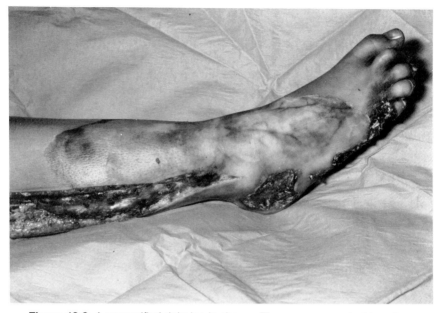

Figure 12.2. A mummified right leg is shown. There were no palpable pulses.

the contact site at the time of injury. Obviously if air is detected in the subcutaneous tissue where none was present on admission, then an anaerobic soft tissue infection must be suspected and immediate surgical exploration undertaken. Finally elevation of the serum enzymes SGOT and SGPT are nonspecific for muscle injury. They are often abnormal in patients with only cutaneous burns.

Fasciotomy plays an important role both diagnostically and therapeutically in electrical injuries (7). Although areas of obviously nonviable muscle may be grossly identified in the early post-injury period, hypotension, vasoconstriction, and low flow to peripheral tissue secondary to hypovolemia often make differentiation between ischemic yet viable and truly nonviable muscle extremely difficult. Therefore, muscle must not be debrided while the patient is undergoing his early resuscitation. Re-evaluation of the gross appearance of the muscle should be done after the patient has been completely resuscitated. Surgical decompression of muscle compartments is mandatory if there is evidence of distal ischemia, i.e., absence or diminished pulses, pain, paralysis, or pallor of distal unburned skin. If a fasciotomy is performed early before the preceding clinical signs and symptoms develop, it would stand to reason that small vessel thrombosis secondary to unrelieved tissue edema could be minimized. This would thereby prevent muscle with marginal blood flow from becoming completely ischemic.

The technique of fasciotomy is as follows: local anesthetic is infiltrated into the skin and underlying soft tissue. An incision can either be made with an electric cautery or cold knife. The electric cautery is preferred because it minimizes blood loss particularly when medial and lateral escharotomies and fasciotomies are performed on more than one limb. The lateral and anterior compartments in the leg must be decompressed because they are located between the long bones (enclosing them in a rigid compartment) and, therefore, are extremely susceptible to ischemia. It is generally not necessary to decompress the posterior and deep compartments. Fasciotomy is often required in an area with overlying unburned skin. This, of course, will leave a permanent scar. In areas with overylying third degree burn, the eschar will slough or require excision and later autografting.

Persistance of gross chromagens in the urine after 12–24 hours of adequate resuscitation portends the presence of a significant volume of nonviable muscle. Although the presence of chromagens does not identify the location nor the amount of muscle, surgical intervention, either débridement and/or amputation, must be undertaken to decrease the likelihood of acute renal failure secondary to the precipitation of pigment in the renal tubules. Debulking of all necrotic muscle in a patient with gross chromagens in the urine very often results in clearing of the pigment 20–30 minutes after the surgery.

Other diagnostic studies that have been recommended to identify nonviable muscle include arteriography (5), xenon[133] wash-out of soft tissue (2), and intraoperative use of frozen sections (8). Arteriograms are not of adequate technical quality to identify any but the largest vessels that are thrombosed. The small intramuscular vessels are generally thrombosed and unfortunately are too small to be easily identified. The xenon[133] technique involves sophisticated technical equipment which is not readily available in most hospitals. If muscle biopsies are performed within 48–72 hours of injury, muscle viability as determined by frozen or permanent tissue sections is difficult to identify histologically by the pathologist. When histological assessment is utilized after the third or fourth post-injury day, diagnostic accuracy is better, but the procedure is time consuming and because of the mixed nature of muscle injury in electrical burns, multiple sections are required. This is not practical when large surface areas of muscle need to be debrided.

A new diagnostic test utilizing the radionucleide technetium[99m] stannous pyrophosphate has proven to be very useful in identifying irreversibly injured muscle (4). This same radionuclide scan has been used to diagnose early myocardial ischemia and infarction. The radioactive isotope is given intravenously. After several hours, during which bone and soft tissue background clearance has occurrred, a scan is performed over areas of suspected muscle damage. Where possible, opposite uninjured areas are scanned for comparison. The radioactive agent can only be taken up in an area of injured tissue that has blood flow, therefore two types of injury patterns are noted on the scans. First, the presence of a "hot spot" is indicative of irreverisbly injured muscle. Second, if there is no blood flow to an area of muscle, then the scan will show no radioactive uptake and consequently, a "cold area" will be noted (Fig. 12.3A and B). The test is so sensitive that scan positive areas, indicative of irreversibly injured muscle, may grossly appear normal. Cold areas on the technetium scan grossly appear nonviable—pale, bloodless, and do not contract to electrical stimulation. Hot areas, on the other hand, show varying degrees of contraction with electrical stimulation, bleed when cut, and are pink to red in color. It only takes several minutes to scan each suspected area. The test can be performed serially to evaluate the completeness of surgical débridement. The test is rapid, noninvasive, and identifies not only the location but the extent of injured muscle thereby aiding the surgeon in planning the operative procedure.

Wound Treatment—Topical Antimicrobial Agents

The topical antimicrobial agent of choice or an electrical injury is mafenide acetate (Sulfamylon[R]). It diffuses through the entire thickness of the eschar, the subcutaneous tissue, and muscle while retaining its antimicrobial potency. This topical agent is particularly effective against both *Pseudomonas aeruginosa*, a common microorganism infecting burns, and anaerobic organisms of the Clostridia species. The latter microbes represent a potential lethal infection so long as nonviable muscle is present. The burn cream

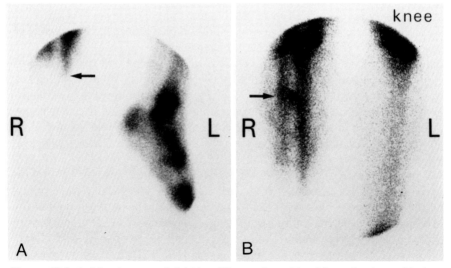

Figure 12.3. A. Muscle scan of right leg (R) reveals no blood flow distal to ankle (see arrow). Left (L) foot is normal. B. Increased uptake in entire right calf. Note very dense area of uptake at *tip of arrow*. Left calf has normal background activity.

is applied every 8–12 hours. Complications arising from this drug include bicarbonate loss in the urine because of the carbonic anhydrase effect of the drug. Pain is also a problem especially when applied to partial-thickness burns because of its hydroscopic nature and acid pH. In small cutaneous burns such as associated with most electrical injuries, the bicarbonate loss causes either no or only very mild metabolic acidosis. The larger the burn, the greater the bicarbonate loss and, therefore, the greater the increase in respiratory rate necessary to maintain a normal serum pH. This physiological response (hyperventilation) has little clinical significance unless the patient has bronchopneumonia or some other type of pulmonary pathology which would preclude the respiratory system from effectively compensating for the metabolic acidosis.

If there is only a cutaneous burn, silver sulfadiazine can be used. This agent has a broad antimicrobial spectrum. Complications associated with this agent are minor and include skin rashes, as with any sulfa drug, and although the cause and effect are not known, a questionable depression of the white blood count. This most often occurs in large burns at 24–48 hours after injury.

Systemic Antibiotics

If underlying deep muscle damage is present or even suspected, an intravenous antibiotic effective against both anaerobic and aerobic organisms is recommended. The antibiotic is administered until the majority of nonviable muscle is debrided. With only a cutaneous burn and no underlying muscle damage, there is no clinical evidence in the literature to substantiate the efficacy of prophylactic antibiotics in the early post-burn period. It must be emphasized that the primary goal in treating electrical injuries is the early débridement of all nonviable tissue—skin and muscle. Antibiotics are of secondary importance and only represent adjunctive therapy.

Early Surgical Excision

Infection continues to be the leading cause of morbidity and mortality in thermally injured patients. The two common organ systems involved are the burn wound (burn wound sepsis) and lungs (bronchopneumonia). Of course, in electrical injuries necrotic muscle represents an additional site for potential infection. Under most circumstances immediate, less than 24 hours after injury, surgical intervention to debride or amputate nonviable muscle is unnecessary. It is paramount that the patient be adequately resuscitated and hemodynamically stable prior to any type of surgical intervention. The greatest threat to the patient's life in the first 24–48 hours is not infection, but hypovolemic shock secondary to inadequate resuscitation. Surgical débridement of nonviable skin and muscle can be carried out safely by the third post-burn day. A positive preoperative muscle scan enables the surgeon to tell the pateint and his family where the damaged muscle is located and whether débridement and/or amputation is necessary. If the muscle scan is normal, surgical exploration of muscle is unnecessary and attention only need be directed at the cutaneous injury.

If an emergent amputation of an extremity is deemed necessary because of massive muscle injury, guillotine amputation or disarticulation of the limb is recommended. The skin and fascia are left open and not sutured closed because the amputation site needs to be inspected 48 hours later to evaluate the viability of the muscle. If complete débridement can be performed at that time, the wound is closed.

A "medical" amputation, performed by applying a tourniquet at the upper level of grossly nonviable muscle and then wrapping the extremity in ice until surgery can be performed, is not recommended. In a leg with a mummified foot and ankle, characterized by charring of the skin and muscle and no palpable pedal blood flow, there is often no clear-cut gross proximal muscle margin between viable and nonviable tissue because of the uneven distribution of the muscle injury. Unfortunately, indiscriminate application of a tourniquet can cause more ischemia to ischemic yet viable muscle. In fact if a medical amputation is performed on an extremity that has palpable or Doppler pulses, even though there is obvious nonviable muscle, viable muscle may be sacrificed. Consequently, limb length may be unnecessarily shortened.

Under nonemergent clinical circumstances it is generally impossible to excise all cutaneous burn and debride or debulk the majority of nonviable muscle at the first operative procedure. A two team approach is used to decrease operative time if more than one limb requires extensive débridement. Tangential excision of deep dermal burn is performed with either a Humby knife or Weck dermatome; the electric cautery is utilized to excise all third degree cutaneous burn. Nonviable muscle is excised with a cold knife and bleeding controlled by ligature or electrocautery.

At surgery it is often difficult to differentiate with the naked eye ischemic yet viable muscle from irreversibly injured muscle. This is made more difficult because viable muscle may be intermixed with nonviable muscle. This injury pattern becomes more pronounced the more distant the muscle is from the contact site. This diffuse or uneven distribution of muscle injury is well documented with the pyrophosphate muscle scan. In fact, the scan is so sensitive that areas of scan positive muscle may grossly appear viable yet histological evaluation of a biopsy in that area clearly identifies a mixture of viable and nonviable muscle. Assessing muscle viability by contractility with electrical cautery gives the surgeon a gross indication of viability but contractility may vary greatly from one area to another depending on the amount of viable muscle. Contractility is directly proportional to the amount of viable muscle.

Where there is complete necrosis of muscle, there is no bleeding, but where there is a mixture of viable and nonviable muscle, there are enough patent intramuscular vessels to produce bleeding, consequently during débridement, tissue becomes stained with blood and it becomes difficult to equate viability solely by the color of the muscle. Multiple operative procedures, ranging from one to ten, are often required to completely excise all nonviable muscle. If there is ever any question regarding viability of muscle, the muscle is not debrided but rather a "wait and see" attitude is taken. It is best to return the patient to the operating room at two- to three-day intervals and grossly reassess viability. Conservatism is the rule regarding surgical débridement particularly in areas over or adjacent to vital structures such as nerves, blood vessels, and tendons. This is particularly true about the hand, wrist, ankle, knee, face, and neck.

It is often very difficult to assess viability of tendons and nerves. Therefore, unless the threat of local wound sepsis demands immediate débridement, a conservative surgical approach is followed. It must be emphasized that once tendons and nerves are exposed, unless they are covered with autograft or some type of physiological dressing, homograft or heterograft, they desiccate, become secondarily infected, and ultimately necrose. All wound surfaces created when excising either the cutaneous burn or debriding muscle must be covered. Although immediate autografting is the procedure of choice, both the additional intraoperative time and extra blood loss necessary to procure skin, or reservation on the part of the surgeon as to the completeness of débridement, may necessitate temporary wound coverage with either homograft or heterograft.

Autograft is meshed at a ratio of one and one-half to one to allow the escape of blood and serum from under the skin thereby preventing subgraft accumulation and possible graft loss. Mesh graft conforms better than sheet to the uneven wound surfaces created after electrical burns are debrided.

To preserve viability of neurovascular bundles or tendons local pedicle flaps are recommended for wound coverage. Pedical flaps are also ideal for covering exposed bone. Anatomical areas ideally suited for flap coverage include the wrist, ankle, foot, knee, and neck.

Complications of Electrical Burns

WOUND

Bacterial control of the burn wound is paramount to prevent wound sepsis. It is very important to monitor the bacterial growth on both partial- and full-thickness burns. Contact plate cultures on partial and quantitative wound biopsies on full-thickness burns are obtained three times weekly as long as intact eschar is present. It is not unusual for moderate to heavy wound colonization on contact plate culture or quantitative counts of 10^3

organisms per gram of tissue to precede the early clinical signs of sepsis—hyperpyrexia, altered sensorium, ileus, or hyperventilation. Obviously a quantitative count must be interpreted in light of the TBSA burn. A quantitative count of 10^6 organisms per gram of tissue on a 10% burn does not represent as great a bacterial inoculum as 10^3 organisms on a 60% burn. During the 48-hour interval between biopsy and culture report bacterial growth obviously continues and an increase in the number of organisms by as much as two to three logs per gram of tissue commonly occurs. These bacteriological findings generally still precede the common overt clinical signs characteristic of sepsis—hypotension, oliguria, bactermia, etc.

Cellulitis adjacent to either a partial- or full-thickness burn is not an infrequent burn wound infection. It is characterized by spreading erythema, tenderness, and swelling. It commonly occurs between the third and fifth post-injury day and wound cultures may be sterile. Cellulitis may represent either only a superficial wound infection or the cutaneous manifestation of underlying infected muscle. A broad spectrum antimicrobial agent administered for five to seven days is generally sufficient to treat burn wound cellulitis, but if either underlying necrotic muscle is thought to be present or the infection does not begin to resolve after 48 hours, immediate wound exploration must be carried out.

SPONTANEOUS HEMORRHAGE

Immediate coagulation necrosis of blood vessels occurs in areas about contact sites. Spontaneous separation of the eschar coupled with local wound sepsis leads to dissolution of the clot and spontaneous bleeding, often in massive amounts, from open ended vessels. The hemorrhage commonly occurs between the sixth and tenth post-burn day. It is best controlled by direct local pressure, followed by careful identification of the bleeding point, and suture ligation. With the institution of early muscle débridement and eschar excision, this complication is now rare.

BONE AND JOINTS

Bone is often exposed at the entrance or exit site or after surgical débridement. Exposed viable periosteum must be covered; otherwise it desiccates and ultimately necroses. The simplest procedure is to cover the bone with autograft; unfortunately this is not ideal because the skin is easily traumatized and prone to breakdown. When possible, a local pedicle flap including skin and subcutaneous tissue or a myocutaneous flap offers ideal coverage. If the periosteum is nonviable, several therapeutic options are available. The bony cortex is dermabraded until bleeding identifies the exact level of cortical viability. If only a few millimeters deep, the necrotic cortex is removed and if anatomically feasible, a pedicle flap is used to cover the area. When either a deficiency of surrounding soft tissue or adjacent burned skin precludes coverage with a flap, a conservative approach is undertaken.

Granulation tissue is allowed to cover the area and then autografting can ultimately be carried out. If it is determined that the entire thickness of the bony cortex is nonviable, dermabrading is not practical particularly in small bones such as the phalanx because an iatrogenic fracture may result. Therefore multiple holes are drilled into the marrow cavity to allow granulation tissue to grow out and cover the surface. This may take from four weeks to two and one-half months. The length of time required to eventually bring about wound closure using the latter technique increases wound morbidity—pain, local soft tissue sepsis, osteomyelitis, and bony sequestrum. Wound closure by any means other than a flap is less than an ideal form of therapy.

Nonviable joint capsule often represents a significant therapeutic dilemma. Débridement of nonviable tissue is mandatory in order to prevent local wound sepsis, but in doing so the joint space may be opened. This enhances the risk of septic arthritis. When possible after all nonviable ligamentous and capsular tissue is excised, the joint is immediately covered with a skin flap. If this is not possible, a conservative approach that includes appropriate splinting to immobilize the joint and wound coverage with a moist dressing to prevent tissue desiccation is followed. Once granulation tissue has formed, the wound is autografted or covered by a pedicle flap.

AMPUTATIONS

The greatest number of amputations in burn patients occur in those with electrical injuries (Tables 12.1 and 12.2). The reader is referred to Chapter 13 entitled Amputations and Prosthetic Fittings for a more detailed discus-

Table 12.1.
Number of Amputations

	35 Patients			
	Single	Double	Triple	Quadruple
Patients	25	9	0	1

Table 12.2.
Site of Amputations

Location	No. of Patients
Shoulder disarticulation	2
Above elbow	8
Below elbow	2
Finger(s)	9
Above knee	5
Below knee	6
Foot	3
Toe(s)	8

sion of this problem. Two troublesome complications associated with amputations include the formation of peripheral neuromas and bony spurs at the amputation site. The former can result in a painful localized swelling that creates a significant prosthetic problem. A painful stump interferes with the comfortable wearing of a prosthesis. Careful identification of all nerves and meticulous surgical technique are paramount to minimize the formation of neuromas when working with nervous tissues during amputations. Bony spur formation at the amputation site is an unpredictable complication. Spurs can occur as early as four to six months after amputation and are characterized by pain and tenderness associated with hard masses in the subcutaneous tissue. Bony spurs form at the tip and edges of the amputated bone. Soft tissue x-rays should be obtained in any patient that has persistent pain about the amputation site. Surgical excision of spurs may be necessary to ensure a pain-free stump.

Neurological Complications

ACUTE

It is paramount that a complete neurological examination be performed on admission and weekly thereafter. Neurological deficits that are present on admission, particularly those that involve nerves adjacent to or directly under contact sites, most often result in permanent deficits. Nervous tissue is never debrided unless obviously necrotic. Every attempt is made either to autograft or cover the nerve with a pedicle flap in the hope that some neurological function will eventually return.

Contact points about the head and neck are commonly associated with cerebral symptoms. A variety of complications including depression, memory loss, blunted affect, transient and/or permanent motor paralysis, and brain stem syndromes have been reported. There is no way to predict if, what type of, or when a neurological deficit will appear and even worse to what degree it will improve. Therefore, the patient and his family must be made aware of this problem. Current that passes from one arm to another arm or from one arm to a leg, or patients that have entrance and exit points around the spine may potentially develop spinal cord syndromes. These include spastic paraplegias, bladder and bowel dysfunction, motor, sensory, and sympathetic nerve involvement. In addition, peripheral nerve syndromes can include radiculopathies and neuropathies.

CHRONIC

The appearance of any new neurological deficits generally occurs within two years of injury. Serial neurological examinations should be performed every four to six months for the first two years after injury. Both the patient and his or her family should be told of the possibility that new neurologic sequelae might occur after discharge. Cerebral symptoms may include chronic memory loss, mental depression, and personality changes. Paralysis and spastic paraplegia or quadriplegia can occur. Peripheral neuropathies are troublesome complications and may result from either direct damage to a nerve, compression of the nerve by scar tissue, or worse yet may occur in patients who had no physical evidence of direct nerve damage. Patients who had current pass through the legs often complain of weakness manifest by inability to stand on the feet for long periods of time and a general lack of stamina. It is worthwhile to evaluate nerve conduction and motor unit potentials in these symptomatic patients to rule out organic lesions causing the patient's symptoms. Very often subtle peripheral neuropathies are identified with these studies.

OCULAR

Electrical contact points about the head and neck and the shoulder girdle are not uncommonly associated with the development of cataracts. Cataracts can be evident as early as one month and as late as three years after injury. Serial ophthalmological examinations should be performed at six-month intervals for a period of two to three years after an injury.

PSYCHOLOGICAL

A variety of psychological aberrations may occur in patients suffering from electrical injuries. Some of these may have an organic basis secondary to the injury and every attempt must be made to document if that is the case. If no organic cause can be identified, the psychological evaluation and support is mandatory. It is imperative that this be obtained early during hospitalization, continued through the entire hospital course, and after discharge.

Summary

In summary, a better undersanding of the pathophysiology of the injury, coupled with early and aggressive fluid resuscitation has virtually eliminated acute renal failure. Improved diagnostic techniques to identify underlying muscle damage plus early surgical excision of the burn and necrotic muscle has markedly decreased the incidence of burn wound sepsis. The temporary use of physiological dressings such as homograft and heterograft have improved the salvage of neurovascular tissue and tendons which in the past would have been debrided. The early creation of pedicle flaps has allowed for salvage of limbs which might otherwise have been amputated. The acute hospitalization represents the shortest portion of the patient's injury time. After discharge, extensive occupational and physical therapy and psychological support are often necessary. Careful attention to the "entire" patient is mandatory by all parties involved in patient care if maximal rehabilitation is to be accomplished.

REFERENCES

1. Baxter CR: Present concepts in the management of major electrical injury. *Surg Clin North Am* 50:1401–1418, 1970.
2. Clayton JM, et al: Xenon-133 determination of muscle blood flow in electrical injury. *J Trauma* 17:293–298, 1977
3. Hunt JL, et al: The pathophysiology of acute electrical injuries. *J Trauma* 16:335–340, 1976.
4. Hunt JL, Lewis S, Parkey R, et al: The use of technetium[99m] stannous pyrophosphate scintigraphy to identify muscle damage in acute electric burns. *J Trauma* 19:409–413, 1979.
5. Hunt JL, McManus WF, Haney WP, et al: Vascular lesions in acute electric injuries. *J Trauma* 14:461–473, 1974.
6. Hunt JL, Sato RM, Baxter CR: Acute electric burns, current diagnostic and therapeutic approaches to management. *Arch Surg* 115:434–438, 1980.
7. Mann RJ, Wallquist JM: Early decompression fasciotomy in the treatment of high-voltage electrical burns of the extremities. *South Med J* 68:1103–1108, 1975.
8. Quinby WC Jr, et al: The use of microscopy as a guide to primary excision of high-tension electrical burns. *J Trauma* 18:423–431, 1978.

13

Amputations and Prosthetic Fitting

ROBERT H. MEIER, III

The tissue insult from a flame or electrical burn is occasionally of such magnitude that tissue viability is lost, necessitating extremity amputation. This occurs more frequently in high voltage electrical burns where bone and neurovascular damage is added to the loss of skin and subcutaneous tissue. While flame burns often involve a specific extremity or body area, electrical burns often involve two or more extremities in addition to the intervening body segments (Fig. 13.1A). Usually, the most severely damaged areas are the points of entry and exit where extremity viability is frequently lost. Even if the extremity can be salvaged, there often remains significant neuromusculoskeletal injury with resulting disability.

The patient with such severe burns that require amputation often has other extremity problems which complicate the rehabilitation process. These additional complications differ in flame and high voltage electrical burns. In flame burns, the usual complicating problems, in addition to amputation, involve the skin and underlying soft tissue. Burned skin will result in scar which may be problematic if this area comes into contact with the prosthetic socket. If there is little soft tissue padding and scar overlying the bone, the integument will poorly withstand the shear and loading forces of the prosthetic socket. Frequently, this combination of factors results in skin breakdown (Fig. 13.1B and C).

In patients with amputation secondary to high voltage electrical burn, the same problems are seen as those discussed above in flame burn patients. However, several other post-electrical burn complications should be assessed. Heterotopic ossification of proximal joints, amputation site bone overgrowth, myelopathy, neuropathy, and cataract formation can produce significant prosthetic function limitations.

The type of amputation performed by the surgeon is extremely important in allowing the best prosthetic function. Most surgeons involved during the acute burn period will be conservative and attempt to debride while salvag-

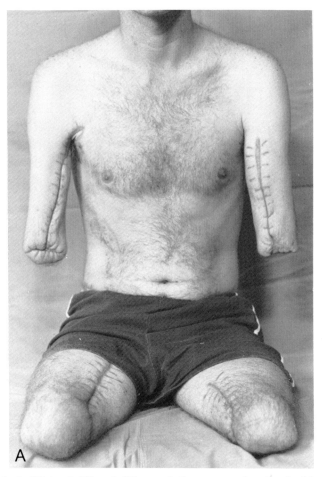

Figure 13.1. A. Bilateral AE and AK amputations secondary to electrical burns. B. Anterior view of BK amputation with split-thickness mesh graft over infrapatellar area. C. Posterior view of same leg with soft tissue loss and graft over medial and lateral areas at the knee.

ing all possible bone length. This is important since tissue viability may not be well demarcated initially. However, definitive amputation should be planned only after discussion with a health professional who understands current prosthetic fitting and function.

An amputated limb which can function well in a prosthesis has the following characteristics (Fig. 13.2):

(1) pain free;
(2) well padded by soft tissue;
(3) full-thickness skin;

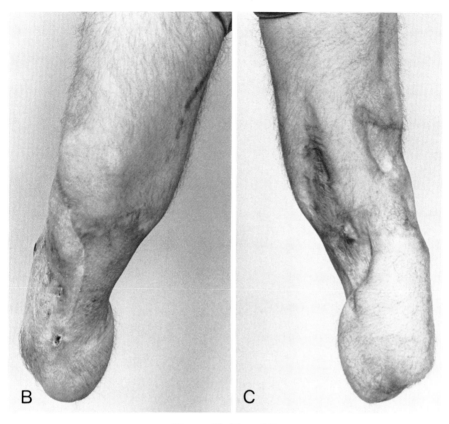

Figure 13.1B and C

(4) nonadherent scar;
(5) cylindrical shape;
(6) greatest bone length to produce prosthetic movement;
(7) normal sensation.

As can be readily observed, the limbs amputated secondary to burns seldom meet all of these ideals; often, a less than ideal stump results.

In addition, there are also several amputation levels which make these characteristics difficult to obtain and special attention regarding selection of these levels should be addressed:

(1) hindfoot—between transmetatarsal and Syme's;
(2) below-knee (BK) longer than tapering of gastrocsoleus muscle bellies may create problems especially if normal full-thickness skin is not present. There is an adequate lever arm to maneuver the prosthesis without this extra length.
(3) knee disarticulation without full-thickness skin;

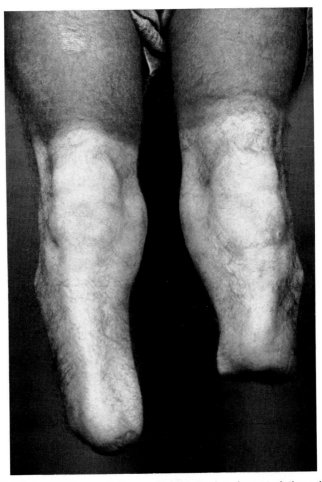

Figure 13.2. Bilateral BK amputations which meet the characteristics which should permit good prosthetic function.

(4) above-knee (AK) without good muscle bulk and nonadherent scar;
(5) partial hand without sensation and useful range of motion;
(6) wrist disarticulation with prominent condyles and adherent scar;
(7) below-elbow (BE) without soft tissue coverage and with adherent scar;
(8) elbow disarticulation with condyles covered with adherent scar or split-thickness skin graft;
(9) long above-elbow (AE) without room for internal locking elbow unit.

Specific prosthetic issues relating to these problematic levels will be discussed under the prosthetic prescription section.

For this chapter, the prosthetic rehabilitation program will be divided into the following phases:

(1) acute postsurgical;
(2) preprosthetic;
(3) prosthetic prescription and fabrication;
(4) prosthetic checkout and training;
(5) functional follow-up.

These are artificial divisions and in practice these phases often overlap. Therapeutic practices do, however, change from phase to phase and what is appropriate at one phase may not be for another. Each of these phases is best approached in terms of short- and/or long-term goals. These goals will precede the discussion of each phase of the rehabilitation program. They are not meant to be an exhaustive list but should provide guidelines from which a realistic and functional program can be designed.

Phase 1: Acute Postsurgical Phase

Time: Amputation surgery to suture removal.
Goals: (1) promote wound healing;
      (2) control incisional and phantom pain;
      (3) mantain joint range of motion;
      (4) promote positive nitrogen balance;
      (5) mobilize entire body;
      (6) explore patient's and family's feelings about change in body;
      (7) obtain adequate financial sponsorship for prosthesis and training.

In the burn patient, this is usually a phase fraught with multiple surgeries and painful procedures necessary to salvage life and as much limb as possible. Debridement, grafting, tanking, dressing changes, and staged amputations cause repeated insult and pain. The patient has little control of these treatment processes and must depend on the local health system to provide the best care possible.

Once the amputation has been closed with adequate soft tissue covering, the focus is primary wound healing. Often, in the burn patient, however, there are surface burns adjacent to the amputation incision. These need to be covered as quickly as possible, usually with a split-thickness graft.

Incisional pain should be controlled with adequate amounts of narcotic or synthetic narcotic agents, preferably given intravenously on a regularly prescribed basis rather than on an as warranted patient request. This is usually helpful for the first three postoperative days. Subsequently, oral analgesics should be adequate if there are no other sources of significant pain. Transcutaneous electrical nerve stimulation (T.E.N.S.) has been used with some success in order to decrease amputation incisional and phantom pain. T.E.N.S. should be tried as an adjunct to other traditional means of analgesia.

Phantom limb and phantom pain should be explained to the patient before they occur since they can occur in the early postoperative period. Phantom pain should be differentiated from incisional pain. The patient should expect the phantom limb and phantom pain sensations to change and usually diminish; they are seldom a long-term problem. Use of oral pain medications for significant phantom pain has not usually produced adequate pain reduction over a period of time exceeding one week. Addiction to analgesics is a significant possibility in problematic phantom pain. In lieu of long-term analgesic medications, some recent success has been achieved using Elavil at doses of 75–150 mg daily at bedtime. This drug is involved in serotonin production and is believed to modify pain perception. Elavil is used in this situation for pain relief rather than for its antidepressive effects.

On the first or second postoperative day, a specific exercise program which has been explained to the patient and which is supervised by a therapist should be started. The program should emphasize active or active assistive motion of the joints proximal to the amputation. This exercise should not produce more than mild discomfort. Isometric exercises of the transected muscles, at this time, only cause the patient pain and put stress on the suture line.

Gentle isometric contractions can be started at the fifth postoperative day and isotonic contractions can be encouraged at 7–10 days postoperatively. These exercises appear to help a patient maintain the kinesthetic sense of residual and phantom limb motions which can later be used in prosthetic training.

Active motion of all proximal joints through the full range of motion should be obtained by 10–14 days following amputation unless grafting procedures preclude exercising. Programs of muscle contraction and joint movement should be repeated several times daily and, once adequately performed, need no supervision.

In the upper extremity amputee, several important functional concerns should be remembered. Any limitation of the motion at the shoulder or elbow may significantly limit the functional placement of the hand or prosthetic terminal device (T.D.). Also, upper extremity prosthetic activation depends on scapular and glenohumeral movement; therefore, the muscles which produce these motions need to be strengthened and scapulohumeral mobility maintained. Full flexion and extension at the elbow, together with maximum pronation and supination of the residual forearm, provide the best T.D. function. Burns involving the axilla and elbow create a special problem for potential scar contracture across the joint (Fig. 13.3) or for the formation of heterotopic ossification. Both of these burn complications can

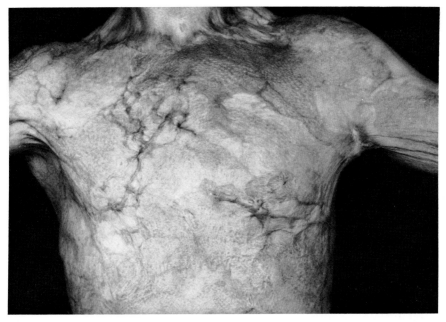

Figure 13.3. Limitation in shoulder abduction because of axillary burn scar contracture.

cause limitation of motion. Careful attention to maintaining full range of motion of these areas may prevent catastrophic loss of function later.

In the lower extremity amputee, the most dread contractures are those of hip flexion and hip abduction. Both can cause an increase in the energy expenditure of prosthetic gait and thereby limit maximum walking function. The maintenance of full hip extension and adduction is essential. Proper bed positioning and active exercise can help prevent these problems. In the BK amputee, a knee flexion contracture of more than 15 degrees will limit successful prosthetic fit and utilization. Likewise, the knee must flex at least 35 degrees from full extension to allow a normal gait. Flexion of less than 90 degrees from full extension may also impair the sitting position of the prosthetic limb.

The nutritional needs of the burn patient have been discussed elsewhere but need to be re-emphasized at this time. Proper prosthetic utilization requires good muscle strength and physical endurance which are dependent on positive nitrogen balance. Not only may the burns place increased metabolic demands on the patient, but so will active exercise with and without the prosthesis. If kidney function is satisfactory, both caloric and protein requirements should be calculated and the patient should be educated about appropriate dietary habits.

The emotional turmoil of the burn patient, who has also had the body alteration of one or more amputations, is usually of such magnitude that the patient hands his body over to health professionals to do with as they wish. There is a significant depersonalization which takes place during this period of survival struggle. The patient usually will give up a part of his body for amputation if he understands his survival depends on this sacrifice. The family, likewise, is usually so emotionally overwhelmed, they can only think of survival and are usually willing to allow anything necessary to this end. Long-term functional considerations usually are of less importance than the maintenance of life. This does not, however, negate the need for careful discussion of the importance of amputation and the plan for useful prosthetic function wherever possible. If the surgeon is not familiar with the realities of prosthetic function, then a health professional with prosthetic experience should be made available to provide information and support for the patient and the family.

An effort should be made to explore third-party sponsorship not only for the acute burn treatment phase but also for the functional phase of rehabilitation. Sponsorship for specialized functional equipment including the prosthesis must be sought so that a comprehensvie rehabilitation program is financially realistic.

Phase 2: Preprosthetic Phase

Time: Suture removal to prosthetic prescription.
Goals: (1) stump shrinking and shaping;
        (2) stump desensitization;
        (3) maintain normal joint motion;
        (4) increase muscle strength in all extremities;
        (5) increase mobility skills;
        (6) maximize independence;
        (7) patient education about prosthesis and training;
        (8) inventory patient's concerns about future life style;
        (9) determine need for revision;
     (10) scar maturation;
     (11) restore patient's feelings of some control of his/her situation.

If healing occurs as usual, suture removal from the amputation incision occurs within two to three weeks of surgery. The wound, if healed primarily, will have maximal tensile strength by the 21st postoperative day and should allow a vigorous program for prosthetic preparation. Any wound healing problems should be treated aggressively since this will delay prosthetic fitting.

With complete healing of the stump incision and maturation of the grafts, shrinking and shaping of the residual limb should be pursued. This can be accomplished by compression from elastic bandage wrapping, a stump shrinker, intermittent positive pressure compression, or with the use of a preparatory prosthesis. Most amputated limbs can be adequately compressed using a figure-of-eight ace bandage wrap which is anchored above the next proximal joint (Fig. 13.4). The proper technique of wrapping should be taught to the hospital staff, the patient, and the family. The wrap should apply more pressure distally than proximally and should never be done in a circumferential manner. Early in the wrapping process, the skin should be closely monitored for signs of excessive pressure. The wrap should be removed and reapplied at least every four hours, or more frequently if it slips or bunches. An alternative method for compression is a prefabricated elastic garment called a stump shrinker which is measured to fit the residual limb. This shrinker should be applied for short periods of time initially with frequent examination of the skin for signs of excess pressure. As shrinking occurs, the shrinker may need to be replaced with a smaller one to continue adequate compression. Shrinkers and elastic wraps are difficult to keep in place on many short AK and short AE stumps. In these patients, a preparatory prosthesis which has an easily adjustable socket has proved beneficial.

Stump desensitization can be hastened with soft tissue compression as outlined above but also the stump can be desensitized by using gentle massage and tapping techniques. These techniques appear to improve the patient's tolerance to the pressure placed on the natural limb by the prosthetic socket.

With good wound healing, a therapeutic program to improve mobility skills, to maintain normal joint range of motion and to increase extemity and trunk muscle strength is essential.

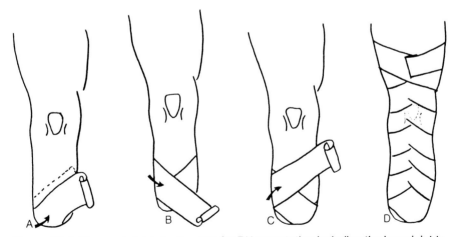

Figure 13.4. Figure-of-eight elastic wrap for BK amputation including the knee joint to help suspend the bandage.

In a unilateral upper extremity amputation, scapular and glenohumeral exercises will maintain full motion and aid prosthetic control motions. Also, teaching one-handed activities and, if necessary, beginning change of dominance skills will enhance functional independence. In the bilateral upper extremity amputee, these same exercises should be taught but additionally, adaptive equipment may allow some activity of daily living function, i.e., feeding, brushing teeth, writing. Often this equipment can be as simple as a universal cuff with a utensil holder and an adapted utensil.

For the unilateral lower extremity amputee, ambulation with gait aids should be taught or a comfortably fitted wheelchair prescribed. Ambulation with gait aids should be started after there is good trunk balance when standing on one leg. Otherwise, use of a wheelchair is safer and will not cause undue stress on weakened hip, leg, and trunk muscles. Although a walker may be a useful ambulatory aid, patients should be quickly progressed to crutch walking since the walker will never allow a normal prosthetic gait. If use of the wheelchair is anticipated for any significant period of time, mobility skills including wheelchair propulsion and transfers should be accomplished. Also, an appropriate wheelchair cushion should be provided to make prolonged sitting as comfortable as possible. The BK amputee should have a wheelchair leg extension under the amputated leg to help keep the knee extended and support the distal soft tissues. Specialized wheelchairs such as a one-arm drive or a motorized wheelchair may be necessary in certain combinations of multiple limb loss.

Because this phase is aimed at preparing the patient and his residual limb for a prosthesis, education about the prosthesis and the prosthetic training programs are necessary. Attention to education begins to include the patient actively in the care decision-making process. He can gently begin to understand the therapeutic process required for prosthetic training and begin to learn the realities of prosthetic function. A careful inventory of the patient's previous life style, his/her support system, and concerns about the future should provide the patient with a sense of caring concern on the part of the health professionals involved in this process. Frank discussion of nightmares, daymares, suicidal ideation, and depression should be supportive rather than confrontive. Helping the patient to be actively involved in his/her own care decisions will help restore the sense of control both in terms of control over his/her own body and over the situations which arise regarding his/her life.

The preprosthetic phase may be prolonged for three common reasons in the burn amputee. These problems are usually (1) a delay in obtaining complete skin healing, (2) immature skin graft, and (3) inadequate soft tissue coverage over bone. A superficial skin defect can usually be closed adequately with a split-thickness graft but a full-thickness defect over a bony prominence is better handled with full-thickness coverage. Either a local flap, pedicle flat, or free island flap should be considered. If a full-thickness defect is allowed to granulate from the base, the resulting scar will not usually tolerate prosthetic use for any length of time. This is especially true when the scar is adherent to the underlying bone or is located over a bony prominence. Scar and adequate soft tissue are of greater importance in a lower extremity amputee than in the upper extremity loss because weight bearing and shear forces at the stump-socket interface are greater in the leg than the arm. Immature skin grafts also will not withstand the pressure and shear generated at the stump-socket interface. Skin grafts should be kept supple and flexible once the burn defect has closed and as the grafts mature. These skin qualities can sometimes be achieved by applying a silicone cream preparation followed by gentle massage at least three times daily.

In spite of all these measures to promote rapid healing and adequate tissue coverage, it sometimes becomes apparent that an amputation revision is the best treatment to assure good prosthetic function. Typically this occurs when there is adherent scar over bone with no soft tissue padding between the skin and bone. In this instance, a scar revision with bone shortening should be planned to provide better scar placement and improved soft tissue coverage (Fig. 13.5A and B). The need for surgical revision may also occur when there is insensitive distal skin with no function across the proximal joint. In light of these circumstances, a major revision proximal to the nonfunctional joint will often be necessary prior to successful prosthetic fitting.

In cases where there is doubt as to whether the patient can be successfully fitted with a prosthesis, a conservative approach applies. This should be done with the patient's understanding that his residual limb may not tolerate even the most gentle prosthetic usage. However, some amputees will choose to proceed with prosthetic fitting and training rather than face additional surgery, even a minor revision.

Phase 3: Prosthetic Prescription and Fabrication

Time: From prescription decision until prosthetic fabrication is completed.

Goals: (1) team consensus regarding most appropriate prosthetic components;

(2) discussion of steps of fabrication with patient;

(3) decision for inpatient and/or outpatient training program;

(4) realistic orientation about artificiality of prosthesis.

When soft tissue shrinking and shaping have stabilized and desensitization has occurred, prosthetic prescription formulation should be discussed. Prosthetic component decisions should be a conjoined effort which includes the patient, the physicians, therapists, prosthetist, third-party payer, and

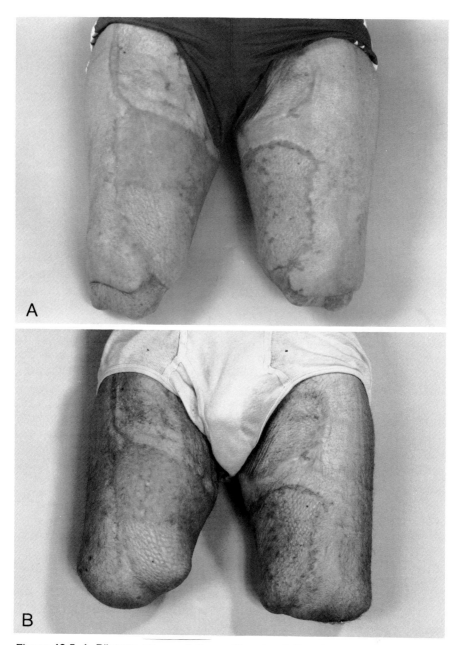

Figure 13.5. A. Bilateral AK amputations with pointed distal femurs covered only with split-thickness mesh graft and would not tolerate prosthetic wearing. B. Bilateral stump revisions with bone shortening and improved soft tissue covering which allows prosthetic wearing.

family. Once again, the patient can only be involved intelligently if he/she has had adequate education regarding the component options. Whenever possible, this educational process should include actual visualization of the component parts and an assembled comparable prosthesis.

In addition to prescribing the prosthesis, the steps involved in the prosthetic fabrication should be explained. An approximate time framework for the process from prescription until final fitting of the prosthesis should be given. Knowing when and how often he will need to visit the prosthetic laboratory will help the patient plan his/her daily schedule.

The treatment options for prosthetic training should be discussed. The entire process may need to be accomplished on an inpatient basis but whenever possible should be done as an outpatient. Most unilateral upper extremity and unilateral BK prosthetic training programs can be successfully completed as an outpatient. However, it is preferable to admit all bilateral upper extremity, bilateral lower extremity, and unilateral AK amputees at least for the initial phase of prosthetic training (usually two to three weeks).

This is an appropriate time to elicit the patient and family reactions to the prosthesis. This is also a time when they have an opportunity to meet other amputees who have worn a prosthesis for some time or who are also being fitted for a new prosthesis. Sometimes, the exchange of reactions to the prosthetic experience, in addition to the discussion of common frustrations and achievements by other amputees, can be helpful for the new amputee. However, it must be remembered that one amputee's experience of success or disappointment may not bear any relationship to the new amputee. These amputee-amputee encounters should be followed by an opportunity to discuss the new amputee's feelings with a psychosocial professional who is experienced in amputee rehabilitation.

In general, the prosthetic prescription is based on a number of criteria which should be accurately assessed and recorded. These criteria frequently include:

(1) length of residual limb;
(2) amount of soft tissue coverage;
(3) presence of adherent scar;
(4) movement of proximal joint(s);
(5) strength of muscle in residual limb;
(6) movement and strength in opposite limb;
(7) adequate vision;
(8) adequate ability to learn and retain new information;
(9) adequate sensation in residual limb;
(10) desire for function;
(11) desire for cosmesis;
(12) vocational interests;

(13) avocational interests;

(14) third-party payer considerations;

(15) family preferences.

UPPER EXTREMITY

Prosthetic restoration following the loss of a portion of the arm, forearm, or hand can be successful if the prosthesis is relatively comfortable and provides meaningful function. Unfortunately, often in the upper extremity, the most cosmetic prosthesis is not the most functional prosthesis. In reality, there are no perfectly satisfactory replacements for the marvelous mechanisms of the human hand and arm.

If the amputation involves the nondominant extremity, the prosthesis can usually provide useful assistance to the normal dominant side. If the amputation has occurred on the dominant side, the patient may learn to switch dominance to the opposite normal side and use the prosthesis to assist the newly dominant side. In bilateral loss, the longer and stronger amputated limb will usually become the dominant side.

A list of prosthetic components which are most commonly used is presented with comments regarding their advantages and disadvantages. The list begins with the most proximal components and expands distally as more lost anatomy requires additional prosthetic restoration.

PARTIAL HAND LEVEL

If a prosthesis is desired for this level, it usually is a passive cosmetic glove replacing the lost anatomy. For certain remaining hand elements, an artificial thumb or palmar opposition device may improve gross grasp of certain objects. A handi-hook may be placed against the palm and the activating cable is attached to a figure-nine harness to allow gross grasp and release when the residual hand is not capable of this prehensile function (Fig. 13.6A and B).

Conversion of a partial hand amputation to a wrist disarticulation should be contemplated under these conditions:

(1) Remaining digits do not provide useful grasp and release or partial hand does not provide assistance to opposite extremity.

(2) Reconstructive surgery will not provide useful grasp and release.

(3) There is a marked amount of insensitive skin or scar which breaks down repeatedly with usage.

TERMINAL DEVICE—PROSTHETIC HOOK AND HAND

Body-powered (cable-activated) T.D.s allow the choice of a split hook or a functional hand covered with a cosmetic glove. Most hooks are lighter weight than the hands and permit the amputee to see more of the object when he is using the T.D. to grasp and release. A hook is also easier to get into a pocket. A hand T.D. provides better cosmesis than the hook but is

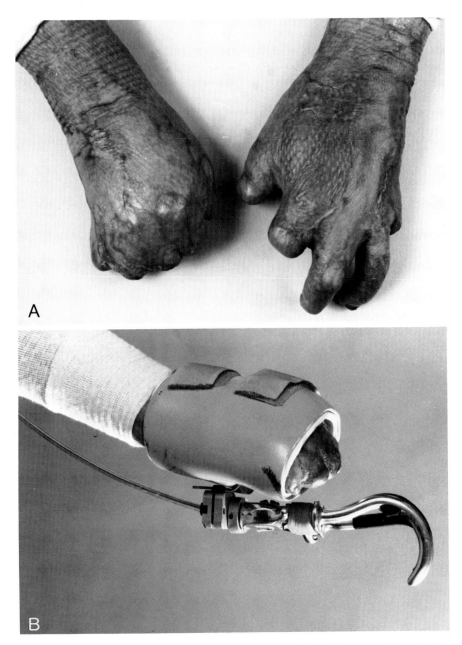

Figure 13.6. A. Bilateral hand burns with almost complete loss of digits on dominant right side. B. Handi-hook worn over residual right hand to facilitate bimanual activities.

bulkier and is usually less functional than the hook. The cosmetic glove for the prosthetic hand frequently stains, tears easily, and is costly to replace.

Myoelectric hands allow greater grasp force than the body-powered T.D.s but are heavier and significantly more expensive than a body-powered prosthesis. Myoelectric prostheses also require a stabilized stump shape and because of the electric components, require more maintenance. Their availability and use should be discussed as an option for the patient. It is preferable to fit, train, and stabilize the amputated forearm for six months before fitting the initial myoelectric prosthesis.

WRIST DISARTICULATION PROSTHESIS

Prescription Considerations

Socket: Single wall plastic laminate which extends part way up forearm.
Suspension: Flexible elbow hinges through triceps pad.
Control: Single Bowden cable with figure-of-eight harness and axilla loop to opposite axilla.
Wrist Unit: Constant friction; wafer unit.
T. D.: (1) Hook or (2) hand.
Alternate Option: Myoelectric hand.

This amputation level retains some residual pronation and supination of the forearm which is translated to the prosthesis allowing more accurate approach of the T.D. to the object to be grasped. One disadvantage to this level is the limitation of using only one wrist unit. Also, if the radial and ulnar condyles remain untrimmed, the distal end of the amputation is bulbous and, therefore, the socket has a greater circumference compared to the opposite wrist. Because of the condylar bony prominences, the prosthesis may cause significant discomfort and skin breakdown especially if burn scar is present.

BELOW-ELBOW PROSTHESIS (Fig. 13.7)

Prescription Considerations

Socket: Double wall plastic laminate with trim lines extending to upper forearm but allowing as much pronation and supination as possible.
Suspension: (1) Flexible hinges in long BE attached to triceps cuff. (2) Rigid hinges in short BE through triceps cuff. (3) Muenster socket providing self suspension from bony prominences at elbow.
Harness and Control: Single Bowden cable with figure-of-eight harness and axilla loop.
Wrist Unit: (1) Constant friction; (2) quick change; (3) locking; or (4) flexion.
T. D.: (1) Hook or (2) hand.
Myoelectric prosthetic restoration can be a good option at this level. A

Below-Elbow

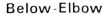

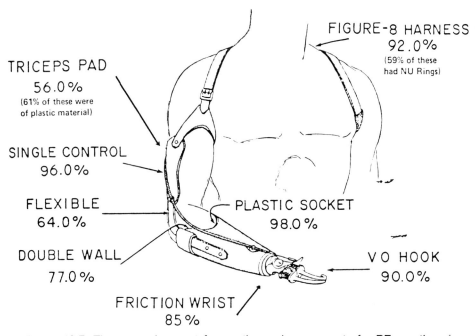

FIGURE-8 HARNESS
92.0%
(59% of these
had NU Rings)

TRICEPS PAD
56.0%
(61% of these were
of plastic material)

SINGLE CONTROL
96.0%

FLEXIBLE
64.0%

PLASTIC SOCKET
98.0%

DOUBLE WALL
77.0%

VO HOOK
90.0%

FRICTION WRIST
85%

Figure 13.7. These are the most frequently used components for BE prostheses. (Reproduced with permission from Davis, et al: Amputees and their prostheses. *Artif Limbs* 14:19–48, 1970).

very short BE amputation will probably require a special elbow unit with polycentric hinges or a split socket with a step-up hinge (Fig. 13.8A and B). An alternative to these hinges can be a Muenster socket which is self-suspending over the olecranon and humeral condyles. The T.D. in this socket design is operated by a Bowden control cable to a figure-nine axilla loop to the opposite arm.

If there is a significant scar or irregular contour to the residual limb, these problems can usually be accommodated by a molded soft socket liner which is placed on the stump prior to donning the plastic socket. In the burn patient with an arm amputation there may be scarring over the thorax or opposite axilla which can prevent use of the usual figure-of-eight harness and/or axilla loop. In this situation a shoulder saddle and/or cross-chest strap can be used, at least temporarily, while the burn scar matures, softens, and becomes more mobile (Fig. 13.9).

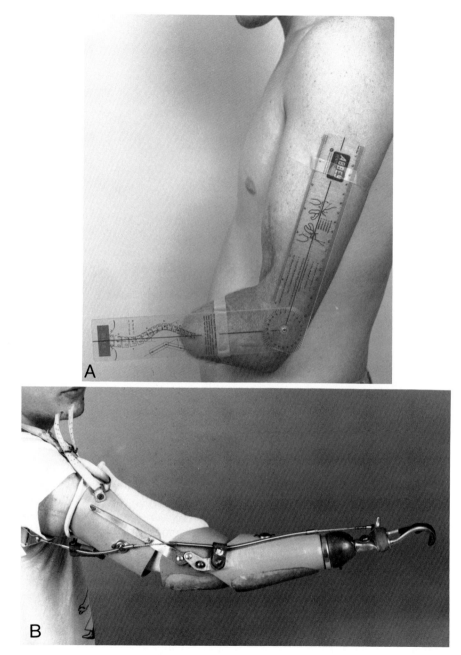

Figure 13.8. A. BE amputation with antecubital burn demonstrating maximum active flexion. B. Left BE prosthesis with split socket and step-up hinge which allows greater forearm flexion.

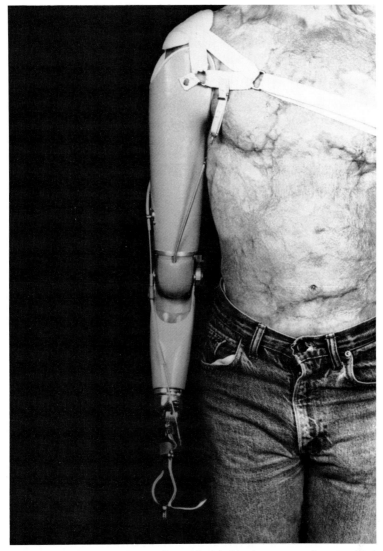

Figure 13.9. Extensive thoracic scarring with shoulder harness and cross-chest strap.

ELBOW DISARTICULATION PROSTHESIS

Prescription Considerations

Socket: Single wall or double wall plastic laminate.

Suspension: (1) Strapping to harness or (2) expandable socket liner which grasps humeral condyles.

Control: Elbow lock strap and dual Bowden control strap to opposite shoulder.

Elbow Unit: External lock on outside of socket. No turntable.

Wrist Unit: See BE.

T.D.: See BE.

There is some disagreement about the desirability of this amputation level. Proponents who recommend this level indicate there is better translation of internal and external glenohumeral rotation to the socket allowing better T.D. placement. Those who recommend against this level of amputation recommend a long AE limb so that an internal elbow lock and a turntable can be provided. The external elbow lock is less durable and enlarges the external diameter of the prosthesis. Detractors also cite skin and pain problems from the prominent humeral condyles which can rub against the socket.

ABOVE-ELBOW PROSTHESIS (FIG. 13.10)

Prescription Considerations

Socket: Double wall plastic laminate. With severe scarring or unusual stump contour, a molded soft insert may better accommodate the stump inside the socket.

Suspension: (1) Straps attached to harness or (2) suction. Short AE levels may require socket suspension which extends proximal to the glenohumeral joint thereby limiting some motion at this joint. Scapular mobility must, therefore, substitute for this limited glenohumeral motion.

Control: An elbow locking strap and a Bowden dual control cable.

Elbow: Internal alternating locking unit with a turntable permitting forearm shell internal and external rotation.

Forearm Shell: Single wall plastic laminate.

Wrist Unit: Same as BE but try to keep as lightweight as possible.

T.D.: See BE but often a lighter T.D. is better with which to start.

The AE amputation should be performed far enough above the humeral condyles so that with an internal locking prosthetic elbow the axis of the prosthetic elbow motion coincides with the axis of the normal elbow. This normally requires the amputation be performed four cm above the distal end of the humerus.

Electrically powered elbow units from switch or myoelectric controls are available. These units are heavier than the body-powered units but do require less strapping. They do significantly increase the cost and require more maintenance than body-powered components.

SHOULDER DISARTICULATION PROSTHESIS

Prescription Considerations

Socket: (1) Plastic laminate or (2) aluminum frame (Fig. 13.11A).

Suspension: From shoulder girdle with cross-chest strap.

Above-Elbow

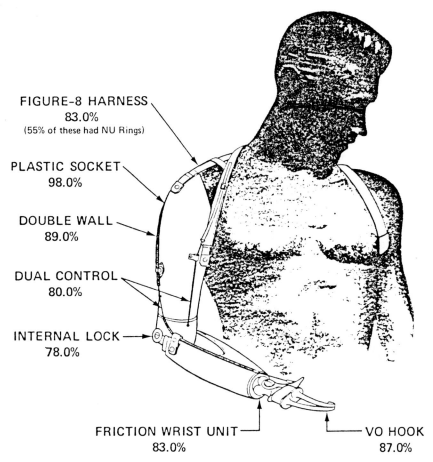

FIGURE-8 HARNESS
83.0%
(55% of these had NU Rings)

PLASTIC SOCKET
98.0%

DOUBLE WALL
89.0%

DUAL CONTROL
80.0%

INTERNAL LOCK
78.0%

FRICTION WRIST UNIT
83.0%

VO HOOK
87.0%

Figure 13.10. These are the most frequently used components for AE prostheses. (Reproduced with permission from Davies et al: Amputees and their prostheses. *Artif Limbs* 14:19–48, 1970).

Control: Often need to have triple controls: (1) Elbow lock, (2) elbow flexion, and (3) T.D. activation.

Shoulder joint: Flexion-abduction unit.

Humeral segment: (1) Endoskeletal or (2) exoskeletal design.

Elbow: (1) Use alternating locking exoskeletal or (2) endoskeletal passive locking unit.

Forearm: (1) Endoskeletal or (2) exoskeletal design.

Wrist Unit: Lightest possible—usually constant friction.

T.D.: Lightest possible—usually 5XA hook.

An alternative to a full prosthesis is a cosmetic shoulder cap illustrated

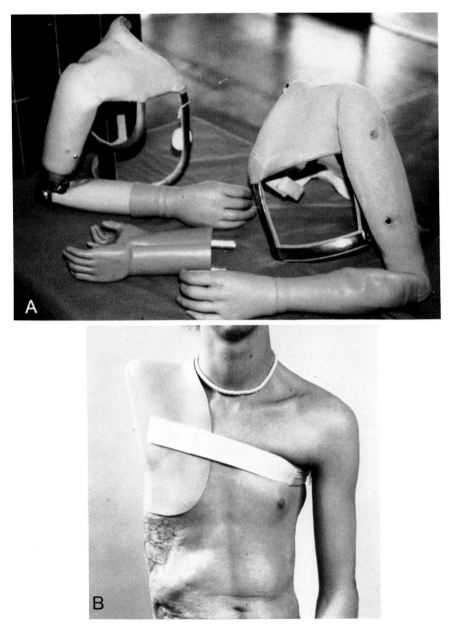

Figure 13.11. A. Aluminum frames for shoulder disarticulation prosthesis are shown. B. Cosmetic shoulder cap is shown.

in Figure 13.11B. A very short AE amputation which is proximal to the lesser tubercle of the humerus will need to be fitted as a shoulder disarticulation level.

INTERSCAPULOTHORACIC DISARTICULATION PROSTHESIS

The same specifications apply for the shoulder disarticulation level except that the proximal trim lines of the socket extend closer to the neck and cover more of the thorax. In both of these proximal levels of limb loss, endoskeletal design with an aluminum frame keeps prosthetic weight to a minimum thereby improving comfort and patient wearing acceptance.

Since control sites are limited at these high levels of amputation, powered components appear attractive but add significantly to the weight of the prosthesis. However, if electric power is chosen, probably only one electric component should be given. A powered elbow can allow for better lifting and T.D. placement while a powered hand can allow for greater grasp than a conventional T.D. If a powered hand is given, a passive locking elbow can be positioned and locked by the opposite hand.

BILATERAL UPPER EXTREMITY AMPUTATIONS

It is very common in burn amputees, especially those secondary to electrical burns, to encounter bilateral arm loss. The immediate imposition of total dependency coupled with the deforming change of body image is usually devastating. Encouraging the grieving process for missing (dead) body parts is often a necessary and an emotionally healing process. All haste should be used to provide adaptive aides which can allow some self-care even if it is just for feeding, phone handling, or writing. The provision of temporary prostheses as soon as the incisions and burn wounds allow, will permit immediate restoration of some function at all levels of bilateral arm loss except the most proximal levels. Even if the stumps are not maximally shrunken or shaped, prostheses should be fabricated within a few days of the decision for prosthetic prescription.

Some special prosthetic component considerations should be mentioned. Split hooks for T.D.s provide better bilateral function than functional hands or myoelectric prostheses (Fig. 13.12). Also because the hooks are more maintenance-free than the other options, the bilateral arm amputee can better depend on these T.D.s for essential daily function. Unless the bilateral loss is at the wrist level, at least one wrist flexion unit, usually on the dominant side, will ease essential midline functions such as shirt buttoning, belt buckling, and toileting. Also, active wrist rotation units make T.D. prepositioning easier. These rotation units add weight and prosthetic maintenance but have been invaluable for many bilateral arm amputees. In bilateral proximal arm loss, switch- or myoelectric-controlled prostheses suspended from aluminum frames may permit some limited self-care activities (Fig. 13.13). With bilateral loss, it is imperative that a spare set of

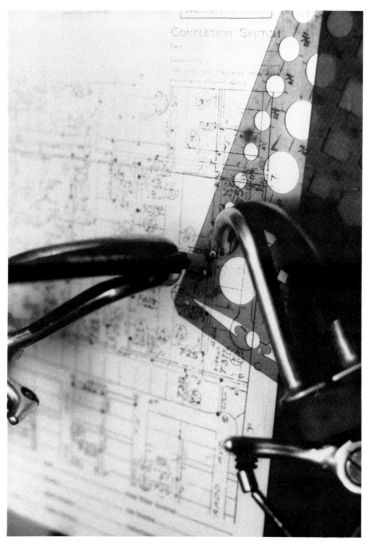

Figure 13.12. Amputee with short BE and elbow disarticulation prostheses using hook TDs for drafting.

functional prostheses be available in case of maintenance problems with the primary set. Also, accessory prostheses, such as shower arms, may make certain functional activities easier to perform.

LOWER EXTREMITY COMPONENTS

In restoring missing anatomy and function, the lower extremity prosthesis is designed to allow the transmission of superimposed body weight through the pressure tolerant areas of the residual limb. Pressure sensitive areas of the stump are relieved from weight bearing by concave contours of the prosthetic socket design. The usual pressure tolerant areas are often compromised in the burn amputee because of scarring, skin graft, irregular stump contour, or insensitive skin. Special prosthetic design or extraordinary component prescription are needed in these cases to allow prosthetic use while the integrity of the skin is maintained and prosthetic comfort is maximally achieved.

In cases where no special prosthesis would appear to allow maintenance of skin integrity or functional comfort, stump revision should be discussed prior to prosthetic prescription. If several specialized prostheses and components have been tried without functional success, revision of the skin and/or bone should be offered to improve the chances of successful prosthetic function.

PARTIAL FOOT AMPUTATION—FROM TOES TO TRANSMETATARSAL

These amputation deficits can usually be treated with the fabrication of a shoe insole with a molded replacement for the area of the missing phalanges and metatarsals. This insole helps keep any residual portion of the foot and toe(s) in normal position while wearing shoes or boots. If there

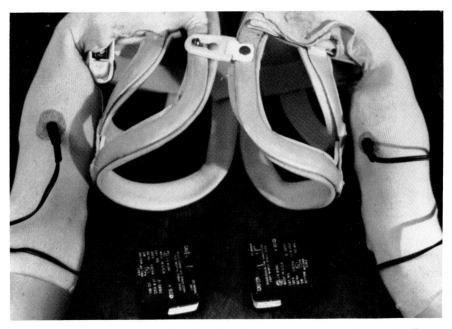

Figure 13.13. Aluminum frame shoulder disarticulation prostheses with electric elbows and hands are shown.

is a significant amount of split-thickness graft or scarring, a gel insert may help to prevent blistering or ulceration. Shoes should be soft and large enough to accommodate any deformity. They should lace over the foot and the prosthetic insert. The heel should not be much higher than the sole of the shoe and the entire bottom of the shoe should be fabricated from nonskid material.

Hindfoot amputations are difficult to fit successfully especially in terms of a comfortable prosthesis which will allow good function. If a foot amputation is required proximal to the transmetatarsal level, a true Syme's amputation usually provides better prosthetic function than a hindfoot amputation will allow.

SYME'S AMPUTATION

Prescription Considerations

Foot: Modified solid-ankle-cushion-heel (SACH).

Socket: (1) Plastic laminate with rear or side window to allow bulbous end of stump to pass into distal socket. (2) An alternate socket is similar in design to patellar tendon bearing (PTB) with an expandable inner lining.

Suspension: (1) Removable window of socket which when replaced into socket fits over the malleoli or (2) self-suspension using expandable inner wall.

In order for this level of amputation to function successfully with the prosthesis described above, the heel pad must be intact over the end of the tibia and fibula to allow some end bearing. Also, some trimming of the medial and lateral malleoli will permit suspension from them but provide less bulk at the ankle. This level of amputation may not provide enough prosthetic cosmesis for a slim male and most female patients.

BELOW-KNEE AMPUTATION

Prescription Considerations

Socket: Plastic laminate PTB design. May use soft insert.

Suspension: (1) Supracondylar cuff; (2) suprapatellar-supracondylar; (3) external knee joints and thigh lacer; or (4) rubber sleeve.

Foot-Ankle Complex: (1) SACH; (2) single axis; or (3) stationary-ankle-flexible-endoskeleton (SAFE).

Ankle Options: Greissinger, rotator.

In the BK burn amputee, if the stump is the desired cylindrical shape and the skin is normal, the usual PTB prosthesis with SACH foot and supracondylar cuff suspension should serve well. However, this idealized residual limb is often not present. With scar and irregularly contoured soft tissue, a molded insert will help distribute pressures more evenly (Fig. 13.14A and B). Also, the prosthetic suspension system with the least

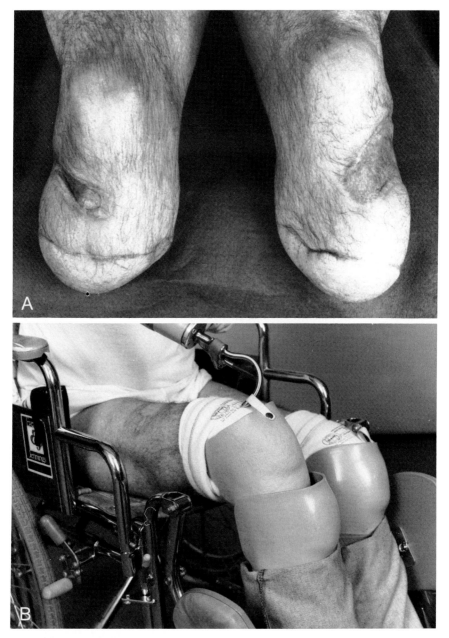

Figure 13.14. A. Bilateral short BK amputations with scar and skin graft in infrapatellar region. B. Molded suprapatellar-supracondylar inserts for bilateral BK prostheses.

pistoning movement in the socket may help maintain skin integrity. This can be provided using suprapatellar-supracondylar design, a waist belt with a suspender attached to the proximal socket, or a rubber sleeve which covers the proximal socket and the residual limb above the socket brim. In addition, shearing force at the stump socket interface may be diminished by using a multiaxial ankle such as the Greissinger or a multiaxial foot such as the SAFE. These special components can help maintain stump integrity.

Lastly, unweighting the troublesome BK stump area may promote prosthetic function. This can be done by crossing the knee using single-axis knee joints which are attached proximally to a thigh corset. A tradeoff in problems may result despite the unweighting of the leg below the knee. Superimposing the single-axis knee joints of the prosthesis over the human multiaxial knee joint increases the amount of pistoning of the stump in the prosthetic socket. This can result in skin breakdown in addition to the disadvantages of the increased weight of the joints and corset themselves.

Another BK problem has resulted from preserving the length of the tibia and fibula at the expense of insufficient soft tissue coverage. There is no significant functional gain in trying to retain bone below the level of the gastrocsoleus muscle bellies. Leaving too much tibia and fibula does not allow for good myofascial closure over the distal stump. The excessively long stump is cone-shaped instead of the desired cylinder shape. This cone-shaped stump produces increased point pressures on the skin of the residual limb at the stump-socket interface.

KNEE DISARTICULATION

As with the Syme's level, this can be a good weight bearing stump if covered with mobile skin, if it is free from excessive scar, and if the stump possesses normal sensation. If any or all of these conditions is missing in the adult amputee, skin problems in the distal stump will result from weight bearing.

Prosthetic Considerations

Socket: (1) Plastic laminate with anterior Velcro closures or (2) molded leather with lacer.

Suspension: (1) Socket self-suspends over femoral condyles or (2) suction.

Knee: (1) Orthopedic Hospital of Copenhagen (O.H.C.) hydraulic knee or (2) single-axis knee joints.

Shank: (1) Endoskeletal or (2) exoskeletal.

Foot-Ankle: Same as BK.

This prosthesis may prove to be unsightly if the femoral condyles have not been trimmed slightly. The distal prosthesis is often larger than the opposite thigh and the distal knee is longer and higher than the normal knee when sitting. These cosmetic considerations often make this amputation level less desirable for slim men and most women. Children with burn amputations through the knee may tolerate this prosthesis even if the distal stump is covered with grafted skin. This usually is not true in older teenagers and adults.

ABOVE-KNEE AMPUTATION

The longer the femoral length, the better the function, if the end of the residual thigh has full-thickness skin and soft tissue covering it. However, a supracondylar amputation of the femur may not allow enough room for the variety of knee units available. The best length above the knee disarticulation level is five cm above the adductor tubercle.

Prosthetic Considerations

Socket: Plastic laminate for definitive limb. Preparatory prosthesis may be formed from polypropylene allowing easy adjustment of socket. Quadrilateral shape can use soft liner or insert for abnormal stump contours.

Suspension: (1) Hip joint and pelvic band; (2) full suction; or (3) partial suction with Silesian band.

Knee: (1) Constant friction with friction brake (safety unit); (2) single-axis with constant friction; or (3) hydraulic. Endoskeletal or exoskeletal units available.

Shank: (1) Exoskeletal (wood) or (2) endoskeletal (aluminium with foam cover).

Foot-Ankle: Same as BK. At this level, the single-axis provides more stability than the other options.

Usually, the three greatest pressure areas on the residual AK level are the ischial tuberosity, the distal lateral, and distal anterior femur. These areas especially need good skin and soft tissue padding with nonadherent scar. In the patient with firm muscles and a properly shaped cylindrical stump, the use of suction or semisuction suspension decreases prosthetic weight and increases wearing comfort (Fig. 13.15A and B). Choice of the knee unit involves a number of factors but in the younger amputee, a hydraulic unit which gives a more cosmetic gait when the cadence varies is preferred. Knee safety units are appropriate for patients with weakened stump muscles. Endoskeletal prosthetic design significantly decreases the weight of the prosthesis with proximal levels of amputation. An endoskeletal prosthesis also can be useful as a preparatory limb for gait training since alignment adjustments are easier to make than with the exoskeletal plastic laminate limb.

HIP DISARTICULATION AMPUTATION

Amputations with less than four cm of femur distal to the lesser trochanter often need to be fitted with a hip disarticulation prosthesis because

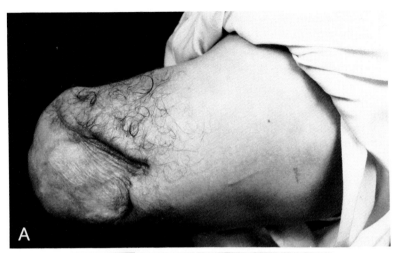

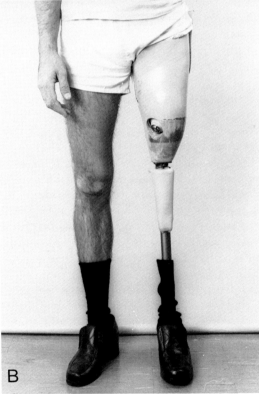

Figure 13.15. A. AK stump with distal anterolateral scar is shown. B. Endoskeletal prosthesis with suction insert and socket fitted over scarred stump is shown.

there is insufficient femoral lever arm to stabilize or activate an AK prosthesis.

Prosthetic Considerations

Socket: Plastic laminate bucket (Canadian).

Hip: (1) Endoskeletal (Bock); (2) exoskeletal (Northwestern); or (3) flexion bias.

Thigh: (1) Endoskeletal or (2) exoskeletal.

Knee: Constant friction with friction brake.

Shank: (1) Endoskeletal or (2) exoskeletal.

Foot-Ankle complex: Same as BK and AK.

In older adolescents and adults the endoskeletal design for this level of loss is preferred. The decreased weight is approximately one-half compared to an exoskeletal prosthesis. In the vigorous, younger person, the additional exoskeletal weight is better tolerated and better withstands the wear and tear to which it is subjected. Endoskeletal prosthetic legs are more subject to loss of alignment and the foam cover tears easily when put to vigorous use.

HEMIPELVECTOMY AMPUTATION

This level uses the same basic prosthetic components as those described above for the hip disarticulation level. The major difference is the socket which must stabilize the abdominal contents and superimposed body. The trim lines of the socket usually extend to incorporate the lower rib cage, the lumbar spine, most of the abdominal wall, both flanks, and the opposite iliac crest. Weight and comfort are major considerations for successful wearing. Endoskeletal design is preferable for this amputation. Young, vigorous ambulators often choose to walk using crutches and no prosthesis because it is faster for them. They often do not like the gait produced with this prosthesis because they consider their walking awkward and unsightly.

BILATERAL LOWER EXTREMITY AMPUTATIONS

Bilateral lower extremity amputees who have lost their limbs because of burns, have greater difficulty obtaining the expected prosthetic function than most traumatic bilateral leg amputees. This occurs because of the need for weight bearing on tissues which are frequently covered with burn scars or grafted skin. Not only is there usually scar which is inopportunely located and insensitive but the scar is often totally adherent to the underlying bone. Shear forces applied to this type of immobile scar cause ulceration. Every attempt must be made in the early postoperative period to prevent the scar from becoming adherent and the soft tissue immobile against the bone.

It is difficult to achieve prosthetic function in bilateral amputations occurring at or above the knee. The energy requirements to use bilateral prostheses at above knee levels is so great that even if the patient can walk with prostheses for short distances, he usually chooses to use a wheelchair for longer distances. This amputee also requires a wheelchair if any prosthetic wearing or maintenance problems develop.

In preparing the bilateral knee disarticulation or AK patient for wearing articulated legs, a period of "stubby" prosthetic training is useful. The short stubby prostheses with quadrilateral sockets, no knee units, and wide rocker bottoms assist the patient in strengthening his hip extensors and abductors (Fig. 13.16). The stubby prostheses also help the amputee to gain balance and endurance. This amputee should use stubbies to the exclusion of the wheelchair for several months or more prior to fitting with articulated prostheses.

Once the prosthetic prescription has been formulated, the casting, fabrication, and fitting processes should be explained to the patient and his/her family. The adjustment to a prosthesis can be aided by showing the patient a finished prosthesis similar to the one prescribed. The basic fabrication steps include: (1) taking a plaster cast of the residual limb, (2) making a negative plaster mold of the stump, (3) laminating plastic over the mold of stump forming the socket, (4) attaching the joints and components to the socket, (5) aligning the components to give the best movement, (6) final fitting and trial use of prosthesis.

A discussion of the prosthetic training portion of rehabilitation should be conducted. The desirability of inpatient and/or outpatient care should be decided. Also, the patient should be presented with an approximate time for prosthetic fabrication and training.

Phase 4: Prosthetic Training

Time: Delivery of finished prosthesis to completion of training in prosthetic skills.

Goals: (1) evaluation of prosthetic components and fit of socket;
(2) relative comfort when wearing and functioning in prosthesis;
(3) improved function with prosthetic use;
(4) good body posture with prosthetic use;
(5) minimal assistive equipment;
(6) verbalize patient's frustration and any disappointment with the prosthesis;
(7) successful transfer of skills from rehabilitation center to home;
(8) education regarding prosthetic maintenance;
(9) explore vocational and avocational options.

The period of time from casting until final fitting is usually one of anticipation for the amputee who is expecting or hoping to once again function as he did prior to his amputation. All too frequently, the finished prosthesis is a disappointment for the patient. It is perceived as being

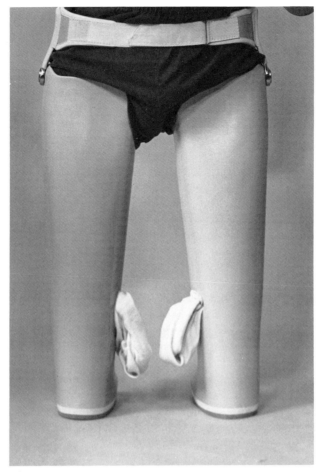

Figure 13.16. Stubby prostheses for ambulation training in bilateral AK limb loss are shown.

"artificial looking", heavy, uncomfortable, and it smells of the chemicals used in its manufacture. Orienting a patient to the realities of prosthetic appearance and the prosthetic differences from the lost extremity help ease the patient into this phase.

Once the finished prosthesis has been delivered to the patient or therapist, the period of prosthetic wearing can begin once an evaluation of socket fit and prosthetic components has been completed. The initial program of prosthetic training should include short periods of prosthetic wearing which are followed by a thorough inspection of all the stump skin. This inspection should indicate any points of excess pressure. The wearing periods can be repeated several times over the day and can be increased rapidly if no skin redness or pain occurs.

When lower extremity prosthetic wearing has reached 15 minutes and if proximal muscle strength will allow, the patient can begin standing in the parallel bars. Static weight bearing begins by shifting weight from side to side with an increasing amount of weight being placed on the prosthetic side. Stepping forward and backward follows. Then actual steps with emphasis on residual limb muscle activation can begin. The amputee should be consciously aware of the feeling of how the muscles in the limb proximal to the amputation are working in order to propel and control the prosthesis. Kinesthetic feedback from the stump-socket interface should be consciously used during the early training period. With practice, these conscious feelings can become automatic so that the amputee does not consciously have to think about what to do with each lower extremity muscle group. Periods of static prosthetic wearing and prosthetic ambulation should be gradually increased within the tolerance of the amputee's skin, muscle strength, and physical endurance.

The skin is most vulnerable during the early prosthetic training period and any blistering or breakdown can delay further prosthetic wearing from days to weeks. Despite adequate muscle strength there is often a significant reduction in endurance. Short periods of wearing should be followed by adequate rest and nonwearing. Also during this time, the patient should continue to wear a compression bandage or stump shrinker. If the soft tissue compression is removed for 15–20 minutes, edema can occur quickly enough to prevent prosthetic wearing until the swelling is sufficiently controlled.

The patient should progress from the parallel bars to crutches. Rarely should a walker be used and then only in older or unsteady individuals with poor trunk control. Walkers are to be avoided whenever possible because they do not allow a normal prosthetic gait pattern. Progression from crutches to canes or a single cane can occur when there is good trunk balance, good hip and leg muscle strength, and good prosthetic control.

Functional skills which should be taught to the patient include walking, ascending and descending stairs, ramps, curbs, and falling to and rising from the floor. Stump hygiene, stump sock care, and prosthetic care should be included at this time.

Operating or driving a car, truck, tractor, or other equipment should be discussed and when necessary, driver evaluation, training and vehicle modification should be prescribed by the amputee team. Occasionally, a new driving test is required by the state and license restrictions may be imposed for the legal operation of a vehicle. Helping the amputee to become a legally qualified driver is the responsibility of the rehabilitation team.

In addition to these usual ambulatory functions, any unique vocational and avocational prosthetic usages should be reviewed whenever possible. Prolonged standing, walking, bending, stooping, and lifting are often necessary in a vocational situation. Occasionally climbing a ladder is useful. Avocational requirements for prosthetic use should be reviewed and practiced whenever possible. Simulations in the rehabilitation setting should mirror the actual vocational and avocational situation as closely as possible.

UPPER EXTREMITY PROSTHETIC TRAINING

Training in the wearing and functional use of an upper extremity prosthesis can usually be accomplished as an outpatient and requires less time than gaining functional use of a lower extremity prosthesis. This diminished training time results from longer initial wearing periods which are more readily tolerated because the upper extremity prosthesis is not used for weight bearing. Also, basic upper extremity prosthetic skills are more easily learned than the more demanding motor skills of bipedal ambulation.

The initial prosthetic wearing periods should consist of short periods (15 minutes) with frequent examination of the skin for signs of excess pressure or poor socket fit. The amputee should first learn how to put on and take off the prosthesis. A basic orientation to the various components and control straps will assist in demonstrating how the prosthesis functions as a useful assist to the opposite extremity. Flexion and extension at the glenohumeral joint together with scapular abduction, adduction, elevation, and depression are motions which the arm amputee should be practicing frequently in the preprosthetic period. These motions when used together with the harness and cable controls produce activation of the T.D. and an elbow unit when present (Fig. 13.17).

Essential principles of early training consist of teaching the patient how to open and close the T.D., how to approach an object to grasp it with the T.D., how to transfer the object, and how to release the object. The period of prosthetic wearing and use can be rapidly increased if there is good skin tolerance. Often an upper extremity prosthesis can be worn for the entire day within a week of fabrication. Also, prosthetic training can usually be completed within this same time framework.

In addition to the basic use skills, homemaking, work-related and recreational skills should be reviewed and simulated whenever possible.

For the bilateral upper extremity amputee a variety of essential activities should be accomplished with the therapist's direction. Special problem areas can arise with dressing, toileting, and hygiene especially if one or more of the amputations is above the elbow. Assistive devices for feeding, dressing, and toileting may add significantly to functional independence.

Continued successful upper extremity prosthetic wearing depends greatly on the functional outcome. If the prosthesis does not add significant function to the amputee's life style, the amputee will frequently choose to

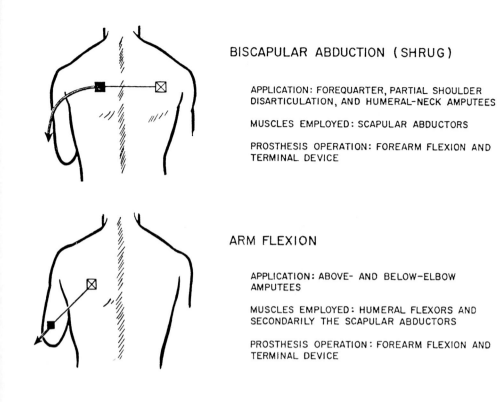

BISCAPULAR ABDUCTION (SHRUG)

APPLICATION: FOREQUARTER, PARTIAL SHOULDER DISARTICULATION, AND HUMERAL-NECK AMPUTEES

MUSCLES EMPLOYED: SCAPULAR ABDUCTORS

PROSTHESIS OPERATION: FOREARM FLEXION AND TERMINAL DEVICE

ARM FLEXION

APPLICATION: ABOVE- AND BELOW-ELBOW AMPUTEES

MUSCLES EMPLOYED: HUMERAL FLEXORS AND SECONDARILY THE SCAPULAR ABDUCTORS

PROSTHESIS OPERATION: FOREARM FLEXION AND TERMINAL DEVICE

ARM EXTENSION

APPLICATION: ABOVE-ELBOW AMPUTEES

MUSCLES EMPLOYED: HUMERAL EXTENSORS

PROSTHESIS OPERATION: ELBOW LOCK

Figure 13.17. Major harness control motions for upper extremity prosthetic function. (After Taylor C: The biomechanics of control in upper extremity prosthesis. *Artif Limbs* 2:4–25, 1955.)

forego wearing a prosthesis. For this reason, it is the responsibility of the rehabilitation team to be certain that the prosthesis provides maximal function, maximal comfort, and that the patient thoroughly understands how he can use the prosthesis to his greatest advantage.

Training with a myoelectric- or switch-controlled electric upper extremity prosthesis frequently requires more time and team effort than the comparable body-powered prosthesis. Separation of muscle activation, weak and strong muscle contraction, and muscle substitution for performing a new activity require concentrated training and re-education. Often, biofeedback is a useful technique to assist the amputee to develop better muscle control.

The prosthetic training period can be a very confrontive experience for the amputee. He begins to feel the discomfort of prosthetic wearing and the demands placed on the remaining body parts to function effectively in the prosthesis. The amputee has formulated in his mind certain expectations about his new artificial arm. The actual prosthesis is often a disappointment for the patient when compared to the prosthesis he has constructed in his mind. These differences between imagined and real prosthetic restoration produce an emotionally traumatic time. Whenever possible, these feelings should be acknowledged and the normalcy of these reactions should be discussed in a supportive manner.

Often, the amputee team views the finished prosthesis in a very positive manner while the amputee is having difficulty dealing with the perceived ugliness of this "artificial contraption." While the team may understand the adaptive process involved in successful prosthetic usage, the patient may not be able to see the functional end point beyond his current feelings of frustration and despair. These feelings should be allowed to surface and be explored. Meanwhile, prosthetic training can be presented in short, frequent sessions where tasks are presented that are within the patient's capability. Successful prosthetic use with positive feedback from the team will often help support the patient so he can work through this period of emotional turmoil.

As prosthetic training continues, a home program of wearing and functional use should be formulated so the patient has some functional goals with which to measure progress outside the artificial therapy setting. This program should be reviewed prior to discharge from the prosthetic rehabilitation facility with the patient and his family. Specific instructions regarding which team member can assist with a problem should also be provided. A follow-up appointment should be arranged and an explanation of what activities the amputee can expect during the follow-up visit is helpful in making the transition from the rehabilitation center to the home environment.

Phase 5: Functional Follow-up

Time: Finish of initial training to end of life.
Goals: (1) maximize prosthetic function;
        (2) maintain prosthetic components;

(3) decrease assistive devices;

(4) resume previous vocation or explore new vocational options;

(5) resume avocational interests;

(6) re-enter family and community environment;

(7) regular periodic follow-up with rehabilitation professionals.

Periodic prosthetic follow-up allows maximal amputee function and minimizes prosthetic frustration and disuse. It is preferable to see all new patients within four to six weeks of discharge following the initial treatment period. Often, prosthetic adjustments are needed soon after initial fitting and these modifications can be accomplished at the same time that a reassessment of the prosthetic wearing and functional goals is made. A check should be made regarding any assistive equipment which may have been ordered but not received. Any functional or fitting problems should be evaluated by the team and appropriate remediation arranged. A discussion of the patient's experience in returning to his/her family and community should occur.

Vocational and avocational plans should be explored so the team can discuss realistic recommendations and expectations (Fig. 13.18). While vocational aptitudes, interests and previous job skills are usually inventoried early in the rehabilitation process, job counseling, retraining, and placement usually are not formally arranged until there is maximal function with or without the use of the prosthesis. Reintegration of the amputee into the family and the familiar surroundings of home is recommended before planning his return to the demands of employment. While reintegration into the family, the community, and workplace can occur simultaneously, this is not the usual experience.

While walking with the lower extremity prosthesis increases, gait deviations should be corrected and gait aids decreased when indicated. Instruction in how to vary the number of stump socks as stump size fluctuates should be reviewed. An assessment of stump and prosthetic hygiene should be made. A new set of prosthetic functional goals should be presented.

In follow-up for the upper extremity amputee, a careful charting of prosthetic wearing and functional use should be performed. Prosthetic functional or discomfort problems should be solved before the patient finishes the follow-up appointment. If these problems are not resolved early in the follow-up period, the prosthesis will probably be put on a shelf in the closet and soon forgotten. This is a crucial time for the upper extremity amputee and patterns of prosthetic use must be very carefully re-evaluated at each visit. Problem solving between the amputee, the physicians, the therapists, and the prosthetist are vital team functions at this time.

After the first visit, follow-up visits are scheduled at wider intervals, i.e., three months, six months, and eventually an annual visit is recommended. Specific goals to be accomplished during the intervals between return visits

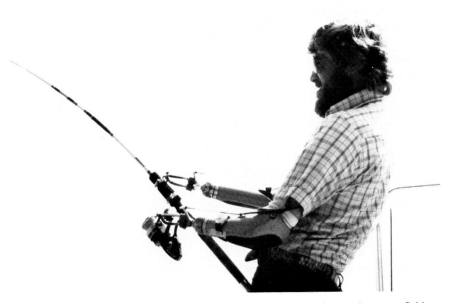

Figure 13.18. Short BE and elbow disarticulation amputee shown deep sea fishing.

should be presented to the amputee by his prosthetic rehabilitation professionals.

Common Burn Amputee Problems

In the burn amputee, skin problems represent the most common complication of prosthetic wearing. These problems range from minor irritations to significant ulcerations and infections. Any minor skin irritation should make one look for a prosthetic fitting or skin organ problem.

The skin problems most frequently seen include:

(1) Folliculitis or infection of a hair follicle is often caused by *Staphylococcal* bacteria resulting in a pustule. This condition is aggravated by prosthetic wear and more commonly seen during hot weather. Constant friction and moisture promote skin maceration and bacteria then invade the skin lesion. This is treated by instructing the patient to wear a thin nylon sheath between the skin and the stump sock. More frequent changing of stump socks can also improve this condition. Prosthetic wearing may need to be discontinued until the folliculitis has subsided.

(2) Furuncles, representing bacterial invasion of the pilosebaceous apparatus, are larger and more painful than the pustules of folliculitis. Treatment usually includes the application of heat until the lesion has pointed and can

be incised and drained. Prosthetic wearing should be discontinued during this acute phase and systemic antibiotics given to hasten local resolution of the infection.

(3) Contact dermatitis may be secondary to skin cream application, soap, wool of the stump sock or the plastic resins used in fabrication of the prosthetic socket. Treatment of this condition includes cool compresses, Spenco Second Skin, antipruritic lotions, or steroid cream.

(4) Post-traumatic epidermoid cysts appear after months or years of prosthetic wear and are most often seen in AK prosthetic users. These cysts are located near the proximal medial portion of the prosthesis near the inguinal region. These cysts enlarge and become sensitive to the touch. Treatment may include local heat and systemic antibiotics. Surgical excision of chronic cysts may be helpful when they are not acutely inflamed.

(5) Nonspecific eczemitization usually appears as a weeping, itching, nonhealing plaque of dermatitis over the distal end of the stump. These lesions may be dry and scaly then suddenly become moist. They can wax and wane over periods of years. This problem may be secondary to edema and congestion of the residual limb often caused by a poorly fitting prosthesis. If this is the cause, the prosthesis should be modified and the chronic plaques treated with a steroid cream.

(6) Intertriginous dermatitis is usually seen in the inguinal region or in any invaginated area of redundant or scarred stump skin. This dermatitis is caused by constant rubbing of the skin surfaces which are in opposition. The presence of salt and moisture from persistent sweating aggravate this condition. Attention to hygienic measures in addition to application of absorbant powders may improve this problem. Also, application of a drying agent such as extra strength aluminum chlorhydrate may help by decreasing the sweating.

(7) Callus formation usually presents as an elevated hyperkeratotic region often appearing at a point of friction or pressure. If the calloused area is sensitive or ulcerated, socket modification should be considered. Also, a change in suspension to decrease pistoning in the prosthesis may be of added benefit.

(8) Ulceration of skin or scar can be caused by excessive socket pressure or excessive motion of the stump in the socket. The pressure or motion may be improved by socket modifications or by adding or decreasing the number of stump socks. A change of prosthetic suspension may decrease pistoning. It is helpful to keep the base of the ulcer clean. If the ulcer is superficial, application of Spenco Second Skin may allow the ulcer to heal while continuing to wear the prosthesis. If the ulcer enlarges or does not heal, prosthetic wearing should be discontinued until the ulcer has completely healed. Resumption of prosthetic wear should be gradual following prosthetic adjustments to avoid recurrence of the ulcer.

(9) A significant decrease in body weight often occurs during the catabolic acute burn period. Once the open burn areas are covered, protein anabolism can begin with the addition of lost pounds. The burn amputee may be fitted with a prosthesis before the preburn body weight has been achieved. This weight gain is more problematic in the lower extremity amputee. This is especially the case at the AK level where a gain of more than five pounds from the time of initial socket fitting may cause a significant prosthetic wearing problem. Of course, it is usually desirable for burn patients to obtain an ideal body weight but the burn amputee must be alert to the need for socket modification if this weight change occurs.

(10) Following prosthetic fitting, limitation of joint motion may increase in the burn amputee for several reasons. Heterotopic bone formation near a joint may enlarge and thereby limit active joint motion. Also, as burn scar matures across a joint, the resultant scar banding may limit previously full joint motion. This banding may need to be revised surgically if the motion limitation interferes with significant joint or prosthetic function. Catastrophic limitation of joint movement may result from immobilization of the joint for a lengthy period of time. If conservative measures such as stretching, paraffin, and ultrasound cannot improve functional movement, then surgical exploration should be considered.

(11) Neuroma formation occurs when any peripheral nerve is transected. It forms as the distal nerve end regenerates into scar tissue forming nodular bundles of axons. When pressure is applied from prosthetic wearing, these neuroma can cause pain. Initially, prosthetic relief can be obtained with socket modifications. Local injection of the neuroma with local anesthetic drugs and long-acting steroids can alleviate the pain. Application of ultrasound for two to three weeks following this injection may provide additional benefit. If injection with local anesthetic drugs and steroids is effective for three to four weeks, longer pain relief can be gained by injecting phenol into the neuroma bulb. Desensitization of the neuroma can sometimes be aided by tapping, massage, and vibration. If these conservative measures are tried to no avail, surgical excision of the neuroma with relocation of the distal nerve ending under soft tissue padding may help this difficult problem.

Persistent, troublesome phantom pain appears more frequently in amputees who have sustained high voltage electrical burns and is more pronounced in upper extremity electrical burn amputees. This phenomenon may occur because of the destructive nature of the high voltage current to the peripheral and sympathetic nervous systems. In severe, chronic phantom pain, all chronic pain treatment modalities should be tried either singly or in combination. However, destructive surgical procedures have not proven to be of long-term benefit and may add to the disability already present.

Problems identified by the patient frequently require assessment by

rehabilitation professionals experienced in amputee and prosthetic management before therapeutic recommendations can be intelligently made. These
professionals must communicate clearly with one another to expedite problem solution. Otherwise, valuable prosthetic function may be lost and the
patient may suffer needless frustration. The amputee should be educated
regarding the cause of the problem and what role he/she can play for future
prevention of a similar problem. Problem areas which are not quickly

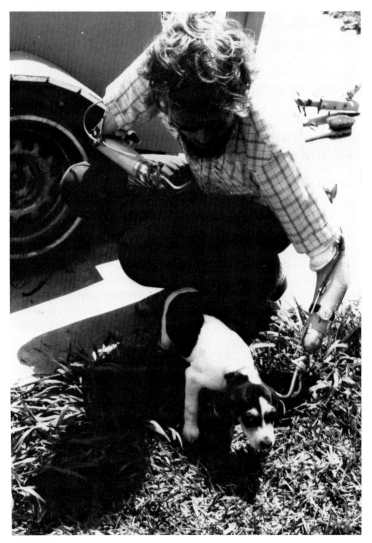

Figure 13.19. Successful prosthetic rehabilitation includes more than wearing and
returning to work.

resolved require multidisciplinary input and close follow-up until they are resolved. If resolution is not easily obtained, major changes in prosthetic components and socket design are necessary. If these prosthetic changes cannot solve the problem, limb revision should be considered and the pros and cons of yet another surgery should be explained to the amputee.

Revision surgery should not be recommended lightly. Further surgery not only carries the risks of any amputation surgery, but often brings up forgotten and unpleasant associations with the original amputation period. A careful discussion concerning the amount of soft tissue and bone revision, in addition to the assurance of good pain control, will often help alleviate some of the presurgical apprehension. Also, an honest appraisal of the time from revision until a prosthesis can be worn helps the patient in planning his life following the revision.

The burn amputee runs the risk of becoming a victim of the famous Latin dictum in medicine "*PRIMUM NON NOCERE.*" Replacement of the lost limb with a prosthesis can often result in harm to the physical body and the psyche. This is found to be the case when a prosthesis is prescribed, fabricated, and fitted with no prior preparation of the amputee's body or mind. It is exacerbated when the patient is handed the prosthesis and summarily sent home to fend for himself. This is a mimicry of rehabilitation and can only result in prosthetic functional disappointment. Maximal prosthetic expectation and adaptation can best be achieved when the needs of the patient are considered and fulfilled as nearly as possible. Meeting these specialized needs requires the experience and knowledge of the physician, the prosthetist, the psychologist, the social worker, and the therapist who are willing to take the time necessary to listen to the patient and try to discern his interpretation of his burn amputation experience. The entire burn amputee rehabilitation process essentially becomes a period of mutual education between the amputee and his prosthetic rehabilitation professionals (Fig. 13.19).

ADDITIONAL READINGS

1. American Academy of Orthopaedic Surgeons: *Atlas of Limb Prosthetics. Surgical and Prosthetic Principles.* St. Louis, C.V. Mosby Company, 1981.
2. Bender LF: *Prostheses and Rehabilitation after Arm Amputation.* Springfield, IL, Charles C Thomas, 1974.
3. Bunnell S: The management of the nonfunctional hand reconstruction vs. prosthesis. *Artif Limbs* 4:76–102, 1957.
4. Carlen PL, Wall PD, Nadvorna H, et al: Phantom limbs and related phenomena in recent traumatic amputations. *Neurology* 28:211–217, 1978.
5. Davies EJ, Friz BR, Cleppinger FW: Amputees and their prostheses. *Artif Limbs* 14:19–48, 1970.
6. Foort J: How amputees feel about amputation. *Orthot Prosthet* 28:21–27, 1974.
7. Friedman LW: *The Surgical Rehabilitation of the Amputee.* Springfield, IL, Charles C Thomas, 1978.
8. Gillis L: *Amputations.* New York, Grune and Stratton, 1954.

9. Gillis L: *Artificial Limbs.* London, Pitman Medical Publishing Co., Ltd., 1957.
10. Henderson WR, Smyth GE: Phantom limbs. *J Neurol Neurosurg Psychiatr* 11:88–112, 1948.
11. Kegel B, Carpenter ML, Burgess EM: Functional capabilities of lower extremity amputees. *Arch Phys Med Rehabil* 59:109–119, 1978.
12. Kerr D, Brunnstrom S: *Training of the Lower Extremity Amputee.* Springfield, IL, Charles C Thomas, 1956.
13. Kostuik JP, Gillespie R: *Amputation Surgery and Rehabilitation. The Toronto Experience.* New York, Churchill Livingstone, 1981.
14. LaBorde TC, Meier RH III: Amputations resulting from electrical injury: A review of 22 cases. *Arch Phys Med Rehabil* 59:134–137, 1978.
15. Levy SW: The skin problems of the lower extremity amputee. *Artif Limbs* 3:20–35, 1956.
16. Munroe B, Nasca RJ: Rehabilitation of the upper extremity traumatic amputee. *Milit Med* 140:402–409, 1975.
17. Murdock G: Amputation surgery in the lower extremity. *Prosthet Ortho Int,* 1977.
18. Murdock G: Amputation surgery in the lower extremity. Part II. *Prosthet Orthot Int* 183–192, 1977.
19. Santschi W: *Manual of Upper Extremity Prosthetics.* Dept. of Engineering, University of California, Los Angeles, 1958.
20. Sherman RA, Sherman CJ, Gall NG: A survey of current phantom limb treatment in the United States. *Pain* 8:85–99, 1980.
21. Slocum DB: *An Atlas of Amputations.* St. Louis, C.V. Mosby Company, 1949.
22. Solem L, Fischer RP, Strate RG: The natural history of electrical injury. *J Trauma* 17:487–492, 1977.
23. Taylor CL: The biomechanics of control in upper extremity prosthesis. *Artif Limbs* 2:4–25, 1955.
24. Tooms R: Amputation surgery in the upper extremity. *Orthop Clin North Am* 3:383–395, 1972.

14

Pain Management

JANET A. MARVIN
DAVID M. HEIMBACK

Have you ever burned yourself on a skillet or iron or spilled hot coffee or hot water on your skin? Have you ever had a skinned knee? We all have and we all know the pain associated with such injuries. Therefore, we imagine that the patient with a 30 or 50% burn must have 50–100 times the amount of pain we have suffered. Have you ever had a headache that was relentless? Was it worse at night when you were alone and could imagine all sorts of awful reasons for the headache such as a cerebral aneurysm or a tumor? Yes, all pain becomes worse when we experience feelings of aloneness, fear, or grief. It is no wonder then that burn patients experience intolerable pain and that friends, family, and staff express great sympathy for the burn patient and his/her pain.

How much pain does a burn patient have? What are the characteristics of this pain? When does it occur? Is it intermittent or constant? Does it vary from patient to patient? Does it vary in the same patient from time to time? Can we measure it or quantify it? Can we prevent it or treat it? If treated, will the patient become an addict? What are the realities of the pain problem and the pain management in the burn patient?

Unfortunately, there are many preconceived ideas about pain and pain management in the burn patient. Many nurses, physicians, and therapists repeatedly tell patients: "There is no way we can relieve all of your pain, you will just have to bear it", or "No, I am sorry, we can't give you narcotics, you will become addicted", or "Now Mr. Jones, it's only been four hours since your last shot, can't you tough it out a little longer?" Also, nurses argue with other nurses, with physicians, and with therapists about the amount of pain the patient has or the amount of relief that the patient gets from a certain therapy. Nurses and therapists also often attribute the reason for leaving burn care to their inability to deal with the patient's pain complaints.

So what do we really know about the burn patient and his pain? What attempts have we made to describe, measure, or study the factors related to

311

pain in the burn patient? What therapeutic modalities have we tried and how effective are they? Can we reduce the patient's pain and the stress on the staff or is this just a "pipe dream?" To examine these questions and to develop a protocol for pain management, the medical and nursing literature for the past 20 years has been reviewed.

Defining Pain

To begin, one must define the problem, the contributing factors, and the latest theories for the explanation of pain. To communicate our ideas about pain and pain relief, it is helpful to look at a few definitions. The Subcommittee on Taxonomy of the International Association for the Study of Pain has recommended the following definitions (22):

Pain: An unpleasant sensory and emotional experience associated with actual or potential tissue damage, or described in terms of such damage.

Analgesia: Absence of pain or noxious stimulation.

Hyperalgesia: Increased sensitivity to noxious stimulation. (This represents a lowered threshold to noxious stimulation not an increased response to suprathreshold stimulation).

Pain Threshold: The least stimulus intensity at which a subject perceives pain.

Pain Tolerance Level: The greatest stimulus intensity causing pain that a subject is prepared to tolerate.

Wall has described the phases or stages of pain perception in response to injury (47). He states that "pain is better classified as an awareness of a need state than as a sensation. Pain serves to promote healing and avoid injury, therefore it is more like the phenomena of thirst and hunger than the sense of hearing or seeing." Therefore, in describing the stages of pain after injury he has divided the experience into three distinct phases: immediate, acute and chronic.

The immediate phase, which may last from seconds to hours, is often characterized by minimal or no pain. This is often seen in men in battle or in any other situation in which the injury may be followed by circumstances in which treatment of the injury does not have the highest biological priority. Medical and lay literature abounds with such anecdotal examples. President Reagan is said not to have realized that he was injured until he was safely on his way to the hospital after the 1981 assassination attempt. Most clinicians caring for burn victims have recorded histories of patients performing heroic tasks after their injury such as rescue of others or walking miles for help. One patient had sustained an 85% mostly third degree burn when his gasoline tanker went off the road and exploded. He walked and hitchhiked 20 miles to reach a hospital for care. Beecher (6), in a study, showed that battle casualties undergoing surgical procedures required much less postoperative pain medication than did a matched group of civilians undergoing elective operations. It was theorized that since soldiers having been injured in battle looked at this as a means of escaping the battlefield area, their perception of their pain was quite different than the civilian who was undergoing an elective procedure. In none of these patients was the patients' perception of pain during the few hours after injury or operation incapacitating because other actions were necessary for their immediate survival or as in the case of the soldiers an injury meant the transfer out of the war zone.

The second stage described by Wall is the acute stage which extends from the first awareness of tissue injury until recovery is assured. Acute pain is a combination of the sensations related to actual or perceived tissue damage and anxiety. Acute pain and acute anxiety are completely coupled and should be treated as one. Both acute pain and acute anxiety are triggered by damage to tissue but are more related to the treatment and the recovery process than to the injury itself. With the burn patient, acute pain continues to occur with each movement of an affected part, with exercise therapy, with debridement, and with many other treatments. Acute anxiety in these patients is a mixture of anxiety about the past, the present, and the future. Many patients experience guilt and anger about how the accident occurred. "Did I cause it? Did someone else cause it? Who is to blame?" They experience anxiety about the present. "What will happen to my house, my car, my family? Can my wife and children manage financially, emotionally? Can I stand the pain, the treatments? Am I going crazy? Will the therapy, the next surgery, the new medicine work? And last, but certainly not least, are the anxieties about the future: will I survive? What will I look like? How will my wife, my family or my friends adjust to my altered appearance?" The patient's awareness of these threats and, therefore, his/her anxiety will "depend on personality, experience, knowledge, information, religion and trust." Acute pain and acute anxiety are coupled to produce the behaviors that we have come to recognize as pain behaviors in the burn patient. The continued or repeated episodes of tissue damage and the prolonged recovery phase in which the outcome is far from predictable contributes to the continuous nature of burn pain. Therefore, acute pain (as defined by Wall) in the burn patient is not just the pain associated with the acute phase of burn care but continues until scar maturation is complete.

The third stage as described by Wall is the phase of chronic pain. This begins after the expected period of recovery and is characterized by unremitting expressions of pain, depression, and periods of inactivity. This is often seen as a mismatch in the amount of pain and the amount of injury. Staff and family become frustrated and suspicious. There is obviously nothing wrong. These patients present special diagnostic and therapeutic challenges to the health care professional. Although few burn patients actually develop chronic pain, as described by Wall, because of the prolonged recovery and scar maturation phase, the pain experienced by burn patients do develop chronic pain problems, but these are truly the minority in that most burn patients will have no pain complaints after complete scar maturation at 12–18 months after injury. For those few patient who do develop chronic pain syndromes, one wonders what if anything could have been done during the acute phase to minimize the occurrence of such problems. Perhaps better pain management, improved psychological support early in the treatment phase, or better explanations of the temporal nature of wound healing could minimize the occurrence of chronic pain problems. This is certainly a fertile area of research even though, of the thousands of burn victims every year, only a few are so affected. Although few burn patients develop chronic pain syndromes as mentioned previously, many have a protracted period of healing which may mimic the patient with chronic pain. These patients are often depressed, go through periods of inactivity and withdrawal and feel isolated and alone which makes the pain associated with scar maturation even more of a problem for these patients.

Neurobiology of Pain

To better understand pain, pain theories, and therapeutic modalities, one should have a concept of how pain is transmitted within the peripheral and central nervous systems (CNS). Casey (8), in a recent review, has shown that the sensation and reaction to pain is a complex integration of responses in the peripheral nervous system and CNS and the modulation of these responses.

Pain receptors found in skin, muscles, and deep tissues are known as nocioceptors and are uniquely sensitive to painful stimuli. The nocioceptors excite afferent discharges in the finely myelinated (A delta) or unmyelinated (C) sensory fibers. The nocioceptive afferent fibers send their messages to the brain primarily through the caudal portion of the trigeminal sensory nucleus, and the dorsal horn of spinal gray matter. This is accomplished when nocioceptive and large myelinated tactile afferents, with cell bodies in the peripheral sensory ganglion, send excitatory presynaptic terminals to the dendrites of deep dorsal horn neurons and to an inhibitory interneuron in the substantia gelatinosa. Within the substantia gelatinosa, the interneurons can suppress the output of the marginal neurons and dorsal horn neurons directly by postsynaptic inhibition of the neurons or indirectly by presynaptic inhibition of nocioceptic afferent terminals. While the marginal neurons and dorsal horn neurons receive nocioceptive input and send axons toward the brain via the contralateral spinothalamic tract, extensive interaction and cross-modulation among neuroelements occur within the substantia gelatinosa. Although the specific dynamics of these interactions are still being investigated, they may explain why rubbing, vibratory stimulation, or innocuous electrical stimulation relieves pain to a moderate degree.

Within the CNS, there are two central pathways; the ascending pathway which mediates pain and the descending pathway which acts to suppress pain. The spinothalamic tract and trigeminal neurons comprise the classical pain pathway projecting directly to the posterior lateral thalamus. Neurophysiological and clinical observations have established that nocioceptive information is transmitted to the posteriolateral thalamus and associated cortex, and there is general agreement that the neurons of this system mediate the discriminative aspects of somesthesis. From our current knowledge it has been suggested that the direct spinothalamic tract system subserves the discriminative aspects of pain, permitting the person to recognize that potential or actual tissue damage has occurred, to localize it in space and time, and perhaps to recognize the physical nature of the stimulus.

Dorsal horn neurons projecting to the medullary or mesencephalic reticular formation form the spinoreticular tract. A substantial proportion of the neurons of the reticular formation within the brainstem and neurons of the medial thalamus respond either differentially or exclusively to noxious stimuli. Experimental evidence with localized lesions indicate that the reticular formation and medial thalamus are an essential part of pain perception. Notwithstanding this evidence, the medial spinoreticulothalamic system cannot be considered an exclusive, specific pain pathway. Many of the reticular and medial thalamic neurons respond to innocuous somatic stimuli and some are activated by visual and auditory input. Observations suggest that the reticular formation is not simply a sensory pathway but undoubtedly mediates motor and autonomic responses as well. The medial thalamus and hypothalamus which receive spinoreticulothalamic tract input, both project to the limbic system forebrain structures, which are known to play an important role in motivational and affective mechanisms. There is evidence that narcotic analgesics act on reticular formation neurons to modulate spinoreticulothalamic activity, perhaps accounting, in part, for the reduction of clinical pain while preserving much of the discriminative ability to recognize noxious stimuli. The neural system mediating motivational and affective mechanisms is not, of course, a specialized pain pathway. Many other inputs are important determinants of affective states and can motivate behavior.

Modulation of pain occurs within the CNS through the descending pain suppression pathways. Sensory experience is thus determined, not only by ongoing afferent activity, but also by activity of sensory control systems in the central nervous system. Research has shown that electrical stimulation within certain parts of the CNS can produce an analgesia which typically outlasts the duration of the stimulation. This stimulation-produced analgesia has been consistently demonstrated by stimulation within the midline raphe nuclei of the brainstem, a group of serotonin-containing neurons forming part of the descending pathway which may attenuate responses to pain. The mechanisms underlying stimulus-produced analgesia appear closely related to the analgesia produced by morphine. Furthermore, naloxone reverses the analgesia of both morphine and stimulus-produced analgesia and repeated exposure to stimulus-produced analgesia or morphine results in the development of tolerance. The possible activation of an active and specific pain suppression mechanism by morphine suggested that there may be endogenous opiate-like substances in the brain which are important for normal, physiological operation of the system.

Through extensive research, opiate receptors have been found at several CNS sites, but are most dense in portions of the limbic system, the medial thalamus, the periaqueductal gray of the midbrain and in the substantia gelatinosa of the spinal cord. Some neurons in these regions are thought to be more important in mediating the affective dimensions of pain. Following the discovery of opiate receptors in the CNS, researchers have found a small peptide with opiate-like pharmacological properties (19). These two pentapetides are called enkephalins; met-enkephalin and leu-enkephalin. The enkephalins are released from the terminals of short-axon interneurons to act as neuromodulators or perhaps neurotransmitters to modulate synaptic transmission between neurons mediating pain. The release of enkephalins from these endings is likely to have powerful effects on synaptic transmission since, like morphine, met-enkephalin has been shown to inhibit cholinergic, adrenergic, and dopaminergic transmission. Decreased monoamine levels in the brain have been associated with depression in man and monoamine oxidase inhibitors have been used successfully to treat depression in man. In experimental animals opiates have been shown to influence amine function and amines have been shown to affect the analgesic actions of opiates (18, 45). For example, many studies show that increasing brain serotonin or blocking cerebral serotonin uptake enhances morphine analgesia (30). There is good evidence to suggest that brain amine mechanisms control pain threshold in part at least by manipulating opiate actions; that brain amines affect mood; and that opiates affect brain amines. It follows that mood alters pain appreciation and that opiates alter mood. Thus, although all of the mechanisms of chemical and physiological modulation of pain, are not well understood, pain is a complex interaction of these integrated biological functions, primarily within the CNS (29).

Pain Theories

Currently there are three major theories of pain: the specificity theory; pattern theory; and the gate control theory. Both the theory of specificity and pattern theory are based on earlier concepts by von Frey and Goldscheider in 1894 and historically are held to be mutually exclusive (44). The theory of specificity holds that pain is a specific modality like vision or hearing with its own central and peripheral apparatus. The specificity theory proposes that a mosaic of specific pain receptors in body tissue projects to a pain center in the brain. It maintains that free nerve endings are pain receptors and generate pain impulses that are carried by A-delta and C fibers in peripheral nerves and by the lateral spinothalamic tract in the spinal cord to a pain center in the thalamus (31, 32). Although this theory may explain the physiological reaction to a noxious agent or tissue injury it does not explain any of the psychological reactions to pain or the perceptions of pain. Furthermore, the pathological pain states of causalgia, phantom limb pain, or peripheral neuralgias dramatically refute the concept of a direct-line nervous system.

The pattern theory maintains that the nerve impulse pattern for pain is produced by intense stimulation of nonspecific receptors since there are "no specific fibers and no specific endings" (41). The theory proposes that all fiber endings are alike, except those that innervate hair cells, so that the pattern for pain is produced by intense stimulation of nonspecific fibers. The physiological research has shown that there is a great degree of physiological specialization. Therefore, the pattern theory of Weddell and Sinclair fails as a satisfactory theory because it ignores the fact of physiologic specialization (41, 49). Built on the frameworks of Goldscheider's concepts also, Livingston (27) was perhaps the first to suggest specific neural mechanisms to account for the remarkable summation phenomena in clinical pain syndromes. He proposed that intense, pathological stimulation of the body sets up reverberating circuits in spinal internuncial pools, or evokes spinal cord activities such as those reflected by the "dorsal root reflex" (3) that can be triggered by normally non-noxious input and generates abnormal volleys that are interpreted centrally as pain. The concepts of central summation and input control explain many of the clinical phenomena of pain but they fail to comprise a satisfactory general theory of pain integrating the diverse theoretical mechanisms of pain.

Melzack and Wall have proposed the gate control theory in which these systems interact to explain the phenomena of pain (31, 32). The systems proposed are that (1) the substantia gelantinosa functions as a gate control system that modulates the afferent patterns before they influence the central transmission cells of the dorsal horn; (2) the afferent patterns in the dorsal column system act, in part at least, as a central control trigger which activates brain processes that influence the modulating properties of the gate control system; and (3) the central transmission cells activate neural mechanism which comprise the action system responsible for response and perception. This theory is a more complete theory and includes not only the theory of specific neuropathways and the concept of summation or modulation but also that modulation can occur from both sensory feedback mechanisms as well as influences of the central nervous system. This theory has been increasingly supported by the latest neurobiological research that suggest a number of integrating functions throughout the CNS which influences the person's perception of pain. The gate control theory and the latest neurophysiological research explain the effectiveness of the many modalities used to manage pain.

Burn Pain

ACUTE OR CHRONIC

According to Loeser (28), acute pain is almost always percipitated by a nocioceptive stimulus and serves as a warning signal to patient and doctor alike. Although environmental and personality factors may modify pain behavior in response to an acute nocioceptive stimulus, they are rarely the predominant factor. In contrast, whatever the course of the chronic pain syndrome, there is little to suggest that the pain is of any value to the patient or the physician as a warning signal and environmental and personality factors play a major role in the genesis of the patients' disability. The literature would lead one to believe that psychological factors predominate in the burn patient's response to pain; yet no one would deny the authenticity of the nocioceptive stimulus in burn pain (2, 3, 39, 43). An attempt to better describe the components of burn pain was undertaken by Charlton et al. (9). Using a series of pain measurement tools and some standard psychological tests to measure anxiety and depression, he observed that each of these psychological factors were apparent at sometime during the test period for most patients. To measure pain in these patients he used the Melzack pain questionnaire and a self-rating on a linear analogue scale. To measure anxiety he used the State-Trait Anxiety Inventory and for depression he used the Zung depression questionnaire.

On the self-rating scale the patients were asked to rate the overall pain experience of their burn injury. It is of interest that the ratings that patients make of their pain were skewed toward the low end of the linear analogue scale with a median pain rating of 1.75 on a 10-point scale. On the McGill Pain Questionaire three subscales were used with these patients. The subscales were: the present pain intensity (PPI), the number of words chosen (NWC) to describe the pain; and the pain rating index (PRI). When burn patients scores were compared with other patients studied by the same investigators the burn patients most closely resembled scores of patients with post-herpetic neuralgia on the present pain intensity scale and the number of words chosen scale. However, on the pain rating index, the burn patient most closely resembled the arthritic patients.

In Charlton's study, burn patients, when compared to other groups of patients, were not especially anxious. In terms of trait anxiety (or proneness to anxiety) the burn patient most closely resembled male college students showing minimal anxiety. On their state anxiety scores the burn patient more closely resembled general medical surgical patients. Trait anxiety is said to be a stable personality factor which predicts state anxiety in ego stress situations, but not in physical danger situations. State anxiety is the transitory anxiety seen when a person is subjected to a temporary emotionally stressful situation. Studies using the State-Trait Anxiety Scale have shown that stable personality factors can not necessarily be used to predict how the patient will function in physical stress situations. Studies by Cromes et al. (11), in burn patients confirmed that trait anxiety did not necessarily predict state anxiety in the real physical threat situation of débridement. Cromes et al. also showed that trait anxiety levels did not change from pre- to post-débridement. In addition, they showed that percentage of the body burned was a better predictor of state anxiety levels in débridement situation and state anxiety levels consistently decreased as treatment progressed. In later work, Cromes et al. (12), using the state anxiety scale, showed that relaxation training was effective in reducing experience of anxiety and pain in a group of burned patients, but that its effectiveness was reduced in the actual débridement situation. Therefore, although burn patients have been described by some as being particularly anxious, other studies have not confirmed this assumption.

Charlton used the Zung scale to measure depression. He found that the majority of patients showed only minimal to mild depression but that a small number of patients showed moderate to severe depression. He also found that patients who were in the hospital more than three weeks all showed increased amounts of depression. Andreasen et al. (2), Jorgensen et al. (23), and Steiner et al. (43) have found variable amounts of depression (ranging from 10% to as much as 50% of patients in some series) in burn patients especially after the second week after injury. Steiner attributed grief and acute grief reactions to what others described as mild depression. As noted by Avni (3), depression often increased the patient's pain behaviors or reactions to pain.

Klein and Charlton (24) studied pain behaviors in burn patients during hydrotherapy and debridement. In this study, they look at pain behaviors, somatic and psychological well-being, criticism and praise of hospital staff, and other patient problems. Their data indicated that: (1) although patients expressed a considerable number of pain behaviors, they expressed a significantly higher frequency of psychological and somatic well-being behaviors (p > 0.05); (2) the frequency of well-being behavior increased more rapidly than the frequency of pain complaints when both were receiving positive reinforcements (p > 0.01); and (3) differences in patient behavior during treatment procedures could not be attributed to size of burn, preinjury psychiatric history, age, or days since onset.

From this review of pertinent literature one could theorize that although much of the patient's perception of pain is derived from nocioceptive stimuli related to movement, exercise therapy, débridement and other pain-producing procedures, the outward manifestation of this perception, i.e., pain behaviors may be related to certain psychological factors such as acute anxiety, helplessness, acute grief reactions and, in some patients, depression. Nevertheless, burn pain should be considered a form of acute pain and should not be confused with chronic pain. Management of burn pain must, therefore, include analgesia for acute severe pain and appropriate management of observed psychological components.

Therapies for the Management of Burn Pain

PHARMACOLOGICAL THERAPIES

Narcotic analgesics remain the drugs of choice for treating severe acute pain. This is the type of pain exhibited by the burn patient during the first few hours after the injury and with each manipulation of the wound. These manipulations may occur each time the patient moves, is exercised or when his/her wounds are cleansed and debrided. The most severe pain occurs with exercise and the daily cleansing and débridement of the wound. Medical and parmedical personnel have acknowledged that these drugs can provide prompt relief when used in adequate doses (33). Because of the fear of producing respiratory depression and addiction, physicians commonly prescribe insufficient amounts of narcotic analgesia for patients with excruciating, acute pain, even though it is well known that pain antagonizes the depressant effects of narcotics. Therefore, with careful titration of dose and frequent evaluation of effect, adequate relief of pain without respiratory depression can be provided. Orgain et al. (35) reported that even when adequate doses of pain medication were prescribed for a group of burn patients, nurses administered less than one-half the daily dose that any patient could have received. This finding was at a time when the nursing staff complained that the physicians were not ordering adequate amounts of pain medication. Addiction is a frequent concern of physicians and nurses alike when prescribing and administering narcotics. Addiction is of no concern when narcotics are prescribed in adequate doses for a few days for acute pain. Tolerance does develop in patients who receive narcotics over extended periods of time and will require increases for effective dosage. A survey of 54 burn care facilities in 1978 showed that the most frequently prescribed narcotics for the management of acute burn pain were morphine and meperidine. Of the units treating adults, 96% reported using whenever necessary narcotics throughout the patient's treatment course. On the other hand, only eight percent of the units treating children used narcotics stronger than oral codeine. Sixty-eight percent used acetaminophen or acetaminophen with codeine and 24% used no routine pain medications.

The following opium alkaloids, semi-synthetic and synthetic derivatives may be used for the relief of acute pain (1, 20):

Morphine Sulfate

Morphine sulfate may be administered intravenously in adults ranging in dosage from 2.5–15 mg diluted in four to five ml of water for injection and injected slowly over a period of four to five minutes. Intramuscularly, the dose should be one-tenth to two-tenths of a mg per kg of body weight. The dose may need to be adjusted upward to produce desired effects in severe pain or when given for longer periods of time. The oral route is rarely used because of the reduced effectiveness of this drug in oral preparations. The desired analgesic effect of morphine is usually seen in approximately 20 minutes when given intravenously and within 30–60 minutes when given intramuscularly. Maximal respiratory depression usually occurs within 7–10 minutes when given intravenously and within 20–30 minutes when given intramuscularly. Respiratory depression may be reversed with naloxone.

Codeine

Codeine offers little advantage parenterally over morphine and has an analgesic equivalent of 120 mg to 10 mg of morphine when administered hypodermically. Orally, a dose of codeine of 32 mg is approximately equianalgesic with 325–600 mg of aspirin. When the two drugs are combined, the analgesic effect equals or sometimes exceeds 65 mg of codeine.

Hydromorphone Hydrochloride or Sulfate (Dilaudid)

Recent control studies have shown that Dilaudid is approximately eight times more potent on a milligram basis than morphine. In addition, hydromorphone is better absorbed orally than morphine. It has been shown to be approximately one-fourth to one-half as active orally as intramuscularly. The recommended dosage in adults is two mg intramuscularly or intravenously (slow) and may be increased to four mg for severe pain. The initial oral dose is two mg but may be increased as necessary. Respiratory depression is similar for equianalgesic doses to morphine.

Meperidine Hydrochloride (Demerol)

Meperidine hydrochloride is less effective than morphine in relieving severe pain. Equianalgesic doses of meperidine and morphine produce a similar degree of respiratory depression; this effect may be reversed with a narcotic antagonist such as naloxone. The usual adult dose is 100 mg (50–150 mg) given either intramuscularly or intravenously (slow). In children, the dose is one to one and one-half mg per kg of body weight (maximum dose, 100 mg) administered intramuscularly or orally. Meperidine is less effective orally than parenterally.

Pentazocine Hydrochloride or Lactate (Talwin)

Pentazocine is both an agonist of the morphine type and an antagonist of the nalorphine type. It is effective for moderate pain but is less effective than morphine in relieving severe pain. The analgesic potency of pentazocine on a milligram basis is approximately one-third of that of morphine when administered parenterally and approximately equal to that of codeine when administered orally. Pentazocine may produce respiratory depression, but it is less marked than with morphine. Naloxone is an effective antagonist in the treatment of overdosages with pentazocine.

Methadone Hydrochloride

Methadone is slightly more potent than morphine on a milligram basis when administered subcutaneously, and it is relatively more effective orally. Maximal analgesic doses depress respiration to a greater extent than do equivalent doses of morphine. The recommended dosage is 2.5–10 mg intramuscularly or subcutaneously in adults and the dose is only repeated when pain returns. Orally, for sustained acute pain, the recommended dosage is 2.5–10 mg every six to eight hours as required. Because it is effective orally and has a longer duration of action, it has become a major constituent of a "pain cocktail", frequently used for chronic or long-term pain problems.

ANESTHETIC AGENTS

Although little is written about the use of narcotic and synthetic narcotics in the treatment of burn patients, much has appeared in the recent literature about the use of anesthetic agents for débridement and dressing changes for burn patients. Of particular interest are the subanesthetic doses of ketamine, methoxyflurane, and 50% nitrous oxide. The experience of Demling et al. (14), Slogoff et al. (42), and others (37, 48, 53) have shown subanesthetic doses of ketamine to produce satisfactory, short-acting (15-minute) analgesia, complete amnesia, and rapid recovery. Most reports indicate that there is no need for long pretreatment starvation and that patients are able to resume eating within one hour of the procedure. All reports indicate that tolerance develops in all patients receiving more than two exposures. The usual initial dose is one and one-half to two mg per kg given intramuscularly or about 15% of the usual intramuscular anesthetic dose. Although frequently touted as a major side-effect, the incidence of unpleasant emergent reactions are relatively infrequent if the patient has received suitable premedication and pretreatment explanation of the dream state that this drug produces. A major advantage to the use of ketamine in subanesthetic doses is that it does not depress respiration and because muscle tone is maintained the airway remains protected.

Oduro (34) has reported the use of methoxyflurane (Penthrane Analgizer) to produce analgesia for burn dressing changes in children. In his experience, the use of this self-administered inhalation analgesic produced excellent pain control. In his study the duration of each exposure was 15–20 minutes with one to twelve exposures per patient. Patients were not starved prior to the procedure and received no premedication. Patients recovered rapidly and resumed eating with no problems. In this group of patients, the Analgizer produced excellent analgesia and amnesia without respiratory depression. Baskett et al. (4, 5), have reported the use of neuroleptanalgesia (dehydrobenzperidol and phenoperidine) and 50% nitrous oxide in the management of burns during débridement and dressing changes. The addition of 50% nitrous oxide to neuroleptanalgesia decreased the incidence of depressed respiratory function and provided a safe, short-acting analgesia. These patients were not given anything to eat for six hours prior to the procedure but resumed normal oral intake within two hours.

Filkins et al. (16), reported on the use of 50% nitrous oxide alone in the treatment of 52 adult patients receiving 632 treatments (range, 1–52 per patient). This was a self-administrated anesthetic and required that the patient hold either a mouth piece or face mask to receive the drug. The safety of this procedure requires that it be self-administered so that the patient does not become anesthetized since 50% nitrous oxide can produce complete anesthesia in some patients. Each patient received morphine and Vistaril pretreatment but none of the patients were starved pretreatment. All patients were able to resume eating after treatment. Of all patients treated, only 3.8% developed side-effects (nausea in one and nonspecific tremors in another) and one patient reported no pain relief. There was no evidence of respiratory depression in this group of patients and the drowsiness seen in some patients wore off in one or two minutes after discontinuing the use of this self-administered anesthetic.

OTHER TECHNIQUES OF PAIN MANAGEMENT

Since the psychological factors such as anxiety, acute grief reactions, and depression have been shown to occur with great frequency in burn patients and since these factors are known to affect the patient's perception of pain, techniques to reduce these factors may also be effective in pain management. In this respect, many behavioral techniques have been used with varying degrees of success. The behavioral approaches which have been used with burn patients include: behavioral modification (operant conditioning or contracting), desensitization, imagery, modeling, stress reduction technique, and hypnosis. The most frequently written about techniques include behavioral modification, stress reduction techniques, and hypnosis.

Wernick et al. (51), Shorkey and Taylor (39), and Zide and Pardoe (54) have presented descriptions of behavior modification procedures and have presented case reports of the successful use of these techniques. Likewise,

Simons and McFadd (40) have reported on the effectiveness of contracting in the management of pain and pain behaviors in the burn patient.

Wernick et al. (52) and Weinstein (50) have reported the use of stress reduction techniques with burn patients. Stress reduction techniques usually require two or more training sessions in which the patient is taught certain physical and/or psychological stress reduction techniques and allowed to practice these techniques before they are actually in a situation to use them, i.e., during débridement. Then usually the patient is coached through one or more treatments in which these techniques are used. These techniques include: deep breathing, autogenic relaxation, muscle relaxation, distraction techniques such as music or other sounds, focusing on environmental aspects or imagery; or a combination of two or more of the above techniques. Wernick et al. (51) reported significant improvement in all nine variables tested (unauthorized request, self-rating physical, self-rating emotional, tank rating subject, tank rating staff, compliance, nurses rating, state anxiety ratings and trait anxiety ratings) from pre- to post-treatment and continued improved ratings in all but three areas (unauthorized request, compliance, and nurses' ratings) in a follow-up study.

Hypnosis was first reported by Crasilneck et al. (10) for management of burn pain. Since then many have acclaimed its effectiveness in some patients. Studies by Dahinterova (13), Finer and Nylen (17), Hartley (21), Pellicone (36), Bernstein (7), LeBau (26), and Wakeman and Kaplan (46) have found hypnosis useful in both adults and children. Schafer (38) noted that after initially establishing rapport and preparing the patients for the hypnotic procedure, treatment could be facilitated by means of a personalized tape to meet the patient's needs when the hypnotherapist is not present. Also, he found that some patients were able to continue the techniques alone and that autohypnosis could be encouraged by the staff with these patients. Wakeman and Kaplan (46) found, as had others, that hypnosis was a useful adjunct to pain management, ego strengthening, and management of psychological crises in the management of burn patients. They also found that the use of hypnosis had a positive impact on the burn unit staff, enhancing their attitudes about themselves as more effective and interpersonally involved caregivers.

In addition, group and individual psychotherapy has been shown to be effective in reducing pain behaviors in some patients (15, 25). Group sessions and peer pressure have been shown to exert a tremendous impact on the control of maladaptive pain behaviors. Unfortunately, as with all other modalities studied, this does not work in all situations. As pointed out by several authors, group pressure only works if the group is relatively cohesive and remains so. The introduction of a new, noncompliant member may disrupt the effect of the group on all group members. This is often seen when introducing a small child or demented patient into the group. For the milieu type of therapy to work, the staff must be knowledgable about the placement of such patients in the unit and the inclusion or exclusion of such patients from the group.

Individual psychotherapy may be needed by some patients. This usually includes patients who have had maladjustment problems previously, demented patients, or patients who are having a particularly bad time with an acute grief reaction or severe depression. Usually if the patient requires individual psychotherapy the patient's family or significant others may need psychological counseling as well.

In addition to the use of behavioral therapy some of these patients will benefit from the use of pharmacological agents to reduce the psychological stressors. Steiner and Clark (43) described a time contingent approach to the pharmacological management of these problems. They divided the injury/recovery process into three stages: stage 1, the stage of physiological emergency; stage 2, the stage of psychological emergency; and stage 3, the stage of social emergency. They related the psychiatric considerations of each of the stages in relation to the patient's grief response. In stage 1, the patient experienced acute grief which is a human response to loss. Stage 2, uncomplicated grief, begins when the patient becomes aware of the full realization of his losses, and stage 3, when the patient accepts his losses emotionally, comes to terms with reality and returns to the best possible level of functioning.

The main complication of stage 1 is delerium, characterized by global but reversible impairment in thinking, memory, and perception. The patient may experience hallucinations, delusions, confabulations, apathy, aggitation, and withdrawal. Delerium is a symptom of cerebral insufficiency often caused by physiological disorders of toxemia, metabolic imbalance, anoxia or cardiovascular insufficiency. The first step in the management of these acute deleriums is to diagnose and correct any underlying physiological problems. To treat the psychological parameters and agitation in these patients, haloperidol and chlorpromazine are most beneficial. Benzadiazepines such as diazepam are of little value, especially in the anoxic or elderly patient. They should only be used in patients with known drug or alcohol addiction during the early phases of care.

During the second stage, the patient becomes aware of the realities of the situation. What makes this the stage of psychological emergency is the fact that long-term adjustment is dependent on how the patient handles his grief or mourning process. Complications at this stage occur when the patient's grief work is arrested in a regressive episode. Patients during this phase often become dependent, hostile, and depressed or withdrawn. Pain becomes a major focus and may become a strategy to negotiate dependency needs rather than a physical complaint. Pharmacologically it is important to provide optimal analgesia for pain. Treating the psychological sequela at this time may be helped with: hydroxyzine, which enhances the effects of pain medication while producing anxiety control or diazapam and chlordiazepoxide for better anxiety control. These drugs are frequently given at bedtime to induce more effective sleep. Antidepressants are rarely needed at this time except in the occasional elderly patient whose depression may interfere with alimentation and sleep.

Stage 3 begins with hospital discharge and is usually characterized by the patient completing the mourning process. In some cases, true depression or post-traumatic neurosis may appear in the patient who cannot complete the normal grieving process. At this stage antidepressants may be helpful in treating depression and minor tranquilizers in treating neuroses.

A Prescription for Pain Management in the Burn Patient

EMERGENT PHASE (72 HOURS)

Narcotic Analgesia

Intravenous or intramuscular morphine in adults administered in small but frequent doses. Intravenous or intramuscular morphine administered to children. (If the child can take oral medications, a pain cocktail of Demerol®, Phenergan®, and Thorazine® (DPT) in cherry syrup may be used.)

ACUTE PHASE (72 HOURS UNTIL WOUND HEALING IS ALMOST COMPLETE)

Narcotic Analgesia

Intravenous or intramuscular morphine may be continued in patients who must remain intubated for pulmonary problems. Oral pain cocktail (methadone, vistaril, and acetominophine in cherry syrup) given every six hours, not on a pain-contingent basis, is an excellent substitute for as warranted narcotics. As warranted narcotics should be given during the first 24 hours of dosage with a pain cocktail to allow the analgesic level to be attained. After this, our experience is that patients usually do not need other narcotics except for the most painful procedures such as débridement.

Intramuscular or orally administered narcotics may be used as premedications in conjunction with 50% nitrous oxide self-administered to provide optimal pain relief during débridement and dressing changes. As noted previously, others have successfully used ketamine in a similar fashion.

In children, the DPT cocktail as described above may be used on a nonpain-contingent basis with the addition of a narcotic or 50% nitrous oxide or ketamine for débridement procedures.

Behavioral Therapies

Behavior modification techniques, stress reduction techniques, or hypnosis may be useful adjuncts to pain management during this phase of care.

Anxiety Reduction Medications

As noted by Steiner and Clark (43), drugs such as Atarax®, Valium®, or Haldol® may help with the anxiety during this phase. Our own experience when using the oral pain cocktail is that these drugs are rarely needed. An occasional patient may need an additional medication at night for sleep; in this case, Haldol® may be used.

After Healing Phase

Prior to discharge, all narcotic analgesics including pain cocktails should have been gradually discontinued. The discharged patient should go home on acetominophine and codeine, or its equivalent, but nothing stronger if his wounds are primarily healed. Antidepressants or mild tranquilizers may be useful in a few of these patients experiencing continued psychological sequela.

Conclusion

Pain management is a significant, complex problem in the burn patient. Our ability to deal with it effectively requires a knowledge of the neurobiology of pain, pain theories, and the techniques of pain management available to us. It also requires a certain amount of relearning on the part of health professionals to accept newer pharmacological and psychological therapies without prejudice. Holding on to old ideas about addiction or being skeptical about hypnosis or imagery or other stress reduction techniques will not allow us to treat the patient in the most efficacious manner. A rational approach to the reduction of pain management problems may significantly effect the psychological outcome of the patient and reduce stress on the staff so that everyone benefits. Therefore, pain management is not only an important part of the patient's management but also in the effective management of our staff.

REFERENCES

1. AMA Department of Drugs: *AMA Drug Evaluations*, ed. 2. Acton, MA, Publishing Science Group, Inc., 1973, pp. 249–260.
2. Andreasen NJ, Noyes R Jr, Hartford CE: Factors influencing adjustment of burn patient during hospitalization. *Psychosom Med* 34:517, 1972.
3. Avni J: The severe burns. *Adv Psychosom Med* 10:57–77, 1980.
4. Baskett PJF: Analgesia for the dressing of burns in children: A method using neurolept-analgesia and Entonox. *Postgrad Med J* 48:138–142, 1972.
5. Baskett PJF, Hyland J, Deane M, et al: Analgesia for patient dressing in children. *Br J Anaesth* 41:684–688, 1969.
6. Beecher HK: Relationship of significance of wound to pain experience. *JAMA* 161:1609–1613, 1958.
7. Bernstein NR: Obervations on the use of hypnosis with burned children on a pediatric ward. *Int J Clin Exp Hypnosis* 13:1–10, 1965.
8. Casey KL: The neurobiology of pain. University of Washington. *Medicine* 7:5–11, 1980.
9. Charlton JE, Klein R, Gagliardi G: Assessment of pain relief in patients with burn. Presented to the Third World Congress on Pain at the International Association for the

Study of Pain. Edinburgh, Scotland, September 4–11, 1981.

10. Crasilneck HB, Stieman JA, Wilson BJ, et al: Use of hypnosis in the management of patients with burns. *JAMA* 158:103–106, 1955.

11. Cromes GF, Hedl JJ, McCallum PS, et al: Hydrotherapy, Débridement, Trait-State Anxiety and Psycho-emotional Intervention. Presented at the American Burn Association. San Antonio, TX, April 1–3, 1976.

12. Cromes GF, McDonald M, Robinson C: The Effects of Relaxation Training on Anxiety and Pain during Burn Wound Debridement. Presented at the American Burn Association, San Antonio, TX, March 27–29, 1980.

13. Dahinterova J: Some experience with the use of hypnosis in the treatment of burns. *Int J Clin Exp Hypnosis* 15:49–53, 1967.

14. Demling RH, Ellerbee S, Jarrett F: Ketamine anesthesia for tangential excision of burn eschar: A burn unit procedure. *J Trauma* 18:269–270, 1978.

15. Fagerhaugh Shizuko Y: Pain expression and control on a burn care unit. *Nursing Outlook* 22:645–650, 1974.

16. Filkins SA, Cosgrav P, Marvin JA, et al: Self-administered anesthesia: A method of pain control. *J Burn Care Rehab* 2:33–34, 1981.

17. Finer BL, Nylen BO: Cardiac arrest in the treatment of burns, and report on hypnosis as a substitute for anesthesia. *Plast Reconstr Surg* 27:49–55, 1961.

18. Genovese E, Zonta N, Mantegazza P: Decreased antinoceptive activity of morphine in rats pretreated intraventricularly with 5,6-dihydoxy-tryptamine, a long-lasting selective depletor of grain serotonin. *Psychopharmacologia* 32:359–364, 1973.

19. Goldstein A: Endorphins and pain: A critical review. In Beers RF Jr, Bussett EG: *Mechanisms of Pain and Analgesis Compounds.* New York, Raven Press, 1979, pp. 249–260.

20. Goodman LS, Gilman A: *The Pharmacological Basis of Therapeutics.* New York, Macmillan Publishing Co., Inc., 1975, pp. 245–283.

21. Hartley RB: Hypnosis for alleviation of pain in treatment of burns. Case report. *Arch Phys Med* 49:39–41, 1968.

22. IASP Subcommittee on Taxonomy: Pain terms: A list with definitions and notes on usage. *Pain* 6:249–252, 1979.

23. Jorgensen JA, Brophy JL: Psychiatric treatment of severely burned adults. *Psychosomatics* 14:331–335, 1973.

24. Klein RM, Charlton JE: Behavioral observation and analysis of pain behavior in critically burned patients. *Pain* 9:28–40, 1980.

25. Kueffner M: Passage through hospitalization of severely burned, isolated school children. *Commun Nurs Res* 76:181–197, 1976.

26. LeBau WL: Adjunctive trance therapy with severely burned children. *Int J Child Psychother* 2:80–92, 1973.

27. Livingston WK: *Pain Mechanisms.* New York, Macmillan Publishing Co., Inc., 1943.

28. Loeser JD: A definition of pain. University of Washington. *Medicine* 7:3–4, 1980.

29. Marsden CD: The emotion of pain and its chemistry. Brain and Mind. ABA Foundation Symposium 69 (new series). New York, Excepta Medica, 1979, pp. 305–313.

30. Messing RB, Lytle LD: Serotonin-containing neurons: Their possible role in pain and analgesia. *Pain* 4:1–21, 1977.

31. Melzack R, Taenzer P: Concepts of pain perception and therapy. *Geriatrics* 32:44–48, 1977.

32. Melzack R, Wall PD: Pain mechanisms: A new therapy. *Science* 150:971–979, 1965.

33. Novoa J: Large-dose Morphine for Pain Control. Presented at the American Burn Association, San Antonio, TX, March 27–29, 1980.

34. Oduro KA: Experiences with the penthrane analgizer. *Ghana Med J* 43–47, 1971.

35. Orgain C, Marvin J, Heimbach DM: Exploring Pain Management Practices. Presented at the American Burn Association, New Orleans, LA, March 15–17, 1979.

36. Pellicone AJ: Hypnosis as adjunct to treatment of burns. *Am J Clin Hypnosis* 2:153–156, 1960.
37. Sadrove MS, Shulman M, Hatano S, et al: Analgesia effects of ketamine administered in subdissociative doses. *Anesth Analg Curr Res* 50:452–457, 1971.
38. Schafer DW: Hypnosis use on a burn unit. *Int J Clin Exp Hypnosis* 23:1–14, 1975.
39. Shorkey CT, Taylor JE: Management of maladaptive behavior of a severely burned child. *Child Welfare* L2:543–547, 1973.
40. Simons RD, McFadd A: Behavioral Contracting in a Burn Care Facility: Strategy for Patient Participation. Presented at the American Burn Association, Anaheim, CA, March 31–April 2, 1977.
41. Sinclair DC: Cutaneous sensation and doctrine of specific energy. *Brain* 78:584–614, 1955.
42. Slogoff S, Allen GW, Wessels JV, et al: Clinical experience with subanesthetic ketamine. *Anesth Analg Curr Res* 53:354–358, 1974.
43. Steiner H, Clark WR: Psychiatric complications of burned adults: A classification. *J Trauma* 17:134–143, 1977.
44. Sweet WH: Handbook. *Physiology* 1:459, 1959.
45. Verdernikov YUP, Aflikanov II: On the role of a central adrenergic mechanism in morphine analgesic action. *J Pharm Pharmacol* 21:845–847, 1969.
46. Wakeman RJ, Kaplan JZ: An experimental study of hypnosis in painful burns. *Am J Clin Hypnosis* 21:3–12, 1978.
47. Wall PD: On the relationship of injury to pain. *Pain* 6:253–264, 1979.
48. Ward CM, Diamond AW: An appraisal of ketamine in the dressing of burns. *Postgrad Med J* 5:222–223, 1976.
49. Weddell G: Somesthesis and the chemical senses. *Ann Rev Psychol* 6:119–136, 1955.
50. Weinstein DJ: Imagery and relaxation with a burn patient. *Behav Res Ther* 14:481, 1976.
51. Wernick RL, Brantley PJ, Malcom R: Behavioral techniques in the psychological rehabilitation of burn patients. *Int J Psychiat Med* 10:145–150, 1980–1981.
52. Wernick RL, Jaremko ME, Taylor PW: Pain management in severely burned adults: A test of stress inoculation. *J Behav Med* 4:103–109, 1981.
53. White PF, Way WL, Trevor AJ: Ketamine—Its pharmacology and therapeutics uses. *Anesthesiology* 56:119–136, 1982.
54. Zide B, Pardoe R: The use of behavior modification therapy in a recalcitrant burned child. *Plast Reconstr Surg* 57:378–382, 1976.

15

Psychosocial Aspects

G. FRED CROMES, JR.

Introduction

Adjustment to severe burn injury is influenced by preinjury individual and family stability, hospital and outpatient treatment environment, sex, age, percentage of burn, location of the burn injury, and community and family support systems. Also involved are the needs, attitudes, and coping behaviors of the patient, family, members of the burn treatment team, and individuals that comprise the extra-family support system. There has been extensive study of these factors which has been summarized by Achterberg-Lawlis and Kenner (1); Bowden et al. (7), and Malt (16). These research studies have suggested some general characteristics of the adjustment process:

(1) Factors which increase the probability of burn injury are family disorganization, personal adjustment problems, substance abuse, life stress levels, carelessness, poor judgment, impulsive outbursts, and unsafe home, work, and transportation conditions (5, 8, 12, 13, 20).

(2) Adjustment to hospital and treatment procedures is related to mental status, severity and location of burn injury, frequency of visitation from family and friends, pain tolerance, attitudes of the members of the burn treatment team and preburn physical and/or psychological problems (4, 6, 9, 14, 21).

(3) Coping with the ramifications of burn injury following hospital discharge is related to the above factors in addition to disfigurement, functional limitations, pending litigation, and availability of family and community support (2, 6, 9, 10, 14, 21).

(4) Approximately 25–30% of adults have some emotional difficulty at one year after burn. Women seem to have more problems related to cosmesis and men with function, but this is debatable. About 50% of children have emotional problems one year after burn, especially when there are unstable family conditions. Adolescents experience more turmoil than children or adults as they deal with the bodily changes that disrupt the already dynamic process of identity establishment during these years (2, 3, 9, 14, 15, 21).

(5) Long-term emotional problems are more frequent in the presence of burns greater than 30% total body surface area, hand or facial burns, and preburn psychopathology (4, 9, 14).

(6) Sexual dysfunction occurs in approximately 25% of adults at one year after burn. Men experience loss of libido more than impotence, whereas women experience orgasmic dysfunction more than loss of libido. Disfigurement is an important concomitant of these problems in both men and women (2, 7).

(7) Approximately 25% of adults experience restrictions in extra-family social participation, with a slight trend for men having more problems than women. Married men tend toward increased family involvement relative to preburn patterns. Divorce rates after burn are no greater than the average for the normal population. About 50% of children experience social withdrawal, especially those older than three or four years of age (2, 3, 6, 10, 14, 19).

(8) Approximately 75% of working adults return to work; but about 50% of them change jobs. Disfigurement of the face is apparently an important factor in these job changes. The interval between burn injury and return to work varies with percentage of burn, but is usually no sooner than six months in burns greater than 30% (6, 9, 18).

Because there is no "typical" burn patient, family member, employer, coworker, or friend or acquaintance, it is essential to be aware of specific and unique patient reactions and behaviors. This enables the burn team to provide psychological intervention that will have the greatest possible positive impact on the person's coping with the treatment and rehabilitation program. It is equally important for the staff to be aware of their reactions and behaviors if this process is to be facilitated.

Issues to be addressed in this chapter focus upon interventions for a variety of emotional-behavioral problems of patients, family, and staff as all work toward the goal of the patient returning to a satisfying life-style. Suggestions are as concrete and practical as possible given the inherent ambiguous nature of dealing with the very unique aspects of each person involved in this psychosocial rehabilitative process. First, two models are described which are relevant to understanding the problems of burn patients. Second, problems and interventions are discussed specifically with respect to adults and children as they progress from acute through convalescent and long-term adjustment stages of burn care. The issue of pain is minimized as it is covered in another chapter.

Two Models for Understanding Problems

Problems experienced by those who have been burned, by their families, and by the treatment team manifest themselves in some kind of overt behavior. Problem behaviors vary along a dimension from passive (silence or noncompliance) to active (screaming or overt criticism).

Behavior is problematic if it interferes with the lengthy process of healing, regaining function, or reintegration into a satisfying life-style. Patients and family may conclude there is a problem if their personal priorities are not being met or if they feel emotional distress. The staff is likely to conclude there is a problem if the behavior interferes with the burn treatment protocol or inconveniences them in some way. Often persons who have been burned do not consider their behavior problematic even when a member of the staff does. This usually produces patient motivation difficulties and conflict between patient and staff.

Although there are many theoretical models for understanding behavior, there are two relatively simple approaches that address the needs of people on one hand and the components of problem behaviors on the other. These models contribute to understanding the nature of the individual problem, a necessary first step prior to initiation of intervention strategies.

A NEEDS APPROACH

People have many needs, i.e., demands to get something from the environment for themselves. For the individual, these needs are demands that must be met or distress is experienced. Even though the burn patient may not be aware of the need, intense distress may be experienced. Needs vary on a dimension from biological to psychosocial. Maslow's conceptualization involves a hierarchy in which needs higher in sequence take precedence over those lower (17). Therefore, if a higher need is in operation, it will dominate a person's behavioral priorities; it must be satisfied in some way as soon as possible before needs lower in the hierarchy can direct a person's behavior. Maslow's hierarchy is as follows:

(1) physiological needs;
(2) safety, physical comfort, autonomy, and nurturing;
(3) belongingness and acceptance needs;
(4) esteem needs;
(5) self-actualization needs.

Physiological needs are those for oxygen, food and water, etc. Safety needs are demands for a secure experience of one's body and immediate environment, and a feeling of being in autonomous control. Belongingness needs are those directed at feeling the acceptance of others and of society in general. Esteem needs are directed at positive experiences such as being successful. Self-actualization needs involve freeing creative energies to allow a person to do things beyond what must be done.

From the moment of the burn injury, needs for safety and comfort are priorities. The patient is in pain, fears dying, is ill, and is subject to the intensive and impersonal process of lifesaving measures. The patient may be stripped of clothing, have tubes in every orifice, and be connected to machines that click and blink. The behavior generated by needs for return to a feeling of safety, autonomy, and security is not usually socially appropriate. The patient may shout, demand, resist, or withdraw. Meaningful conversation designed to help is not likely to be effective because it requires attention to social nuances which are lower in the hierarchy. It is important for the staff members to realize that the patient is not concerned with listening, congeniality, or cooperation, but rather with his existence as an autonomous person.

As the patient improves, safety needs become less a priority. Needs for belonging begin to appear as the patient considers how he might be accepted by others given disfigurement, functional loss, and perhaps, amputation. The patient may become anxious, depressed, and/or hostile. Guilt may become manifest regarding some element of the burn circumstance or an intra-family issue that had persisted for some time. The patient desperately wants signs of acceptance and love as before injury, but fears that no one could possibly provide that acceptance.

As these acceptance needs are satisfied through support from treatment staff, from regular visits from family and friends, and perhaps short trips out of the hospital, issues of being successful in preinjury activities become a priority (esteem needs). These might include working, managing a household, and socializing. As rehabilitation proceeds, a motivated patient who enjoys continued acceptance from others can reach a level of functioning which approximates his/her preinjury level. Functional limitations may require developing new skills which can result in new vocational, social, and recreational pursuits.

A COGNITIVE-BEHAVIORAL LEARNING APPROACH

This model for understanding behavior is based on the writings of Ellis (11) and Maultsby (18). It involves a systematic consideration of the components of a given behavior sequence. Behavior is always the result of an increase in internal energy. In this model, problem behavior is considered energized when a negative emotion reaches a level of intensity sufficient to result in action.

This model consists of describing behaviors with four components that occur in sequence very rapidly as follows:

(1) An event is perceived.
(2) This perception stimulates all the beliefs and attitudes about the event that the person has learned throughout life.
(3) This results in an emotive response which is consistent with those beliefs.
(4) If that response is intense, it causes a behavioral reaction.

Many believe that the emotive response is exclusively caused by the occurrence of an event. Thus, a burned patient may perceive his/her disfigured face and attribute anxiety or disgust almost solely to the perception of that face. If it is true that a perceived event is the sole cause of an emotion, it is logical that all persons would then feel the same emotion in response to that event. This does not occur. All people do not become intensely anxious when they experience pain; all people do not become angered by the same event. The factors that cause different emotive responses and behavior are all the things a person has learned to believe about that which is perceived. For example, all people have learned to value apperance in different ways. Consequently, each person will react uniquely to the perception of a disfigured face. Likewise, people have learned unique beliefs and attitudes about functional capacity and how it is important in every day activities.

Understanding this behavior sequence facilitates understanding the patient. This is a necessary first step in providing an intervention that can result in the patient feeling less distressed, and thus, behaving in a manner which is productive rather than destructive.

It has been stated that emotive responses are consistent with the beliefs and attitudes that are manifest in a person's thinking. Thus, certain habits of consistent thinking produce certain emotions. A simplistic summary of associations between thought content and emotion are presented in Table 15.1.

Behavior in response to these emotions can be varied. When a problem behavior is observed (crying, shouting, lack of compliance, or inappropriate comments), an intervention approach sensitive to both models involves the following basic communication rules:

(1) Respond to the emotion suggested by the behavior.

(2) Ask "open-ended" questions.

Table 15.1.
Thought-Emotion Relationships

Thought (Belief)	Emotive Response
1. I can't It's hopeless I am worthless I will never	1. Depression
2. They must like me It is terrible I'm a freak They must approve of me	2. Anxiety, fear Embarrassment
3. It should be It shouldn't be	3. Anger, hostility
4. I should have I shouldn't have	4. Guilt

For example, if a patient is observed to be crying and staring out the window, one might say, "You seem really sad about something" (response to the feeling). This communicates an attitude of concern, understanding, and willingness to take the time to talk about it. When the patient acknowledges the distress, one might say, "What is happening that makes you sad?" or "What are you thinking about?" or "Tell me about it" (open-ended questions which may reveal the beliefs and attitudes involved). Often learning what the patient is thinking suggests intervention strategies. These might include providing accurate information or reassuring statements, changing a procedure, or referring for more in-depth counseling. Thoughts elicited may suggest which needs are operative, provide understanding of the patient's turmoil, and suggest possible interventions to satisfy those needs.

These models also relate to the important concepts of body image and motivation. If body image is defined as a set of beliefs about appearance and ability to function, then it fits neatly into the cognitive model. When these cosmesis and function beliefs are related to intimate, social, and/or vocational aspects of living, body image is the contributor to emotive responses and behavior reactions. When beliefs are related to the chances of succeeding at a task, the importance of the task, or the cost factors involved (pain, emotion, time, money), then they affect motivation (analogous to emotion), which consequently affects behavior. Avoidance of anticipated discomfort, whether physical or emotional, can be as powerful a motivator as is striving for a desired goal, and may sometimes overpower the incentive to gain a desired objective. For example, a person with a severe hand burn may want to gain maximal function for working or recreation (such as bowling), but may resist therapy for fear of pain or anger at the time required for the program.

Problems and Interventions

The goal of burn rehabilitation is to assist and direct the patient toward a maximal level of functioning in the physical, personal, social, and vocational spheres of life. This requires the coordinated efforts of physician, nurse, physical and occupational therapists, social worker, chaplain, and psychologist or psychiatrist. It must be emphasized that communication among team members is essential in order to integrate psychological management with the demands of the total treatment process.

Problems and interventions are discussed as they occur in acute, convalescent, and long-term phases. There are certain problems generally associated with each phase of treatment; however, any problem can occur in any phase, and some problems may not occur at all. Phases of burn treatment are not mutually exclusive but rather overlap. An acute or convalescent phase problem might occur after a reconstructive surgery procedure when the patient is technically in the long-term phase.

ACUTE PHASE

The acute phase is defined as the interval from the onset of burn injury to the time when fluid resuscitation is complete, initial burn shock is resolved, and the patient is not delirious or disoriented from sepsis or other complications. Specific problems to be discussed include shock/disorientation and fear and anxiety.

Shock/Disorientation

The immediate reaction to a burn of sufficient severity to require hospitalization is one of psychological shock. This reaction is usually short-lived, lasting a few days or weeks, and generally resolves spontaneously with the aid of consistent medical management and support from staff and family. The reaction may involve delirium, emotional instability and lability, nightmares of being burned, sleeping problems, and disorientation.

Fear and Anxiety

There is little question that the burn patient experiences fear and anxiety during this early stage. Massive levels of anxiety contribute to the psychological shock reaction, and often result in overt hostility, withdrawal, and/or resistance to treatment. The patient's behavior is energized by intense, self-centered needs for safety, security, autonomy, and nurturance. Beliefs concerning self-control, survival, comfort, and treatment procedures strongly influence the level of fear. At the same time, the family may experience emotional shock which is associated with anxiety, fear, panic, and perhaps guilt. These emotional reactions can result in behaviors which are disruptive to the staff and treatment requirements. Family members may argue with each other, demand excessive time from the physician and nursing staff, become highly critical of the care of their loved one, and disturb other patients.

A variety of intervention strategies are likely to be effective in dealing with these acute phase reactions of the patient and family. A logical step involves alleviation of the fear and anxiety experienced by the patient. This can be achieved by some combination of the following:

(1) medication;
(2) provision of as much comfort as possible for the patient;
(3) provision of orienting information;
(4) provision of relaxation training after orientation is established;
(5) provision of consistent and accurate information concerning patient status and planned procedures;
(6) early involvement of family;
(7) emphasizing patient control over problems.

If there are no medical contraindications, psychotropic medications may be useful; it is impossible to utilize behavioral relaxation methods when a patient is disoriented or unable to follow instructions. When anxiety is reduced, orientation usually improves. Pain and sleep medications contribute to patient comfort and help with orientation. All burn team members can provide orienting information. This involves greeting the patient by name, mentioning the date and time of day, and describing the activities planned for the day. The family should be instructed to provide similar input, and the patient should be asked if the information is remembered.

As the patient becomes oriented, relaxation training can be instituted. Relaxation training involves a variety of techniques, including deep breathing exercises, autogenic training, progressive muscle relaxation, biofeedback, imagery, or a combination of these procedures. These complement medication because they put the patient in control. As the patient learns to relax and experience autonomy and independence, the probability of medication dependence decreases. As relaxation training becomes effective, medication can be reduced.

The patient's uncertainty regarding the severity of the burn and the treatment procedures is a source of disruptive anxiety. The patient and family should be consistently provided with accurate information, which should be repeated as often as is necessary. The staff must resist the temptation to become irritated with frequent requests for information, especially that which has previously been provided. The patient and family need reassurance and it is important that similar information is provided by all team members.

Establishing communication with the family as soon as possible is crucial to ensure their involvement in the program. Their trust and cooperation are essential. Ideally, the initial meeting with the family should involve the burn physician and at least one other team member. The meeting should allow time for the family to vent feelings, have questions answered, and for the team to enlist their help.

Prior to the initial patient visit, the family should be provided some detail about the patient's appearance and ability to respond. Even though this is difficult to provide, it will reduce disruptive emotional outbursts by the family, and they will realize the support and concern of the burn team which helps establish open lines of communication. For example, the family might be told: "Your son was seriously burned and is not going to look like he did when you last saw him; his face is swollen to the extent that he cannot open his eyes, but he can hear you. His skin is discolored. He is connected to monitors and IV tubes. He has been medicated so he may not be able to respond to you. He has white bandages over much of his body and there may be blood on them. It is important for him to hear your voices and to know that you are here and concerned. Even if he is unresponsive, remember that he can probably hear you. I'll go in with you, and after a few minutes, I'll leave. I'll be available to answer any questions you might have."

If the family is reluctant to visit at this very stressful time, that is all right, but it is important to initiate visitation as soon as possible.

Regular education classes to inform family about burn injuries and treatment are invaluable. Not only do these teach families, but they also provide an opportunity for support from families of other burn patients.

Early in the course of treatment, the family should be interviewed by the social worker, nurse specialist, or psychologist/psychiatrist for information concerning the patient's preburn life-style, coping habits, and reaction patterns. This facilitates the understanding of problems that may arise, the development of strategies for approaching the patient, and the eliciting of patient cooperation with the treatment process. Important content areas include:

(1) recreational interests;
(2) social ability;
(3) educational attainment;
(4) vocational history;
(5) possible legal difficulties;
(6) drug or alcohol intake habits;
(7) marital history;
(8) attitudes about health, illness, independence, and authority-subordinate realtionships;
(9) other serious medical problems.

This information is gathered not for mere curiosity, but rather to learn what may contribute to patient management. It is sometimes more effective to obtain the information in several short sessions as opposed to one long session.

Other problems which may complicate resolution of shock/disorientation are alcohol or drug intoxication at the time of the burn, suicidal etiology, and/or concomitant other injuries, especially of the head. These problems may lengthen the course of reorientation and complicate the entire rehabilitation course. Often, assistance from other specialists is needed for these difficulties.

CONVALESCENT PHASE

The convalescent phase is that time interval between resolution of the initial shock/disorientation of the acute phase and discharge from the hospital. As the patient becomes increasingly more oriented and fears of survival subside, concerns surface regarding appearance and function, and their effects on life-style. During this phase pain, sleep disturbances, fear of long-term consequences, and cooperation with the burn treatment staff become important.

Pain

There is an automatic association between pain and being burned. Although full-thickness burns are not inherently painful, partial-thickness burns are painful from injury onset. In addition, there is pain associated with debridement, positioning, and exercise programs. Pain may be a significant contributor to disorientation in the acute phase and to sleep disturbances during all phases of treatment.

There are few generalizations that can be concluded from studying pain, other than that it is uncomfortable and has various meanings for different people. Some patients seem able to tolerate severe pain while others seem unable to cope with what appears to be minimal pain. Regardless of the opinion of observers as to the severity of the pain, there is little question that the patient hurts.

The very subjective nature of hurting makes pain management a difficult task. It is the individual's attitudes about pain which cause emotional reactions that lower or raise pain thresholds. Also involved are physician and staff attitudes about pain and about patients who complain of pain. These attitudes are based upon ideas concerning whether or not pain is real, how patients are supposed to act, and the potential for addicting a patient to pain medication.

It is important to discriminate between the pain itself and the patient's pain behaviors, which result in potential problems for the staff. These behaviors are a manifestation of the patient's needs for comfort and security, and attitudes about treatment while in the hospital. They are also a result of well-learned coping behaviors for stressful situations. Examples of pain behaviors are facial grimacing, complaining, whining, crying, shouting, demanding medication, refusing to cooperate with treatment, and insisting on staying in bed.

Combinations of medications, relaxation training, counseling, and behavioral management are effective for pain control. The goals are to maximize patient comfort, minimize disruptive pain behavior, and increase patient cooperativeness and productivity. Critical factors are an understanding of the program by the entire staff, and consistent and persistent effort in implementing the procedures. Complicating factors for such a program include history of addiction to alcohol or drugs, psychiatric problems, and medical complications.

A special pain problem involves amputation of a body part. The anxiety contributing to reduced pain tolerance is often exacerbated by body image attitudes involved in the loss of a limb. Further complicating this issue are the presence of intense grieving over the lost body part and phantom limb sensation. It is important to distinguish between phantom limb sensation and painful phantom sensation. Often a patient will mention having sensations in the amputated extremity, and the staff will conclude that it is painful when it is not. Grieving is almost universal among patients who have experienced an amputation. Treatment should be directed at providing emotional support, reducing phantom sensations, and discussing prosthetic devices. In addition, the family may require help in adjusting to their reactions regarding the amputation.

Sleep Disturbance

Most hospitalized burn patients have difficulty sleeping. Reasons are that burn wounds hurt, dressings and splints are confining and disruptive to normal sleeping positions, high metabolic rates cause agitation and feelings of extreme cold or heat, and the patient may be preoccupied with eventual consequences of burn injury. In addition, if one patient in a multibed room is not sleeping, the other patients are often disturbed. Consistent lack of sleep results in disorientation, fatigue, irritability, and reduced tolerance for almost any inconvenience. Sleep difficulties are probably the most important factor contributing to emotional disruption of the patient, both in the hospital and after discharge; the resolution of this problem should be a priority. In the absence of medical contraindications, medication is the treatment of choice. Relaxation training and counseling are useful adjuncts to medication. Sleep can also be facilitated by a busy daily activities program. In addition to dressing changes and exercise programs, the patient should be encouraged to stay out of bed and to participate in recreational activities. This will decrease boredom and interfere with the desire for daytime sleep.

Fear of Consequences

As the disorientation of the acute phase resolves, patients begin noticing other patients, their own burned skin, and perhaps, an amputation. A new set of reactions becomes apparent as the patient emotionally responds to these perceptions. Behavioral reactions that cause problems include emotional lability, acting out, and helplessness. Family reactions to the patient's behavior may cause further difficulties.

These problems can be understood by use of the two models described earlier. The patient's needs that are emerging, when survival is no longer an issue, include those for acceptance by others and self-esteem in addition to a continuation of those needs for safety and comfort. Dependent and demanding behaviors continue, but the primary focus becomes the emotional turmoil relative to anticipated consequences in personal, social, and vocational spheres caused by cosmetic and functional deficits. These emotions and consequential behaviors will vary among patients; however, they are almost always an expression of strong demands for assurance of acceptance by others and an expression of their ability to care for themselves and their families. Although it represents an oversimplification, one can conceptualize such attitudes in terms of the following chart:

	COSMESIS	FUNCTION
Personal		
Social		
Vocational		
Sexual		

Eight combinations are possible, each reflecting the interaction of personal priorities about appearance and function as they may affect different life situations. Personal refers to those close relationships that exist, usually with family and other relatives, while social refers to more casual relationships including encounters with strangers. Vocational involves productive activity regardless of whether or not money is involved, and sexual is self-explanatory. One can also conceptualize that personal, social, vocational, and sexual are not independent of each other, nor are cosmesis and function. Therefore, more complexity than is apparent exists.

An example will clarify this conceptualization. A woman with a right above-knee amputation secondary to an electrical burn injury was fitted with a prosthesis and became a functional ambulator. During a follow-up counseling session it was learned that she never wore her prosthesis at home, but would not venture outside her home, even to get the newspaper, without it. Further inquiry revealed that she could get around in her kitchen faster, and care for her children and her home easier using crutches; she wanted to appear as a person with two legs to anyone outside her immediate family. Function was a priority in the vocational sense (productivity in her house), and cosmesis in the social situation (outside her house).

Among the common emotional problems of burn patients are depression, anger, guilt, and fear or anxiety. Behavioral reactions to these responses are variable but can include crying, poor cooperation in treatment, shouting and/or swearing, manipulation of staff, helplessness, excessive sleep, and a variety of rebellious behaviors. Patients and families, as well as staff members, may manifest such behaviors. It is important to understand that these emotional-behavior problems are usually reactive and are not signs of personality instability or mental disease.

Depression is often observed in burn patients. A patient can be depressed one day but not the next, and it may reappear without an obvious cause. Symptoms of depression may be withdrawal, crying, staring aimlessly, showing disinterest in treatment or eating, and a sad facial expression. When confronted with a depressed patient, it is important to determine if there is medical illness or if what appears to be depression is a normal fluctuation of mood. If depression persists for four to five days, more than routine emotional support may be necessary. Medication may be helpful by allowing counseling to be more effective, but in some cases, psychotherapeutic counseling alone may be sufficient.

Emotional support means that the staff should spend time with the patient, even if the patient is unresponsive. The staff's physical presence, supportive statements, strokes of the patient's head or hand, and even silence do much to provide reassurance. It is important to remember that the patient may need a time to grieve a loss, and therefore, may gain emotional benefits from depressed episodes. It is important not to overreact to depression since it can resolve spontaneously within days. Sometimes a patient appears agitated or tense when depressed. One way to make the distinction between anxiety and depression is to listen to what the patient says. Table 15.1 can provide some assistance in this regard, but in general, if a patient is frequently saying "I can't" or "It is hopeless", he/she is probably depressed, despite anxious affect. This distinction is important because there is a tendency to provide relaxing medication for agitation which can exacerbate depression.

Counseling should be directed at patient understanding of the role that needs and attitudes play in causing depressed affect and behavior. This is followed by attempts to get the patient to become more realistic about the content and pattern of beliefs, which, if successful, impact emotional response, motivation, and behavior. For example, a male patient with burned hands and face may believe that he will never be able to play with his son again, take him fishing, or provide for his emotional needs. He may also be thinking that his wife will be disgusted with his appearance, refuse to have sexual intercourse with him, and that divorce is certain. Perhaps he also believes that he will never work again and, therefore, become financially destitute. These beliefs would most likely cause depression. A counseling approach would be to guide this man in his thinking toward the ideas that (a) there is a high probability that his hands will become functional with time and hard work; (b) it is nonsense that he will not be able to play with his son, even though it will take time before full function is obtained; (c) it is in his best interest to wait and deal with problems of work, intimacy, and recreation if they arise; (d) his thinking was almost totally focused on his losses and fantasized difficulties; and (e) it is in his best interest to think about his condition and the future in terms of probable outcomes as opposed to possible outcomes.

Another important issue is "who" learns about the patient's real concerns. Often the most valiant efforts by the well-trained psychiatrist, psychologist, or social worker to relate therapeutically with the patient are unsuccessful. The nurses, therapists, and family members are often the first to gain the patient's confidence. Daily contact with these professionals results in trust and closeness that are precursors to open and honest communication. Willingness to take time to talk with patients (even if a part of the treatment must be neglected) and a sensitive and caring attitude can facilitate patient adjustment and, perhaps, provide the stepping stone to more intensive intervention by counseling personnel.

The *angry and hostile* patient is a particularly difficult problem for the staff. This patient most likely has a history of attacking problems and frustrations and being overly independent (which may be a facade covering extreme dependency with fear of anyone learning about it). The angry patient desperately wants to be in control, to be respected, and yet does not want to be inconvenienced by anything or anyone. Attitudes about physicians and other authorities and fairness are likely to be involved.

Management includes reacting impersonally to the hostility (a sometimes difficult task), understanding the patient (talking with the patient), and being self-secure. It is important to rule out psychosis or sociopathy, associated head injury (sometimes very subtle), history of substance abuse, illness, and normal reaction style. If there is a psychotic history or a head injury, medication can often be effective in calming the patient. If substance abuse is involved, the problem is difficult, but medication may be helpful to assist the patient to detoxify. If it is a normal reaction style, it will probably continue, but can be somewhat regulated with firmness, consistency, allowing the patient as much control as possible, and discussion in an uncritical and undefensive manner. Firmness involves telling the patient, for example, "I know you are very angry and that is fine, but screaming and throwing your food tray are not acceptable. If you have questions, ask me and I will answer as best I can. All of us are here to help you get well and out of the hospital as soon as possible. You can help a little bit." The staff member must then keep any committments made. Further angry outbursts should be ignored, if feasible, and most importantly, any cooperative and pleasant behaviors should be reinforced with a smile, a comment, or an extra privilege.

There are times when anger masks depression. Again, the content of what is said becomes important in determining the problem. It is also important to remember that despite the difficulty in dealing with hostility, the rebellious patient often progresses more in the long run than the compliant, helpless, depressesd patient.

Guilt is another emotional reaction that may characterize a patient or family. It is usually related to circumstances surrounding the burn injury, and is often associated with depression. Behavioral reactions to guilt may involve self-incriminating remarks, comments about what one should or should not have done, self-defeating behavior, or poor compliance with treatment. Management requires the same attitude of wanting to understand what is occurring and intervening into the beliefs and attitudes that are contributing to the difficulty. Important is the idea that even though it is unpleasant, reality cannot be altered. Therefore, it is a waste of energy to wish it had been different and to take personal responsibility. It is especially difficult to deal with guilt because of considerable resistance to the idea that what occurred could not be any other way. A breakthrough occurs when the patient realizes it is possible to influence tomorrow's events, but not yesterday's. This is also a turning point for the depressed patient.

Anxiety and fear are as prevalent during the convalescent phase as during other phases, but are more related to potential consequences the burn injury may have for everyday living. There is also an anxiety/fear component to each of the emotional problems discussed. In depression, there is fear of helplessness; in hostility, there is fear of losing control; in guilt, there is fear of punishment and rejection. These feelings may be expressed in the hospital or after discharge, when they usually are more reality based. Behaviorally this anxious patient may be very apologetic, demand attention and reassurance, and be overly sensitive to the comments of others. He/she may refuse to look in the mirror and be hyperactive, agitated, and very preoccupied with relatively minor circumstances. He/she may hyperventilate and demonstrate pain behaviors and low pain tolerance. Anxious persons are often manipulative in order to get what they want or to avoid what they do not want, and may passively express hostility and anger. Thought content often involves relationships with others; the patient may behave more to please others than to please him/herself. Anxiety may be related to being inactive, unproductive, and beliefs of worthlessness if not working and making money. Concern about paying bills, feeling self-esteem from work and recreational pursuits, and dealing with family members and friends add to this anxiety reaction.

Management of anxiety includes understanding, providing accurate information, training in relaxation, psychotropic medication, and counseling directed at the basic attitudinal structure that is contributing to the level of discomfort. An important management step is to learn the preburn anxiety and activity levels of the patient. It may be that the level of tension is not elevated beyond what would be predicted by the history.

The issue of appearance is an important one. The patient is often concerned about present and expected future appearance. Treatment staff are often anxious about addressing this issue. Honesty, in the absence of value judgments, should characterize responses to the patient. Questions should be answered in an objective manner. For example, in response to a question regarding appearance, a patient might be told: "Your face is swollen; you have scabs on your forehead and chin; it is quite red over your nose and left cheek. As treatment proceeds, your appearance will change. Your skin will look different after healing than it did before you were burned. It takes several weeks for the redness to fade, but eventually your skin color will be close to its preburn color. There may be some changes in your skin texture. Would you like to see yourself?" If the patient does decide to use the mirror, the staff members should stay to answer questions and provide support. Mirrors should be available for patients and the staff should be available to deal with the emotionality that may occur when the patient first takes this step.

Functional concerns should also be addressed in an honest manner with considerable information about the length of time required to gain physical capacity and what is necessary to reach that goal. Questions from patients concerning return to preinjury work and play activities should be answered cautiously. It should be explained that obtaining relatively full function depends upon their own efforts and persistence and the patient alone has control over this. If the nature of the burn injury suggests permanent disability and it is unlikely that the patient will return to former functional levels, recommending the patient choose from among other activities may be helpful.

These convalescent reactions of depression, hostility, guilt, and anxiety have two foci: how the person is treated in the hospital and what living will be like after discharge. Ideally, as time for discharge approaches, weekend passes should be arranged. This experience allows the patient and family to test in reality many of their expectations and fears as well as the necessary new routine of dressing changes and exercises at home. Immediately after return from a pass, a lengthy discussion with the patient and family is a priority as problems will be fresh on their minds and most amenable to successful intervention. Continuation of support as the patient enters the post-discharge rehabilitation phase is essential.

LONG-TERM PHASE

The long-term phase is the interval from hospital discharge until all treatment programs are completed and the patient has settled into a satisfactory living pattern. When the patient goes home, the issues that were important in the hospital continue; however, there is the opportunity to test the validity of fears and expectations further and to take steps to deal with them. In addition, family problems may increase as the stresses of a new, but temporary life-style are experienced. Problems may appear, such as rejection of the patient by family members or friends, overprotection of the patient, overt conflict between family members, poor cooperation with dressing change and splinting or exercise programs, pain or itching, impatience with the time required for rehabilitation, and others. If a base of trust and concern has been established, and if there are provisions for regular follow-up, the vehicle for dealing with such problems exists. The needs that are primary during this post-discharge phase are those for acceptance and self-esteem. Although needs for safety and comfort may continue, these usually have subsided. The attitudes involved increasingly relate with capacity to work and support family, intimacy and sexual adjustment, and recreational activities. Another complicating factor involves the presence of litigation which may affect motivation and protract the rehabilitation course.

Management during this phase is more difficult because of less direct contact with patients, but the management principles are the same. Behavioral techniques may be ineffective unless the family can consistently follow the behavioral contingencies in the home situation. This is often very difficult, and if it cannot be consistently accomplished, it can cause more problems than it solves. The use of self-control behavioral strategies can be used to counteract this problem.

Overprotectiveness by family is a special problem that may compromise the patient's progress and result in disruption for the rehabilitation staff. Such overprotectiveness may result from guilt or anxiety regarding expectations about long-term outcomes. Patients can become quite comfortable with the pampering and extra attention afforded them, or quite the opposite can occur. A patient might believe he/she is worthless if unable to take care of him/herself; another might think he/she is important if others care for him/her. Responsibility for care is the issue and self-control strategies may be very helpful. Management of such problems requires intense involvement with the patient and family.

It is important, in dealing with what is perceived as overprotectiveness, to determine the preburn pattern of interaction between patient and family. It may be that the overprotective or indulgent pattern was characteristic, and if it was, interfering may create problems. In this case, emphasis can be placed on the patient taking responsibility for exercise, eating, and grooming, but allowing other indulgent behaviors. Incorporating recreational or avocational activities into the exercise program may help the patient work more independently. The usual manner of dealing with overprotection is to suggest not doing things for the patient. This may mean that the family member's needs to care for the patient are frustrated, as well as the patient's need for attention and nurturance. Two rules of thumb are, first, when something important is taken from the patient, it must be replaced; otherwise, the patient may replace it in a destructive manner. Second, a satisfied need is no longer a motivator, and therefore, it no longer causes behavior.

As the rehabilitation process proceeds, the issue of return to work arises. If there is a physical disability that interferes with return to a former occupation, or with effectively performing other tasks, it is necessary to pursue a vocational alternative or modify tasks. Concomitant with dealing with the attitudinal, need, and emotional issues, a vocational evaluation to assess cognitive and physical aptitudes, motivation, and interest may be helpful. When strengths and weaknesses are identified, they facilitate generation of a useful vocational rehabilitation plan. Referral to a state vocational rehabilitation agency or to an insurance company rehabilitation program may be the treatment of choice. Occupational therapy is also a useful resource for task modification or provision of equipment to allow easier accomplishment of tasks. It is also important to advise patients about the most appropriate time to pursue vocational planning.

Another source of tension for the person who has been burned, treated, and discharged is how long it takes for maximal functional and cosmetic recovery. The patient and family should be informed consistently throughout the treatment phase that a lengthy recovery time can be expected. Recovery time can contribute to marital discord because of "too much" husband-wife togetherness. This discord is a result of established patterns being disrupted and attitudes about inactivity, getting attention, and vocational pursuits that contribute to anxiety, depression, or overt hostility. In some cases, this requirement of time results in closer family and marital ties. When this occurs, the patient may delay return to work and fear it will bring about preburn patterns that were less fulfilling. Ultimately, the quality of family functioning preburn will become manifest in post-discharge functioning, either productive or problematic.

The Burned Child

When a child is burned, the psychosocial problems often involve the family more than the child. This is not to say the child has no difficulties, but the family may have intense problems because of their needs, attitudes, and beliefs about family, child rearing, the future, and the circumstances surrounding the burn injury. Many childhood burns are a result of covert neglect or overt abuse. Dealing with the family in these cases, and the potential legal and guilt ramifications, can be very difficult. The staff must deal with their anger at the family before approaching the problem.

The difficulties families have adjusting to the ramifications of a burn injury to their child are similar to those previously discussed, and the management strategies are the same. However, the problems of the child must be approached differently, depending upon developmental factors. For purposes of understanding these very complex issues, children will be discussed in three groups:

(1) *Zero to six years*—This child is very parental dependent and has not developed propositional language skills, rigid coping habits or defenses.

(2) *Seven to puberty*—This child is less parental dependent and more peer dependent. Language development is more sophisticated, but no long-term future planning and understanding exist. Coping habits, defenses, and self-concepts are emerging.

(3) *Adolescence*—This person experiences independence-dependence conflicts as a personal identity develops. Full propositional language and thought are present as are more rigid coping and defensive strategies.

Young children (zero to six years) probably have less in-hospital and after-hospital problems. Dependency needs are met, in most cases, by staff and frequent parental visits. These children are very "here and now"-oriented. Their major problems are dealing with pain and discomfort. They tend to forget such episodes rather quickly although they may maintain associations with the hospital and/or particular staff uniforms and other cues which cause fear. Very young children may develop severe withdrawal or acting out symptoms as a result of basic security needs being frustrated by abrupt separation from home and family, and the concomitant pain experiences of burn treatment. These experiences may have long-term implications, especially as adolescence emerges.

Children from seven years to puberty may act out more in the hospital, but they are likely to experience more problems after discharge because of dependence on peers and the importance of peer influence on developing self-image. Therefore, any of a variety of acting out episodes or withdrawal might be observed. The influence of family support at this time is very important.

Management of burned children involves meeting basic needs and especially assisting with family turmoil. Children need to be held, preferably by parents. Thus, frequent and liberal visitation hours are important as long as they do not interfere with treatment routines. The child has been taken from familiar, secure surroundings, and is frightened. Allowing familiar items from home, such as a stuffed animal, a favorite blanket, or a pillow, can help alleviate fear of the strangeness of the hospital. Also, favorite foods and treats can be brought by the family. In the family's absence, the nursing and therapy staff become substitute sources of emotional support for the child. The frightened child may demand much attention and support which should be provided as routinely as possible. A soothing voice, stroking the head lightly, and other physical contacts are effective strategies for calming the burned child while in the hospital.

Provision of toys, games, books, and an attitude of willingness to participate with the burned child in these activities facilitate cooperation and emotional comfort. In some facilities, recreational, music, or art therapists are available to assist with these activities. Play is also a resource for helping children vent feelings and learn about procedures that are forthcoming, like surgery or splinting.

The child who is burned is sometimes tense and has sleeping problems. Relaxation techniques have not been widely used with children, but can be very effective. Soft music, biofeedback, a tape of mother's voice reading a favorite story, and soft stroking of the forehead are suggestions which may be effective. Learning of the child's preburn priorities may allow for creative solutions for tension and fear-related problems.

Many children will act out, rebel, and disobey with the stress of burn treatment. These are more likely to occur in the seven years to puberty group and among adolescents. Management of these problems involves:

(1) staff monitoring and dealing with their own frustration and anger;
(2) learning from parents whether or not the child was rebellious and undisciplined prior to the injury;
(3) soliciting family assistance with the behavioral problems;
(4) consistent and firm implementation of behavioral contingencies.

It is also important to minimize pain. Some children may withdraw as opposed to acting out. If a child was abused, withdrawal may appear which is an indicator of potentially severe problems. This child may not even cry during a dressing change. Children may also withdraw if they fear punishment; and burn treatment processes may be perceived as punishment.

A firm approach by the parents may be effective if there was consistent discipline prior to the injury. The parent may tell the child the behavior is not acceptable and that the staff does not like it. Important is that the staff support this position. The most crucial ingredient, however, is avoiding the tendency to notice only disruptive behavior. Even the rebellious child loves attention; productive and pleasant acts should be rewarded with extra time, a treat, a compliment, a smile or laughter, or an extra privilege. If there was inconsistent discipline at home prior to the burn, the parent's words may be ineffective. In this case, more strict behavioral management procedures and family counseling to elicit support are necessary. Behavioral management strategies should include consistent withdrawal of privileges or treats when problem behavior occurs, and reward of productive behavior with attention and reinstating privileges. To be effective, these strategies must be consistently enforced by family and staff. Another consideration involves who does the treating. A problem child may be frightened by being approached by two or three nurses or therapists. Sometimes a male therapist will receive a better response, and sometimes, vice versa. Ethnic matching of patient and nurse or therapist may also be productive.

The withdrawing child may be helped by involvement in play techniques, and by consistent support and quiet attention at times when painful procedures are not planned. Rewards should be provided for approach behavior, like eye contact or any noise, from the silent child. Rewards may include candy, gum, or more social approaches like smiles and soothing words.

Family members need information about burns, their treatment, and what to expect, as well as reassurance and perhaps, counseling. If guilt is expressed by a family member, or anger exists about the burn injury circumstances, counseling intervention is essential to deal with the potentially destructive nature of these difficulties. Financial concerns and disruption of family routines are another source of problems that require intervention.

The adolescent reaction to a burn injury is less predictable except in the sense that the injury will create significant turmoil in an already conflict-ridden stage of development. Identity problems may become manifest in poor vocational, social, and sexual adjustment patterns. The reactions of others to the adolescent who has been burned are especially emotionally charged experiences that may or may not contribute to the development of an effective identity.

The adolescent who has been burned is a special problem because of emerging sexuality, distrust of authority, and strong needs for privacy. Eliciting parental support and providing counseling are important strategies for dealing with the myriad of unpredictable behavioral reactions likely to be observed. The adolescent usually appreciates being treated like an adult, but with a little extra attention and concern. If there were conflicts between the adolescent and parents, parental support may produce anxiety. Thus, counseling with parents may be a necessary precursor to effective parental support. Confidentiality in dealing with the adolescent is also a most important consideration.

The Staff

The burn team members are involved in activities that are demanding, somewhat unpredictable, and stressful. They must confront the intense medical management and physical rehabilitation demands of the patient. And, they must deal on a day to day basis with the behaviors of the patient who is in extreme distress and the problems of the family. The staff may sometimes experience the same grief and agitation as the family with respect to the mutilation of the patient's body, the death of a patient, and perhaps, the circumstances under which the patient was burned. As the staff works, they may perceive other members as not doing their share, being careless, or maintaining a callous or negative attitude about the treatment program. So, staff become frustrated and angry with patients, the families, and each other. They become tired, stressed and irritable, and experience "burn out." Not only do these problems affect the staff personally, but they can interfere with the effectiveness and efficiency of treatment, and communicate extra tension and anxiety to the patient. Many of these difficulties relate to the high ideals burn personnel have about how to proceed best with saving life and maximally enhancing eventual quality of life. Other sources of difficulty are institutional administrative policies that affect number of personnel, merit pay incentives, equipment and supplies, and emotional support of personnel in stressful environments.

Complete resolution of these difficulties is not a realistic goal. There will always be unpredictable events that must be addressed. The reality of the burn unit demands that circumstances occur which interfere with treatment and create stress, anxiety, emotional outbursts, and fatigue of staff. Patients will die; physicians will become angry and irritated with nurses, therapists, patients, and each other. Nurses, therapists, and families will become irritated with each other and with physicians. Patients will become demanding, critical, argumentative, and/or withdrawn.

Developing skills to deal with these circumstances requires provision for the staff:

(1) to talk and vent feelings in a noncritical and accepting environment, and

(2) to learn effective means of dealing with difficult patients, families, and intrastaff conflicts.

The best mechanism for dealing with staff stress is a regularly scheduled meeting, preferably during working hours, with voluntary participation. It could easily be argued that participation should be mandatory, but effectiveness may be enhanced if attendance at such a meeting is on a voluntary basis. Ideally, a physician and administrative person should be in attendance. It is also necessary that a person trained in counseling or interpersonal group communication attend regularly. These meetings should conform to the following rules:

(1) Nothing said is discussed publicly outside the meeting, only privately with the specific person or persons involved.
(2) No one is criticized for something over which he/she has no control.
(3) What is said should deal with work-related issues rather than non-work issues.

Another possibility is that such meetings occur off the burn unit, perhaps in a more social setting. However, that implies that they occur during off-hours when many staff members want nothing to do with work problems, and are consequently unlikely to participate.

A second source of opportunity to express feelings and discuss problems is during impromptu private conversation with friends, coworkers, or the psychological team member. It is important that such discussions take a productive direction rather than a "gossipy" one. In any case, there is some value in expressing frustration; it can relieve emotional pressure. However, there is far greater value in finding a solution.

Coping skills are learned by understanding reasons for problems and developing appropriate strategies. A problem arises when negative emotional experiences increase with resultant ineffective and critical behavior. Anger, irritability, and frustration are caused by the beliefs that other people are not functioning optimally. These beliefs cause anger as well as unproductive behavior, and wastes energy and time. It is more appropriate to notice imperfections, to react in an appropriate manner, and to implement proper action to avert a recurrence. All workers make mistakes and need support and understanding coupled with a desire to learn how to better deal with new problems as they arise.

An important final comment relates to the ultimate goal of burn treatment and rehabilitation. The goal for the staff is to do the best possible job, not the perfect or ideal job, to help the burn patient and family adapt to the realities of the burn injury and develop a fulfilling and satisfying life-style. To do this best job, it is crucial for the staff to help each other without expecting perfection or infallibility from anyone.

REFERENCES

1. Achterberg-Lawlis J, Kanner C: Burn Patients. In Doleys DM, Meredith RL, Ciminero AR: *Behavioral Medicine, Assessment and Treatment Strategies.* New York, Plenum Press, 1982, pp. 499–525.
2. Andreason NJC, Norris AS: Long term adjustment and adaptation mechanisms in severely burned adults. *J Nerv Ment Dis* 154:352–362, 1972.
3. Andreason NJC, Norris AS, Hartford CE: Incidence of long-term psychiatric complications

in severely burned adults. *Ann Surg* 174:785–793, 1971.

4. Andreason NJC, Noyes R, Hartford CE: Factors influencing adjustment of burn patients during hospitalization. *Psychosom Med* 34:517–525, 1972.

5. Benians RC: A child psychiatrist looks at burned children and their families. *Guy's Hospital Reports* 123:149–154, 1974.

6. Blades BC, Jones C, Munster AM: Quality of life after major burns. *J Trauma* 19:556–558, 1979.

7. Bowden ML, Jones CA, Feller I: *Psychosocial Aspects of a Severe Burn: A Review of the Literature.* Ann Arbor, MI, National Institutes for Burn Medicine, 1979.

8. Caudel PR, Potter J: Characteristics of burned children and the after affects of the injury. *Br J Plast Surg* 27:63–65, 1970.

9. Chang FC, Herzog B: Burn morbidity: A follow-up study of physical and psychological disability. *Ann Surg* 183:34–37, 1976.

10. Davidson TM, Bowden ML, Thalen D, et al: Social support and burn adjustment. *Arch Phys Med Rehab* 62:274–285, 1981.

11. Ellis A: *Humanistic Psychotherapy, the Rational-Emotive Approach.* New York, Julian Press, 1973.

12. Goldston R: The burning and the healing of children. *Psychiatry* 35:57–66, 1972.

13. Helm PA, Achterberg-Lawlis J, Peyton S: Psychosocial impact of burn injury. *Final Report of a Demonstration of a Regional Burn Care System* (contract 240–77–0161). Washington, DC, Health Services Administration, 1980.

14. Johnson MA: A study of the effects of percentage and locus of burn on body image, self concept, and social perception for an adult burn population. *Dissert Abstr* 3886-B, 1977.

15. Kibboe E: Life after severe burns in children. *J Burn Care Rehabil* 2:44–47, 1981.

16. Malt U: Long-term psychosocial follow-up studies of burned adults: reviewal of the literature. *Burns* 6:190–197, 1980.

17. Maslow AH: *Motivation and Personality.* New York, Harper, 1970.

18. Maultsby M: *Help Yourself to Happiness.* New York, Institute for Natural Living, Inc., 1975.

19. Mlott SR, Lina FT, Miller WC: Psychological assessment of the burn patient. *J Clin Psychol* 33:425–430, 1977.

20. Noyes R, Frye SJ, Slymen DJ, et al: Stressful life events and burn injuries. *J Trauma* 19:141–144, 1979.

21. White AC: Psychiatric study of patients with severe burn injuries. *Br Med J* 284:465–467, 1982.

16

Nursing Care

VERNA CAIN

The Burn Rehabilitation Team

As a result of the physiological and psychological changes which occur, the severely burned patient experiences a multitude of problems which require individualized, specialized attention. Specific medical and nursing management in the area of fluid replacement, nutritional support, wound care, and physical therapy demand strict attention. The socioeconomic changes which may occur within the family structure, as well as the patient and family's response to the injury, give rise to emotional factors which must be dealt with in order to rehabilitate the burn patient appropriately.

It is obvious that no one discipline could possibly provide all the varied needs and requirements of the burn patient. Facilities which specialize in burn management recognize and utilize the services of diverse health care disciplines in the care of these patients. Interacting as a cooperative team, each discipline brings an additional area of expertise to enhance burn care and rehabilitation. It is essential that the team members function in harmony with one another to provide optimal therapy.

The composition of the burn team members may vary within the individual units depending upon the organizational structure, size, and, in many instances, the budgetary constraints of the facility. Although the nucleus of the team generally consists of physicians, nurses, and therapists, there may be a variety of other members. These may include social workers, nutritionists, vocational counselors, recreational therapists, psychologists, and consultant staff. Regardless of composition, the contributions of each member of the team are vital to overcome the many obstacles the patient and family will face. Close cooperative teamwork is essential to allow individual members to function at maximal capabilities. Although it is inevitable that there may be some overlap in roles, each member of the team has a specific function which must be understood by the other members.

PHYSICIAN STAFF

The physician is not only responsible for the medical management of the patient but also has complete authority for the moral and legal aspects of

353

the patient's care. The physician has to deal with grave decisions related to life and death and even the quality of life on a daily basis.

In most facilities, the physician is the recognized leader who directs the burn team. The composition of the physician staff will depend largely on the institution. In designated burn care facilities, the director may be either a general surgeon or a plastic surgeon. In teaching institutions, the resident staff may assume care of the burn patients under supervision of the attending physician. Orders for drugs and other therapy as well as consults are frequently written by the resident physician. The physician staff must be well acquainted with burn pathophysiology and treatment. It is the responsibility of the physician-in-charge to provide adequate teaching and direction to the resident and paramedical staff caring for these patients. Knowledge of prevention and treatment of deformities, as well as acute burn therapy, is essential. This is most often accomplished in rounds and conferences where goals and treatment therapies are discussed. Conferences which include the entire burn team provide a source for exchange of information and knowledge.

Although the final authority in the patient's care rests with the physician staff, success of the care requires the participation of each team member. It is important that the other members of the team understand the medical approach and goals of therapy. The physician relies on the support and cooperation of the entire burn team to provide the diverse therapies required for care of the burn patient.

SOCIAL WORKER

The multitude of socioeconomic issues which accompany the burn patient and family are within the realm of the social worker. The social worker serves as an invaluable member of the burn team, as an advocate, providing patient and family support, and as a counselor assisting the patient and family to cope with the personal, social, and economic devastation caused by the injury. Although in some institutions other members of the team may be involved, large facilities caring for complex burns have incorporated psychosocial teams which may include the social worker, psychologist, psychiatric nurse, recreational therapists, or other members of the burn team. Tasks within this area may be divided among the members to assure that individual patient and family needs are met. Initial assessments of family relationships, financial status, support systems and community resources provide the necessary information on which to base not only patient care planning but the beginning of discharge planning.

Immediately after the injury, families of burn victims present in the emergency room or on the burn unit in a state of shock with a multitude of issues requiring immediate attention. It is primarily the responsibility of the social worker to assist the family in sorting out these issues enabling them to cope. Providing counseling and directing the family during this period requires the expertise of professionals trained in crisis intervention. Although some burn units may utilize the nursing staff or public health nurse for discharge planning, in other facilities the social worker may be primarily responsible, particularly in arranging for visiting nurse services, nursing home placement and other community referrals.

"THERAPIST"—PHYSICAL, OCCUPATIONAL AND RECREATIONAL

The role of the therapist in burn care cannot be overemphasized. Severely burned patients require intense therapy and monitoring. Therapists provide range-of-motion exercises and make orthotic devices for positioning. Burn therapists are concerned with maintaining joint function, preventing contractures, and providing the patient with activities which promote independence. They are responsible for setting up exercise programs which utilize activities to strengthen and enhance functional coordination. The recreational therapist may arrange activities both inside and outside the hospital which not only provide entertainment but assist the patient in developing realistic views of what to expect following discharge. The physical therapist may also be responsible for hydrotherapy and wound care of the hospitalized patient, as well as the outpatient. The number of therapists in a given unit varies and may include physical, occupational, and recreational therapists. Although the physical and occupational therapists have specific functions, roles will vary in different facilities. In a small unit, one therapist may provide all the therapy function, while other units may have two or more physical and occupational therapists.

Burn therapists as a rule are able to work with the patient only during the day. Frequently, the patient may require additional exercise periods, as well as splint replacement and periodic monitoring. Furthermore, due to the pain and discomfort, burn patients need continual encouragement and assistance to exercise. Cooperation from the rest of the team is essential in reinforcing the therapy program.

NURSE

The burn nurse is the key member of the team who functions to provide and maintain continuity of care for the patient. Nursing the burn patient comprises all the fundamental techniques of general bedside nursing care, such as taking vital signs, measuring urine outputs, regulating intravenous fluids, inserting intravenous lines, drawing blood and gathering information to provide guidelines for patient care planning. The nurse must be able to incorporate critical care skills, as well as those of acute and rehabilitation nursing. In addition, certain specialized knowledge, skills, and attitudes must be learned and practiced. Delivering quality wound care and débridement is essential in burn care. Inherent in the nurse's ability to apply good principles of care is the nurse's knowledge of burn wound healing and scarring. Utilizing effective techniques in wound care may decrease infection and enhance early wound closure to decrease scarring. The nurse also must have a good understanding of the psychological effects of scarring and disfigurement in order to respond appropriately to the patient's needs during the various stages of adjustment.

In many settings, the same nursing staff will care for the patient from the acute phase throughout the recuperative period. During the acute period, care is frequently directed at survival of the severely burned patient. Much of the nurse's energies are oriented to technical equipment which monitor fluids and the patient's vital systems. Because the burn wound is an environment for many microorganisms, infection control is of primary concern. Strict isolation techniques, including mask and gown with good hand washing, is emphasized during patient contact to decrease cross-contamination. Wound care, including hydrotherapy, débridement, and dressing changes, is directed at preservation of tissue and expedient wound closure. Not only must the nurse be cognizant of the problems of acute care but must also be familiar with the principles of rehabilitation.

Maintaining joint functions and preventing contractures are essential elements which must be incorporated into the patient's care plan during the initial period. Certain skills and techniques must be learned and mastered by the burn nurse in order to implement these measures. It is essential that the nurse understand and practice the principles of range-of-motion exercises, splinting and positioning to prevent contractures, as well as teach and assist the patient in self-care activities. Position changes are essential to prevent deformities and pressure sores. These activities are a vital part of the patient's daily therapy.

Having a thorough understanding of burn pathophysiology not only increases the nurses awareness of potential problems but also enhances the nurse's ability to deliver effective physical therapy when the therapists are not available. It is essential that the goals of the therapist for the patient be fully understood and reinforced by the nursing staff.

The nurse not only must be able to deal with the physical aspects of care but also must be capable of providing support for the emotional well-being of the patient. The pain and disfigurement experienced by the burn patient are factors which the nurse encounters and must deal with on a daily basis. The nurse must also be aware of the interrelatedness of psychosocial and economic problems. Radical changes within the family structure as a result of the injury, as well as economic problems and vocational issues, may present obstacles to the treatment plan during and following hospitalization. In addition, the nurse must identify and utilize appropriate community agencies in assisting with and providing effective follow-up care. Referral agencies such as visiting nurse services, community mental health, public assistance, nursing home placement, or alcohol rehabilitation will need to be considered appropriate. Such planning should be coordinated with the social worker.

Furthermore, nurses must be aware and capable of dealing with their own feelings and attitudes towards pain, disfigurement, and death. To provide the appropriate support to the patient, they must recognize when a particular situation, other staff members, or a patient is a source of frustration. The burn nurse must be patient, understanding, and sensitive to the patient's needs. In addition to being expert burn technicians, the nurse must learn patient assessment and teaching skills, provide direct patient care and, at the same time, provide emotional support and care to the burn patient.

Nurse as a Team Member

As a member of a burn team, the nurse performs various functions, assuming a variety of roles dictated by the specific needs of the individual patients. Those needs will be altered as the patient progresses through the various phases of adjustment. The American Nurses Association Policy Statement provides a simple definition of nursing which is all inclusive, encompassing every facet of nursing care: "Nursing is the diagnosis and treatment of human responses to actual or potential problems." Nurses are committed to treating the total individual; therefore, the burn nurse must be capable of providing a broad spectrum of services—those which deal with the emotional, spiritual, social, and vocational needs, as well as those which deal with the physical needs of the patient. Nurses must be good organizers with the ability to plan patient activities and provide direct care. It is obvious that all the needs of the burn patient cannot be met, nor all the problems resolved; therefore, the nurse must be able to assess the needs of the patient accurately and select those which must be or can be dealt with most effectively.

PATIENT CARE PLANNER

To meet the needs of the burn patient adequately demands a systematic approach to care. Development of a *Nursing Care Plan* suited to the specific needs of the individual is an essential ingredient in nursing the burn patient. Early resolution of those issues viewed as important by the patient can often decrease much of the anxiety and frustration which impede the treatment program. Patient needs may frequently be unmet for a variety of reasons: lack of information, inaccurate identification of needs, inadequate evaluation of the patient's responses to therapy, and lack of patient participation. The burn nurse not only must *collect information* but also must assess and relate it appropriately to patient needs. Information may be obtained from various sources: the patient, family members, close friends, as well as other members of the burn team. Data collection must be in an organized format to ensure the information will be used. Although various forms of checklists are used for gathering information, a data base nursing history that includes pertinent information regarding the patient and significant family members enables the nurse to develop an in-depth nursing care plan. The information obtained must be complete and accurate. Also, the nurse must possess excellent skills in *assessment*. Nursing approaches to care are based not only on the information gathered but also on the nurse's ability to interpret and assess the data accurately. A good understanding of burn pathophysiology and medical therapies is necessary for the nurse to identify properly current and potential problems and implement appropriate nursing measures. Problems diagnosed in the care plan should be those which nursing can effectively treat. Nursing intervention and approaches to care should be separate and independent of physician's orders. Diagnosing potential nursing problems and implementing preventative nursing measures does not necessarily involve physician input. Initiating such therapies as turning schedules, positioning techniques, and comfort measures are independent nursing functions.

Methods of *communicating* the patient's needs should be incorporated into their care plan. Written care plans provide continuity to the patient's care, enabling other disciplines to be aware of the patient's problems and goals.

Evaluation of nursing intervention is of the utmost importance, allowing the determination of the effectiveness of the treatment plan. The patient's response to therapy should be observed on a daily basis enabling new goals and approaches to be identified. The care plan should be continually updated and modified accordingly. The entire burn team, including the patient, benefits from a well-developed nursing care plan.

PATIENT CARE PROVIDER

The patient care nurse has direct contact with the patient on a daily basis. Although it is desirable to have one nurse primarily responsible for the delivery of each patient's care, that may not always be possible. Nursing care of the burn patient demands a great deal of physical and emotional energy from the nurse. Delivering intense care for long periods of time can be extremely exhausting for one person. Although some burn facilities utilize "primary care nursing," others may use a modified version, whereby the nurse is primarily responsible for developing and maintaining the patient's care plan but does not necessarily always provide direct care. What is more important than "who" is that someone "specific" be designated to maintain the continuity of the individual patient's care. Many burn units utilize hospital assistants, burn technicians, or other auxiliary personnel as the patient care provider. In this case, it is essential that a professional nurse develops clear and concise care plans and sees to it that they are continually updated.

The nursing care plan is a tool which provides the patient care nurse with guidelines to assist in delivering effective nursing care to the burn patient. Implementation of the nursing care plan rests primarily with the direct patient care giver. Knowledge and expertise in burn care and treatment must be acquired and practiced by the patient care nurse to assess and evaluate accurately the effectiveness of the care plan. Being in direct contact with the patient enables the patient care nurse to make critical observations of the patient's responses to treatment and therapy. Other members of the burn team rely on the nurse to make interpretations and recommendations based on sound nursing principles. Recognizing limitations in knowledge and abilities enables the nurse to enlist the assistance and expertise of other members of the team.

Providing daily care to the burn patient can often be frustrating for the patient care nurse. The magnitude of the work involved in completing the daily assignment may often be overwhelming. Taking vital signs, delivering wound care with débridement and dressing changes, assisting with personal hygiene, meals and exercises are routinely part of the burn patient's schedule. In addition, appointments for laboratory tests, consulting services and visits from family and friends are daily occurrences which are essential to the burn patient's welfare. The nurse learns very quickly that including the patient in developing the daily schedule is very often the key to a successful day. In addition to performing routine duties, the nurse must be able to prioritize and *organize* the daily schedule to allow for unplanned events, such as nonroutine x-rays, laboratory tests, changes of intravenous lines, or changes in the routine schedules of other team members.

Furthermore, the patient care nurse must be attuned to incorporating preventative nursing measures to maintain optimal function and decrease deformities into the basic nursing care of the burn patient. The results of prolonged bedrest and inactivity are well known and require early and continued intervention. The importance of prevention becomes acutely evident when physical changes, such as contractures, muscle atrophy, or pressure scores, occur due to lack of adequate intervention. The level of nursing care and intervention provided must be scrutinized whenever decubitus ulcers occur. Frequently, adequate turning schedules and positioning techniques will resolve the issues. Sometimes special equipment, such as Circo-electric or Roto-beds, may be indicated to provide adequate turning. Understanding the implications of wound healing, scarring, and immobility enables the nurse to use independent judgment in making decisions pertaining to implementation of those nursing measures which will enhance patient care.

PATIENT CARE EDUCATOR

A major role of the burn nurse is that of *patient and family teaching.* The burn patient usually has much to learn. Scarring, skin discoloration, joint contractures, blisters, and severe itching are common areas which require a great deal of information and instruction. The patient who has experienced loss of a body part, decreased sensation, or a fixed contracture must learn new ways of performing daily activities, such as bathing, dressing, and eating. The nurse must be able to instruct the patient and family thoroughly in home care procedures, such as washing and debriding the wound, dressing changes, and application of topical ointments, splints, and pressure garments. As an educator, the burn nurse must be able to determine the timeliness of teaching and instruction. Too much information too soon may be worse than no information at all. Teaching needs will vary during the various stages of the patient's progress. Teaching should be a gradual process to avoid overwhelming the patient and family. Teaching is a vital process which affects the success or failure of the patient's rehabilitation. To ensure that teaching is carried out in an effective manner, it must be incorporated into the patient's daily care plan. The patient and family should be included in developing the teaching goals. Areas of teaching and instruction must be specifically identified to clarify and provide direction, not only for the patient, but also other team members. To accomplish the goal of successful patient and family teaching, the nurse must incorporate the information and teaching of other members of the burn team into the patient's daily activities. It is essential that the nurse monitor the need for further information and instruction.

In addition to patient and family teaching, the burn nurse must be qualified to *teach other nurses*, supportive nursing staff and students. The nurse will need a thorough understanding of burn pathophysiology and wound healing upon which to base those teachings. The nurse's ability to transfer knowledge and information is vital to the total care of the burn patient. Inservice education programs, as well as patient care conferences, should be offered on a regular basis. Increasing knowledge and improving the skills of the staff caring for the burn patient lends continuity and stability to the treatment program.

PATIENT CARE SUPPORTER

The burn patient will require emotional support throughout and following hospitalization. The nurse must be able to provide support to both the patient and the family, assisting them to deal with an altered body image and frequently a change in life-style. The nurse must be able to recognize and assist the patient and family in resolving any social and emotional conflict that may impede progress. Being a good listener and observer is essential. Consistency, understanding and trust are the key ingredients to alleviating much of the patient's anxieties. This may sometimes be difficult due to the burn nurse's dual role of inflicting high levels of pain during wound care, dressing changes, or other painful procedures, while at the same time attempting to provide relief from pain and discomfort. The patient will need honest information regarding treatments and procedures. Although answers and explanations should be thorough, they should be simple, direct, and oftentimes repetitive. Providing adequate information and paying attention to the patient's requests provide the structure for trust to develop. The nurse must be alert in observing the patient for clues that additional information is required regarding the injury and disfigurement. Continued reassurance related to progress will be required throughout the patient adjustment.

The ability of the nurse to interpret accurately the goals and treatment therapies for the patient tend to decrease misunderstandings and frustrations so apt to occur at various stages of the patient's progress. A tremendous amount of reinforcement and encouragement will be needed for optimal support. The burn nurse must be capable of conveying caring, understanding, and acceptance of the patient's feelings.

The burn nurse spends a great deal of time in close contact with the patient and family members. The continued day-to-day emotional interactions may often become a source of stress for the nurse. The nurse must be aware of personal anxieties which interfere with the welfare of the patient. It is essential that the nurse's own feelings regarding pain, death, and disfigurement be continually evaluated. The burn nurse becomes involved in the anguish, as well as the joy, experienced by the patients and families. Feelings of anger, frustration, and despair can be consuming, stifling the nurse's ability to provide support when the patient and family need it most. Emotional conflicts must be resolved as soon as possible. The nurse with unresolved frustrations may tend to respond to the patient in an adverse manner, thereby reinforcing the patient's fear of rejection. Adequate resources must be available to the nurse to deal with these issues.

Burn nurses frequently tend to receive the greatest support from each other; however, the support of the entire team is often needed to analyze and resolve conflicts. Professional counseling, either in groups or individually, should be available to all burn team members when necessary.

PATIENT CARE COORDINATOR

Coordination of the team effort is a vital function of the burn nurse. Optimal care and support of the burn patient requires that the expertise of the various disciplines involved be utilized to maximum potential. Coordination of the activities of the burn team is essential, not only to minimize duplication of efforts, but also to facilitate the incorporation of information and teachings of the team into the patient's daily activities. Other members of the burn team rely on the nurse who spends the greatest time with the patient to *reinforce* specific information during daily contact; therefore, the nurse must know what teachings and therapies have been instituted. Furthermore, the nurse must understand the goals and be able to work in harmony with the rest of the team. Frequently, the patient with severe burns over joints have specific exercise and splinting programs with which the nurse must be familiar. The inconsistent approach of one nurse to exercises set up by the physical therapist can markedly impair the patient's progress. It is essential that the information and instructions provided by the nurse be consistent with the teachings of other disciplines. Otherwise, the patient may become confused and discouraged. Information regarding goals, plans, and teaching should be included in the nursing care plan to be shared by the entire staff.

To integrate the team's activities, the nurse must maintain open lines of *communication* with other team members. In order to provide continuity of patient care, the nurse must have access to avenues which permit a systematic exchange of information. While it is true that informal systems such as phone calls or daily contact with individual team members are somewhat beneficial, they may prove to be unreliable in consistency. On the other hand, interdisciplinary patient care conferences, such as Burn Rounds and Rehabilitation Rounds, permit the nurse to interface with the entire team. Conferences such as these prove to be an excellent means for the nurse to share information related to the patient's concerns, fears, and goals, as well as the goals of the rest of the team. The patient is further benefited by the exchange of information between individual disciplines.

What Keeps the Team Functioning Together?

Cooperative teamwork is the fundamental ingredient in the successful care and rehabilitation of the burn patient. The multidisciplinary approach to burn care brings together many health care professionals with individual personalities, goals, and ideals. These professionals must learn to function as a cohesive group working in harmony to benefit the burn patient effectively.

Goals for the individual patient must be defined clearly to facilitate the entire team, including the patient, working toward a common end. A clear understanding of the team goals for the individual patient is essential to decrease confusion and frustration which can arise from conflicting goals. Utilizing such tools as the Kardex, the patient care plan, team conferences, and patient and family conferences helps not only to identify and clarify goals but also to re-evaluate goals periodically.

It is essential, therefore, that team members understand and respect each others' roles to accomplish the integral relationship required to care for the burn patient. Recognizing the patient as the most important team member is the first step toward a smoothly functioning team. Including the patient and family in developing plans encourages patient participation and cooperation. The nurse, being the most consistent factor in the burn patient's environment during hospitalization provides the framework around which the other disciplines function. The contributions of each member must be viewed as vital to the patient's care and recovery. A certain amount of conflict is inevitable when so many disciplines are involved in the patient's care. The enormous amounts of energy required to care for the burn patient places additional stress on the entire burn team. The team must be aware of conflicting forces which might affect its ability to function effectively. Individual members must be able to recognize and identify sources creating conflict. Effective methods of resolving conflict must be available to the entire team. Developing trust in the knowledge and capabilities of the team members is a prerequisite for sharing and resolving the feelings of anxiety and frustration so common to burn unit personnel.

Prescription for Nursing Management of the Burn Wound

This chapter will not attempt to discuss the merits of the various wound care techniques as they will be dealt with at length in Chapter 7. The wound care issues reviewed here will be those pertaining to specific nursing areas and activities which may influence the patient's rehabilitation.

While nursing techniques and approaches may vary from one institution to another, the issues and problems related to wound management and care tend to be universal. Conscious of the patient's potential for disfigurement and scarring, the burn nurse strives to prevent further tissue damage, maintain maximal joint function and adequate activity level, and restore the patient to a useful life in society. Diligent wound management is a crucial component in the overall care of the burn patient and may indeed be the area which impacts the greatest on the patient's ability to respond to therapy and rehabilitation. Nursing efforts must be directed at methods and techniques which prevent infection to facilitate wound healing, promote patient comfort and, at the same time, maintain optimal function and minimize deformities.

PREVENT INFECTION

Wound infection is of major concern in severely burned patients. The extensive loss of skin protection increases the patient's susceptibility to invasive organisms and provides an excellent medium for bacterial growth. Burn units across the country employ a multitude of isolation techniques in caring for burn patients which may range from strict closed isolation with Laminar air flow to an open unit with closed dressings to protect the wounds. Regardless of the method utilized in any given unit, the goal is to decrease the incidence of infection. The extent to which isolation is carried out will be determined by the severity of the burn injury as well as the local habits and successes of the individual units. The following areas of infection control in burn wound management tend to be routine issues which create generalized concern in most burn units.

Environment

Burn wound infection may be contracted in a variety of ways; however, cross-contamination remains a leading concern. The wound is susceptible to invasion, not only by the patient's own flora but also those of other patients, personnel, and contaminated equipment; therefore, an aseptic environment should be maintained during wound therapy to provide protection to the burn patient. The area should be free of extraneous materials and equipment which might collect dust. Equipment should be thoroughly cleaned between patients with an antiseptic agent. Dirty supplies and equipment should not be left for long periods in the patient areas. Religious hand washing by personnel who come in contact with the patient is essential and may indeed be the key to decreasing the incidence of cross-contamination between patients.

Hydrotherapy and Debridement

Daily cleansing is a vital component of wound care which removes accumulated exudate and loose nonviable tissue. The removal of devitalized tissue as soon as possible is essential to rid the wound of the persistent bacterial threat to infection. Hydrotherapy may be accomplished in a variety of methods. The use of Hubbard tanks, whirlpools, lowboys, or spray tables will vary with each unit depending on the facilities available and on the individual patient needs. Whereas the spray table, whirlpool, or a bed bath may be used for washing large extensive wounds, the bathtub, shower or sink may be just as effective for small wounds. Regardless of the methods employed, the effectiveness of therapy requires that the objectives of wound care be maintained at all times. Wound *débridement* generally carried out during hydrotherapy to facilitate the ease of removing loose eschar is accomplished most frequently on the ward by the mechanical use of forceps and scissors. Care must be taken to avoid introducing organisms into the patient's bloodstream. Wound débridement carried out by the nurse or other personnel on the ward should not cause excessive bleeding. The removal of thick, adherent eschar must be avoided, not only to decrease bleeding but to prevent exposure and dessication of underlying tissue prior to the development of granulation tissue. Extensive débridement is a function of the medical staff whereby the eschar is excised, usually in the operating room, with a definitive plan to cover the wound with a biological dressing. Mild bleeding is to be expected when washing and debriding superficial wounds and granulation tissue due to the vascularity of those areas. The bleeding incurred should cease after applying pressure for a brief period.

Although antiseptic agents are effective in removing large numbers of bacteria from the wound surface, they are limited in their ability to destroy many disease-producing organisms or to inhibit their growth. Therefore, the use of antiseptic solutions which are frequently used during the bath should in no way alter the use of aseptic techniques.

Aseptic techniques and basic principles of wound care must be observed to decrease cross-contamination from personnel and the patient's own organisms. Gloves, mask, and gown are essential when extensive wounds are exposed or when providing direct wound care. Cleansing of the wound should be performed with a firm, straight stroke rather than a circular motion to avoid transferring organisms from one area of the wound to another. All cream or ointment should be removed from the wound prior to débridement. Antiseptic agents applied should be allowed ample time for contact with the wound to decrease introducing bacteria during débridement. Following débridement, the wound should be rinsed thoroughly of any solution. Many of the agents used contain iodine which is not only drying to the wound but is readily absorbed through the wound when left on for prolonged periods of time.

Wound Assessment

Daily inspection and accurate wound assessment is crucial to the timely implementation of appropriate wound therapy. Medical management of the wound is largely determined by the inherent conditions which change from day to day. Frequently, the physician relies heavily on information received from the nurse or other personnel providing the wound care. Wound assessment can most effectively be accomplished immediately following hydrotherapy or when dressings are removed. Proper burn wound assessment requires thorough critical examination. Changes, although frequently subtle, are occurring on a continual basis. The nurse must recognize and appropriately communciate those observations. Observations related to the general appearance, such as color, depth, exudate, odor, and extent of the wound, are an ongoing process and must be communicated and documented daily in the nurse's notes. Additionally, any adverse changes in the wound must be brought to the attention of the physician whereby appropriate therapy may be implemented.

Topicals and Other Therapy

A wide variety of topical and bacterial agents are used in the treatment of burn wounds. The nurse must be cognizant that antimicrobial agents alone are not the entire answer to infection control of the burn wound. Most agents, although effective against a wide variety of Gram-negative and Gram-positive organisms, may be limited in their spectrum and tend to be selective against specific organisms. Therefore, contamination of creams, ointments, and solutions may allow the proliferation of bacterial growth. While silver sulfadiazine is generally the agent of choice in most burn units, frequently other agents are used, including Sulfamylon and silver nitrate. As with any drug therapy, frequent observations of sensitivities and reactions to therapy are important. Unexplained temperature with rash, whether localized or generalized, should be explored. However, particular attention must be given those agents which may have deleterious effects on the patient's general condition and even threaten survival.

It is extremely important that the nurse has some knowledge of the potential adverse effects, as well as the desired therapeutic effects, of the topical agents being applied. Sulfamylon, which is readily absorbed through the burn wound, inhibits carbonic anhydrase which may result in acidosis. Close monitoring of the patient's metabolic status is necessary, particularly when covering large wound surfaces. Silver nitrate, applied as a liquid in conjunction with dressings, tends to leach sodium, potassium, and chloride from the wound causing electrolyte imbalance. Metabolic or electrolyte changes can occur rapidly. Therefore, the nurse must be able to anticipate potential problems to facilitate early detection. The physician must be notified immediately of any adverse changes in the wound or patient status. Careful observation and documentation of the patient's vital signs, particularly respiratory status, blood chemistries, and wound appearance, is of the utmost importance to facilitate appropriate medical and nursing intervention.

Systemic antibiotic therapy is extremely important in the treatment of burn wound infection and the systemic complications. Therapeutic blood levels must be achieved for the antibiotic to be effective. The nurse must be cognizant of the expected therapeutic actions from these drugs and the various methods of delivery which affect absorption in the burn patient. Antibiotic medication must be administered at appropriate intervals to assure adequate levels are maintained. Along with observations of drug sensitivities, periodic wound cultures and evaluation of therapeutic levels will facilitate appropriate antibiotic therapy being maintained.

Dressings

Dressings are used in various facets of burn wound treatment and are frequently used in conjunction with topical therapy. The type of dressing will vary according to the desired outcome. The proper applications along with adequate dressing changes may often be as important to overall therapy and infection control as other aspects of wound care. Sterile techniques, utilizing cap, mask, and gloves should be maintained when applying dressings to large open wounds. When used in conjunction with wet agents, such as normal saline or silver nitrate, it is crucial that the outer layer remains dry to minimize invasion of external organisms. Dressings should not constrict; on the contrary, they must be loose enough to prevent pressure and friction which could result in tissue damage, often converting a partial-thickness burn to full-thickness. Dressing changes will be determined largely by the condition of the wound. However, they should be frequent enough to minimize saturation and excess accumulation of purulence on the wound. The need for joint mobility must be considered when applying dressings in conjunction with topical therapy, particularly when used over large body portions. Dressings are frequently used in small burns to facilitate ambulation. They should be applied loose enough to allow ease of motion, yet secure enough to decrease friction.

Dressings used in conjunction with splints to position burned joints require special attention. Adequate padding of splinting devices is essential to prevent tissue damage. Observations for signs of pressure, decreased sensation, and increased edema are imperative.

Following grafting or spontaneous healing, pressure dressings may be required. Frequently, there are small, open wounds as a result of graft loss or blistering. Dressings which absorb the secretions and adhere to the wound often disrupt the surrounding newly healed or grafted skin causing larger open surfaces when removed. The nurse will need to be aware of what the dressing is intended to accomplish. Disastrous results can be produced when dressings are improperly applied or used inappropriately.

PROMOTE PATIENT COMFORT

Providing adequate patient comfort may be the most difficult task facing burn nurses. Unfortunately, the procedures necessary for the patient's recovery in many instances cause a certain amount of pain and discomfort. Furthermore, the daily activities, such as bathing, dressing changes, range-of-motion exercises, laboratory tests and examinations, may all tend to contribute to the patient's discomfort.

Maintaining the patient's physical and emotional well-being is an ongoing endeavor which often requires all the ingenuity the nurse can muster.

Physical

The very nature of the burn injury with the loss of skin protection and exposure to pain compromises the patient's physical comfort. Normally, when heat or cold is detected, regulatory sensors in the brain respond to and adjust the body temperature accordingly. The severely burned patient, having lost large surface areas of skin, is unable to respond normally to sudden temperature changes. Therefore, it is necessary to maintain an environmental temperature which is comfortable to the patient. Any drafts in the patient area may cause chilling which permits the loss of large amounts of body heat. Heat shields, placed directly above the patient, may frequently be used to provide additional source of heat for the patient with extensive wounds. Prolonged wound exposure while doing treatments should be avoided whenever possible.

The length of time the patient is exposed during débridement, which generally should not exceed 30 minutes, can frequently be reduced, particularly with children or patients who have small burns or wounds in which the eschar is tight and unyielding. The discerning burn nurse will recognize that five minutes of firm cleansing may accomplish the same results as 30 minutes of hesitant dabbing at the wound. Time spent in the tank room should be utilized effectively to prevent overexposure and to decrease patient discomfort.

Pain Management: Pain, the focal point of the burn patient's anxieties, generally becomes heightened with preparations and activities related to physical contact with the wound. Following wound closure, those patients with severe joint involvement may experience extreme discomfort during exercise periods. The task of the nurse is to implement methods to minimize pain as much as possible during painful procedures. *Accurate assessment and evaluation of the burn patient's pain is extremely important. Analgesia for tanking and exercises is generally prescribed in graded dosages and ordered on an as warranted bases.* The frequency of the medication and the dosage given is often up to the discretion of the individual nurse. The nursing staff must be constantly on guard that their biases and frustrations with the patient's behavior do not interfere with proper assessment and delivery of adequate analgesia for pain relief. The patient who has difficulty adjusting to the treatment regime frequently has numerous pain complaints, hence, the label "problem patient" may arise. In such situations, the nurse may have a tendency to be influenced in a negative fashion, clouding the ability to evaluate the patient's pain accurately. Medication, which is either withheld or delayed due to inappropriate assessment, tends to cause antagonism and create an unending cycle for the patient and the nurse.

Frequently, pain in children tends to be minimized or ignored for various reasons, some of which are: pain is a learned experience, children forget very quickly, medication causes lethargy and the child is unable to participate in the treatment program. The latter of those statements may indeed be a legitimate concern. However, daily observations and assessment of the individual child's pain and analgesic therapy are essential. Children, as do adults, respond in various fashion to medication. While the behavior of children initially returning to the burn unit following discharge certainly supports the statement that "pain is learned", it belies the issue of children "forgetting very quickly." It leads one to wonder, how much of the pain response is taught on the burn unit and how soon, if ever, will it be forgotten? Pain medication, while by no means alleviating the need for implementation of other techniques, should be administered at adequate levels and well in advance of planned procedures.

Emotional

The burn injury itself is an extremely stress-provoking experience for the patient. Along with the various emotional responses and reactions produced by the injury, the patient often experiences additional stress brought on by varied treatments. The nurse must recognize that many of the lifesaving measures and therapeutic techniques employed to treat the burn patient may indeed contribute to extreme fear and apprehension.

The severely injured patient may be hospitalized for many weeks in a strange environment, frequently much of that time in the intensive care area. *Isolation*, although crucial to infection control, may tend to add to the disorientation experienced by the patient during the acute phase of illness.

The environmental constraints limit the level of positive external stimuli available to the patient. In addition, the buzzers and alarms from the various pieces of equipment in the room, such as ventilators, cardiac monitors, and fluid pumps, may often have adverse affects on the patient's ability to sleep, as well as to determine reality. The patient who is dependent on the respirator may experience extreme fear and anxiety, particularly if the nurse in the room rarely communicates what is happening. Frequently, bizarre behavior in the form of anger, hostility, confusion, and complaints of extreme pain may be exhibited by these patients. The nurse must attempt to discern and differentiate between physiological and psychological disorders to best benefit the patient. Reality orientation is essential. This should include diversionary activities and techniques, which will assist the patient to maintain contact with the environment. Radios, television, calendars, and conversation are frequently used to provide additional stimulation. A neuroleptic may be required to control the patient's agitation. Sleep deprivation is a real concern in the intensive care area; therefore, it is important that the noise level in the patient environment be mimized as much as possible.

Anxiety Management: Although pain cannot be completely eliminated, it is essential that measures and techniques be employed which decrease the patient's fears and apprehension. Performing wound care places the burn nurse in the unique position of having to inflict pain, while at the same time providing a certain measure of pain relief. Débridement of the wound is recalled by many patients as the most agonizing experience one can undergo. The tank room, frequently referred to by burn patients as the "torture chamber," generates a considerable amount of apprehension. Fear and apprehension may create any number of problems. Providing *adequate information* and explanation regarding wound care prior to entering the tank room will alleviate much of the patient's anxieties. Explanations should be simple, reassuring, and repeated often. Attempts to prepare the patient after the therapy is initiated are often futile due to heightened anxiety. The burn patient frequently becomes highly apprehensive when approached by a new nurse or changes in the daily schedule. Although it may be difficult for the same nurse to care for the patient each day, patient cooperation can be greatly enhanced by some *consistency* in the nursing staff providing the care.

Anxiety and apprehension may be decreased by allowing the patient to be involved in planning the bath schedule. Altering the tank schedule to incorporate the patient's requests may require some ingenuity on the nurse's part, particularly since it must be arranged around the various other patient activities which are equally important to the patient's care. It must be remembered that, although the bath may be a technical procedure to be completed by the nurse, it remains an extremely important experience in the day of the burn patient. Developing a *daily schedule* provides consistency and allows the patient a certain amount of control over when certain events occur.

Some burn patients experience nausea and vomiting after meals which immediately precede wound care. This phenomenon can generally be reversed simply by holding the patient's meals until the bath is completed. Allowing an adequate rest period following the bath will enhance the patient's ability to enjoy the meal. *Family* and friends also should be incorporated into the patient's daily schedule to allow for leisurely uninterrupted visits. Although a certain amount of flexibility should be built into the schedule, it should be adhered to as much as possible. Inevitably unforseen incidents, such as emergency admissions or laboratory examinations, will occur requiring changes in the schedule. Anticipated changes should be discussed with the patient. The wise nurse soon discovers that all of the fiascos of the entire day may be attributed to excluding the patient from important planning. The schedule is only effective if it is consistent. Constant conflicts which interfere may imply that re-evaluation of the schedule is necessary.

In instances of continued high levels of anxiety, the patient may be incapable of cooperating with the therapy programs. *Stress reduction* techniques may be required, whereby the patient gains some measure of control over the intense emotions. Music therapy, imagery, and hypnosis are examples of such techniques. Measures and techniques which are effective in promoting the comfort of the patient should be documented in the nursing notes and care plan. Patient anxiety surrounding wound care can be greatly decreased by providing adequate pain control, information and emotional support.

MAINTAINING FUNCTION

Severely injured patients frequently have multiple burned joints which may be threatened by contracture deformities. It is imperative that adequate measures to decrease joint limitations be implemented upon admission and continued throughout the patient's hospitalization. Maintaining optimal function of these areas is a goal which warrants constant vigil by the nurse and therapist. Limited joint mobility may severely hamper the rehabilitation of the burn patient. During the course of the patient's recovery, the nursing staff will need to be wary of the various obstacles presented which interfere with delivering effective therapy. The patient's complaints of pain and discomfort, the inability and sometimes unwillingness to participate may often present deterrents to adequate therapy. During the resuscitation period, an enormous amount of time and effort is devoted by the nurse to stabilizing the patient's fluid requirements, delivering wound care, and providing other lifesaving measures. Adequate positioning and splinting may be difficult to manage and often overlooked. Needless to say, the loss of joint mobility during the early phase may be extremely difficult to correct.

The severity of the patient's condition must not preclude the implementation of a diligent positioning, splinting and exercise program.

Positioning

Deep dermal burns or areas which have been grafted tend to contract, forming scar tissue as they heal. Joints involved in this process are usually pulled in the direction of least resistance. The nurse will need to be acutely aware of the potential for scarring and contracture formation while delivering daily care to the patient. The potential hazards of immobility often become a sudden reality, as the staff views the patient who has been in bed for an extended period in a flexed, contracted position. Recognizing that contracture formation is commonly associated with the position of comfort obligates the burn nurse to incorporate adequate positioning techniques into the patient's daily therapy schedule.

Splinting

Splinting must be considered whenever there is difficulty maintaining range-of-motion in major joints. The contractile ability of scar formation over joints may require the use of splints and conformers on a 24-hour basis. It must be remembered that scar formation is a continuous process; therefore, splinting devices are effective only when in use and when applied appropriately. Continuous assessments must be made by the nurse and therapist to monitor the effectiveness as well as proper fit of these devices. An improperly fitting splint or conformer may result in additional injury to the extremity. Therefore, it must be removed and reapplied only after readjustments have been made. The nurse should observe for indication of undue pressure, increased edema, or decreased sensation whenever splinting devices are used.

Range-of-Motion Exercises

Exercises, in conjunction with positioning and splinting, are an essential element in the burn patient's therapeutic regime. Active or passive exercise must be initiated immediately to maintain joint mobility and to diminish potential muscle wasting. Severe muscle shortening and atrophy occur with prolonged periods of immobility. Any functional losses incurred during the early phase of care may be irreversible.

The nurse must be able to supervise, encourage, and reinforce the exercise program set up by the therapist. Passive range-of-motion should be performed whenever necessary, keeping in mind that optimal joint function is maintained by the active participation of the patient. Independent exercises should be encouraged periodically during the day. In addition to tight and unyeilding scar tissue, open wounds which are dry or covered by bulky restrictive dressings may be extremely difficult and painful to exercise. Accurate knowledge of joint limitations and any contraindications to active or passive range-of-motion is essential. Pain is a powerful inhibitor and usually is the cause of the burn patient's inability to comply with therapy. Implementing measures to decrease pain and promote muscle relaxation prior to the exercise period will enhance the patient's ability to cooperate.

The nurse and therapist must be able to convey to the patient the need for continuing exercise in the presence of discomfort and the setbacks caused by decreased range-of-motion. Frequently, the success of maintaining function may very well lie in the patient's ability to understand the significance of immobility of burned joints. Initiating exercises early in the course of the injury with an ongoing preventative program is essential to enable the burn patient to return to a state of optimal function.

ADDITIONAL READINGS

1. Artz CP, Moncrief JA: *The Treatment of Burns*, ed. 2. Philadelphia, W. B. Saunders, 1969.
2. Artz CP, Moncrief JA, Pruitt BA: *Burns: A Team Approach*. Philadelphia, W. B. Saunders, 1979.
3. Fuller I, Jones C: *Nursing the Burned Patient*. Ann Arbor, MI, The Institute for Burn Medicine, 1973.
4. Wagner M: *Care of the Burn-injured Patient—A Multidisciplinary Involvement*. Littleton, MA, PSG Publishing Co, Inc, 1981.

17

Vocational Aspects

SUZANNE C. TATE-HENDERSON

Introduction

Vocational rehabilitation counselors have only recently joined the inter-disciplinary burn rehabilitation team. With the advances in treatment methods in the past two decades, an increasing number of burned persons are returning to their communities. Their need for vocational rehabilitation services has been recognized, but counselors have found that this population has special problems and that traditional approaches and methods in vocational rehabilitation are inadequate. The purpose of this chapter is to describe strategies that are needed to return the burned person to work and to present in detail a model for the vocational rehabilitation of the burned person.

One major problem with the traditional vocational rehabilitation approach, as applied to the burned persons, is the assumption that only patients who could not return to their former job needed vocational rehabilitation (43). Counselors are finding that burned patients returning to the same job need special counseling and ongoing support once they return to their job. In addition, the counselor may need to negotiate adjustments in the former job with the employer. This type of counseling cannot be carried out effectively as long as only those patients with retraining needs are referred for vocational counseling.

Related to this view of limiting services to retraining is a tendency among workers in the vocational field to turn to a reactive, crisis-oriented intervention program, rather than a planned approach to extended rehabilitation. The injured patient's adjustment to and performance at work is not systematically monitored. The traditional view produced a vocational rehabilitation theory and method that ignored the special problems of burned persons, such as disfigurement, pain, contractures, and dismemberment, with regard to functioning in the workplace. The patient who would benefit little financially from working, who faced great emotional stress and conflict in the workplace, or who had little self-confidence was not considered in the general vocational literature. The effects of this limited conceptualization

373

of vocational rehabilitation on the understanding of the needs of burned patients has become clear. We now need a systematic model for returning a burn injury patient to work. We cannot continue to assess these persons solely in terms of retraining needs, ignore the process of returning to a job and keeping it, and reserve intervention for situations in which a problem develops on the job. Our present approach to burned patients has been perpetuated by state and federal regulations and by the expansions and reductions in funding for services to burn patients. It is my view that assessment should systematically take place in the context of what is known about burn patients in general and the burn rehabilitation process. This chapter is intended to be a first effort at a comprehensive approach to the vocational rehabilitation of the burned patient.

Background

ADVANCES IN BURN TREATMENT AND THE EFFECTS ON THE BURN POPULATION

In 1975, 80,000 persons 15 years or older were discharged from short-stay hospitals with burn as the primary or partial diagnosis (47). More persons are surviving severe burns and treatment methods are advancing (9, 16, 22, 66, 72) and the numbers of burn victims returning to society are expected to grow rapidly. This is a new population, and we do not yet fully appreciate all its special problems. It is clear that the needs of burned persons will place heavy demands on public programs and health services in the coming decades. Because of limited research we cannot quantify the economic impacts of burn injuries but these impacts are major and will grow. One dated study (1972) reported that some 8.9 million work-days are lost and $300 million in medical costs are incurred as a result of burn injuries (21). Psychosocial costs, though more difficult to quantify, are also great and include marital disruption, changes in family structure, unemployment, and dissolution of the patient's social role as a major wage earner.

There is an enormous investment of health care manpower, time, money, and facilities in the acute treatment of burn patients and in restoring them to health (20). The treatment process, however, is long and arduous, demanding, complex, and expensive. Patients spend on the average 18.3 days in acute care (47) undergoing painful and incapacitating procedures such as débridement and dressing changes. The healing process extends well beyond this acute stage, and additional hospital admissions are often needed.

Given this enormous and increasing public, professional, and individual investment devoted to saving burned patients, what quality of life can these persons expect? And what can society expect of them? If most burn patients remain dependent, fail to hold gainful employment, and have lasting emotional, social, and psychological problems, the question becomes, are we saving these persons or merely preventing death? One important objective measure of successful recovery is return to work. Unfortunately, we have no good data on return to work for burned patients. However, the importance of return to work goes beyond providing a quantifiable measurement. The recovery of ability to undertake and maintain employment is a major personal goal for most patients undergoing rehabilitation.

BURN RECOVERY: REVIEW OF THE LITERATURE*

The burn trauma almost always represents a sudden change in the individual and his family. Burned persons are thrust into a crisis situation, and it is unlikely that they will ever be able to return to their former lifestyles. The wage earner's position is precarious, and he/she is bound-up in a process of recovery and rehabilitation. The latter involves working toward an optimal match between level of recovered function and extent of physical and psychological residual capacities. The rehabilitation period begins early after the accident (64), at least during the acute hospitalization stage, but the end point cannot be so easily defined.

Biomedical problems and systems of treatment and interventions in the severely burned population have attracted a great deal of attention in research, but we have little written information on the impact of burn recovery during and following rehabilitation, and in particular, on employment (15). Nevertheless, in order to address vocational issues specific to burn injury, it is necessary to review the burn recovery literature to understand the potentials of social, psychological, and economic factors as they relate to employment. Studies of recovery have been limited to the hospitalization or immediate post-discharge period. These studies, reviewed in some detail below, support the assumption that the consequences of a serious burn injury are drastic and prolonged. This review will concentrate on psychological adjustment, emotional milieu, and common behavior patterns in burned patients. These variables and interventions to affect them are a central element in understanding the vocational needs of the burn patient (64). The physical injuries and recovery of some measure of physical function are less amenable to generalization and need to be evaluated on a case by case basis.

In-hospital Condition

Investigators have found a wide variety of psychological disturbances in burned patients (2, 15, 27, 37, 67). Delirium, regression, and depression are among the serious general conditions identified (4–6, 29, 39, 48, 50, 51, 62).

---

* This section is based on "Determinants of Recovery among Seriously Burned Adults," a research grant proposal authored by Salisbury et al., 1981.

Specific diagnoses that recur throughout the literature are the acute grief reaction and extremely uncooperative and rebellious behavior. Bowden et al. (15) list the following reactions: "loss of appetite, insomnia, emotional constriction, withdrawal, nightmares, conversion or somatic symptoms, wittiness and mild euphoria."

Although the conclusions are tentative, studies of inpatient adjustment have singled out certain populations with poor prognoses: older patients, females, more severely burned, and those with prior physical or psychiatric disorders (15, 49). Some studies comment on the remarkable capacity to endure and accept an injury in some patients. Hamburg et al. (29) and Schlichtman (56) present a discussion of coping with disability.

Functioning After Discharge

As reported in several studies, a significant percentage of burned patients develop or retain emotional problems once they have returned to the community (4, 12, 18, 38, 62). However, these can be avoided, as two cross-cultural projects suggest (1, 8), and some workers indicate that disturbances recede slowly and may resolve after the first year. Nevertheless, 19% of burned patients followed by Steiner and Clark (62) sought help from a mental health professional in the first year after injury. There seem to be distinctive factors inherent in the burn injury that affect psychosocial influences and problems in these persons. Earlier reports give vivid accounts of the special pain and struggling that burn patients experience with respect to both physical problems and debilitating psychological conditions (3).

There is not much reliable information about how discharged patients function in the family and in interpersonal relationships generally and more research is needed in this area. Descriptive studies about family life and marital relations suggest some patterns and generalizations (4, 18, 38, 58, 68, 69). Andreasen et al. (4) and Williams (68, 69) looked at social life beyond the family. There is evidence that some patients develop closer family ties while avoiding contact with friends and the community at large. Others, however, become alienated from even their families. Overall adjustment within the community has been treated in several empirical studies (10, 13, 42, 44). These studies also looked at the continuum of the patient's emotional status before, during and after hospitalization. Bowden and Feller (14) analyzed the effect of a severe burn as measured by self-esteem and social support and found that the burn patient needs emotional assistance for a longer period than has been previously reported. An extensive study has treated development of psychosocial, socioeconomic and functional aspects of burn care (30). The important area of patient attitudes has been overlooked in the literature, with the exception of a 1966 study by Korlof (38). He found considerable patient dissatisfaction about skin grafts, personal appearance, and temperature sensitivity.

Vocational Functioning

The research on work patterns of burned patients in the community is limited. From the available information it appears that most burned persons return to work, although many encounter major vocational problems (4, 18, 38, 58). There are comparatively few publications on specific vocational interventions and their effectiveness. Other areas critical to the recovery phase and not well represented in the literature are organization of services, approaches to vocational problems, and conceptualization, planning, and evaluation of psychosocial programs.

Status of Burn Recovery Research

In general, burn recovery research has been descriptive rather than scientifically designed, static rather than spanning all phases of recovery, and marred by use of subjective data. Previous descriptions of burn patients' recovery have been useful in that they established the importance of psychosocial factors that may become problems in burn recovery. Unfortunately, long-term physical recovery is not covered in a comprehensive way. Also, minimal attention is given to the interaction of these psychosocial factors and the physical aspects of burn injuries and recoveries. In addition, the distinction between psychosocial factors and psychosocial problems is not clearly stated in the literature and needs to be addressed. This distinction needs to be made so that the burn team may be able to anticipate the transformation of a normal reaction to trauma into a problem which adversely affects rehabilitation. As noted, most articles address problems that develop in only one of the phases in burn injury—predominantly the inpatient phase. A patient's progress or lack of it is often not evaluated by taking into consideration the relationship of the preinjury, acute, and rehabilitation periods.

With this brief literature review it is apparent that this is a developing field. This put vocational counselors in the difficult position of having to provide services to an ever-increasing number of burned patients without a complete context and without the benefit of others' reported experiences. It is in response to this need that this model is presented. It draws on the literature when relevant and recommends a stepwise approach that is rational and practical. Its underlying bases in past literature and principles of vocational rehabilitation and counseling, as well as the lack of an alternative comprehensive approach, strengthen its usefulness.

A Model of Vocational Rehabilitation for the Burn Patient

The model is a synthesis of: (1) the Simons et al. (58) partial model of patient adaptation to a burn injury; (2) previous burn research; and (3) vocational rehabilitation theory. The existence of a comprehensive model may help focus future research, as well as direct ongoing services to the burned person. A comprehensive science of burn vocational rehabilitation must incorporate the numerous factors that affect patient outcome. Crucial components of vocational rehabilitation, their interrelationships and the ways in which they influence return to work have not been addressed in a single approach. The model (Fig. 17.2) presented in this chapter attempts to address these needs. This model is designed to be implemented early in the burn treatment process (64). The model provides professionals in the field of burn rehabilitation with a program for vocational rehabilitation for burn patients. It can also be used to direct public policy and funding decisions for cost-effective vocational interventions.

An underlying assumption of this model is that the delivery of vocational rehabilitation services should be done within an interdisciplinary burn rehabilitation team. The use of the team approach provides the patient with optimal participation in decision making and a greater opportunity to participate in an appropriate range of rehabilitation services (43). The burn rehabilitation team approach has been refined and systematized by many of the specialists in burn rehabilitation to begin immediately upon admission and to continue until the patient has reached maximum potential physically, psychologically, and socially. The team approach enhances the participation of the medical staff in the vocational rehabilitation process. This proposed interdisciplinary model is designed to anticipate, identify, and modify the multiple psychosocial, attitudinal, physical, and industrial barriers that hamper vocational rehabilitation. Finally, this team process of rehabilitation planning allows the physician, therapists, employer, and rehabilitation specialist to collaborate directly on the removal of vocational barriers in the rehabilitation process.

PREINJURY STATUS

Figure 17.1 represents the model of Simons et al. (58), which includes consideration of preinjury patient status, extent and nature of the injury, and psychosocial reactions to injury. Preinjury status is probably very important in adjustment (64) but there is little evidence to support this assumption because of the paucity of studies done in this area. It has been suggested that pre-existing medical problems (5, 6, 62) and prior psychiatric difficulties (5, 6, 62) interfere with a patient's hospital adjustment. By implication, patient return to employment would also be affected. Helm et al. (30) have stated that a patient's motivational background and belief system have a major impact on outcome. Therefore, the staff interviews the patient and family to understand what the patient was like before the injury. Patient and family interviews include the elements of cultural and family background, personality factors, and work history.

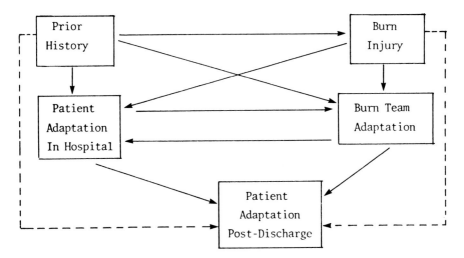

Figure 17.1. A model for adaptation to a burn injury is illustrated. Reproduced with permission from Simons et al. (58).

Cultural and Family Background

A patient's response to trauma and dramatic changes in image and life situation may be determined largely by his/her cultural, social, and family milieu, but there is little information about the family composition and living situations of adult burn patients. Successful recovery may be determined by how treatment is shaped in the knowledge of these milieu (64). For instance, does the patient live in a crowded environment? If so, he/she may become frightened and apprehensive when left alone in the intensive care unit. These intense fears may divert the patient's energies away from healing. Factors such as this are also of key importance in understanding a patient's response to injury and his/her potential for return to work.

Personality Factors

The counselor needs to know as much as possible about the patient's premorbid personality (64). This can usually be done by interviewing the patient and his/her family. Factors such as a self-motivation, excessive dependence on others, or the strength of a faith or belief system affect a patient's ability to return to work. Character defects such as alcohol or drug abuse are especially important to identify. The treatment team should specifically question the family about behaviors that suggest that the patient may have been suicidal.

Work History

The vocational process is predicted on the assessment of the worker's potential capacity to perform vocationally-related behaviors. One of the best sources of information about a worker's capacity (although it should not be relied upon as the sole source of information) is the assessment of his vocational history (64). A work history is an excellent way to uncover any psychosocial barriers to employment. The following case illustrates this point.

> Mr. X, a 43-year-old white male, was burned on the job in a saw dust and propane explosion. He was employed as a general maintenance man for a brick company. His job consisted mostly of welding and electrical tasks. Mr. X had an excellent work history until five years ago. He had held responsible jobs, made a satisfactory income, and achieved advancement in each job. However, in the last five years he had four different jobs. Further discussion into the reasons for the different jobs revealed Mr. X's son had been killed five years ago in an automobile accident. Mr. X began drinking heavily and became very irresponsible. He lost his family and all his assets.

A work history can give the patient as well as the counselor a good, although incomplete picture of personal skills and abilities. The individual may come to recognize some qualities that will lessen the effect of injury on the same job and discover undeveloped talents that have vocational relevance for a different job. Specific skills that have been learned through either formal education, formal vocational training, or on-the-job training experiences should be listed. Some patients with the right match of psychological and physical skills may find a job quickly, despite residual disability (52). Therefore, valuable information about employment can be obtained by assessing the patient's preinjury status.

NATURE OF BURN INJURIES

A second patient attribute that may affect employment is the nature of the burn injury and its complications (Fig. 17.2). The exact effect of a burn on employment and career planning has only recently received attention. Helm et al. (30) have stated that percentage of total body surface area burned is one of the important data on which to predict a return-to-work date. Other studies also reflect the complexity of reliably predicting reemployment. Korlof (38) studied patient assessment of work adjustment and found that most (65%) said the injury had not affected their work. A little under 25% felt choice among job types had been limited by the injury. Of the 120 working men in this study, 45% had changed occupation after the accident and 29% felt the change was dictated by the injury. Women's lives seemed less disrupted. Only six of the 29 working women changed occupations and only three of them regarded this as due to the injury.

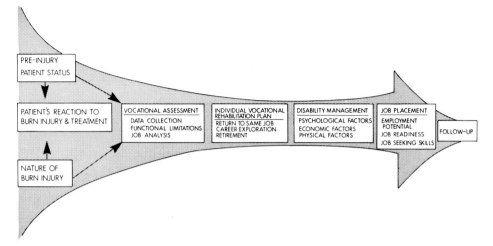

Figure 17.2. Vocational rehabilitation for the burn patient is diagrammed.

Although 29% of the respondents reported their income was lower as a result of the accident, the overall distribution was spread normally both before and after injury. This distribution may have been biased by such factors as additional income in the form of disability payments or the high preinjury income in the study group. Andreasen et al. (4) studied a group of 20 patients in which only one was unable to find suitable work. Four were still undergoing physical rehabilitation when the study was concluded.

Return to work may depend on the manipulative skill and physical strength required of the former jobs as well as extent of the burn. Williams (68) found that 36 of the 46 men in her study were skilled or semiskilled workers who had flame burns, and nine of them had stopped working after their injury. She did not explain this finding. Of the 23 patients questioned by Chang and Herzog (18) who were working at the time of their injury, 22 were working at the time of the study. However, about half (10 of the 22) required a change in jobs. About the same percentage of those burned on the face, on the hands, or in neither area required a change in jobs. These studies indicate that the size and location of a burn is not the sole determinant of job change.

Disfigurement has been suggested by others as a major factor in return to work and job change. Goldberg (25, 26) reported on the vocational aspirations and career planning of adolescents with visible disfigurement. In one study he compared children with facial burns aged 11–15 with children with congenital heart disease on 10 measures of adjustment. He concluded that the heart group had better adjustment in all 10 categories. Statistically significant differences between the two groups were obtained on vocational aspirations, career plans, self-image, and work values. In his second study, Goldberg looked at the relationship between facial disfigurement, career plans and rehabilitation outlook in 34 adolescents. Goldberg (25) states, "Unlike previous studies of chronic physical disability conducted by the author, the severity of disfigurement was as important as previous values, interests, and plans in predicting future careers planned. A visible physical disability with functional limitations may have a more profound effect upon vocational and educational adjustment than an invisible physical disability with moderate limitations." Bernstein (12) also showed that facial disfigurement causes long-term continuing emotional problems among burned patients. Not surprisingly, Williams (68, 69) showed that men with visible scars, severe burns, and physical disabilities seem to limit their community social interactions.

An important factor to consider in a burn patient returning to work is the need for long-term and periodic treatment. According to the National Burn Information Exchange, procedures may be needed for as long as 20 years after the injury, and counselors need to recognize that interruptions of employment are probable. Consideration of this interruption of employment, as well as the well-documented systematic and anatomic abnormalities (7, 40, 53, 66), must be recognized. Similarly, the length of time before the patient returns to work, as determined by the size and depth of the original burn injury, the complications that occur during the treatment, the age of the person, as well as environmental factors, need to be assessed. According to the National Burn Institute Exchange, 20–30% of the survivors of a moderate to critical burn will require at least one readmission to hospitals for functional and cosmetic reconstruction. Many of the procedures will be done in the first several years after a burn injury. Temporary changes in strength and appearance must be accounted for in a rehabilitation plan. As scar tissue develops, burn injured areas may become dark and coarse prior to softening and resuming a more normal color. Scarring causes fingers to contract, neck and shoulders to stiffen and distort body appearance, and also affects functional ability. Some patients may be required to wear splints, inserts, and elasticized garments to help minimize scarring.

Finally, changes in physical abilities, whether temporary or permanent, need to be addressed. Many burn patients have to adjust to amputation, or at least limited range-of-motion caused by scar tissue or heterotopic bone formation. Many patients have neuropathies that can extend beyond impairment of fine motor abilities and a loss of tacticle sensation to impairment of gross motor skills such as walking. A few patients become partially blind or deaf. Most patients have decreased stamina and strength after the long and arduous hospitalization. Even relatively minor problems such as itching, tingling, tight skin, discomfort with hot and/or cold temperature, and aching muscles are factors in return to work.

PATIENTS' REACTIONS TO BURN INJURY AND TREATMENT

This complex and important area of how emotional adjustment affects burn recovery in the hospitalization stage is well documented. However, emotional adjustment and return to work have not been well studied. Another complicating factor in the use of this type of information by the vocational counselor is the wide variation seen among individuals (4, 6, 29, 48, 50, 62). For example, pain is closely associated with behavioral and psychological well-being and the experience of pain is also highly variable (1, 6, 8). Coping behavior is essential for recovery (3, 29, 56). Systematic research on these specific behaviors has caused researchers to speculate about adjustment at various phases of hospitalization. It is suggested that behavior after discharge is related to hospital adjustment (2, 4, 5, 29, 35, 50, 51). Psychological functioning, a significant employability factor, can either restrict or enhance a patient's changes for re-employment, whatever the assessments of physical capacity and acquired vocational skills may be. Research has revealed the importance of the individual's psychological interpretation of the trauma to long-term adjustment. Reactions by family and peers are also important and should be considered in vocational counseling (52).

The psychosocial assessment can be extremely important to the burn patient, who is often permanently impaired (64). Depression, anxiety, hostility, regression, and other negative responses to stress are not unusual in the burn patient. Their origins and expressions may be determined by (1) the severity of the injury, degree of disfigurement, presence of dismemberment; (2) the intensity of the associated pain; and (3) the presence or absence of premorbid psychological factors. The important concept for the counselor is not the presence of negative emotional reactions but how these affect his or her care, progression to recovery, and return to work. Thus, while accepting the therapeutic premise that a patient must be allowed to set his/her own pace for coming to terms with the injury, the counselor must be aware of emotional patterns that inhibit full recovery. Specifically, the counselor's responsibility is to help the patient understand that despite the severe injury he/she will ultimately be expected to return to work. To assure this, the idea of vocational rehabilitation needs to be introduced early in hospitalization (64).

The rehabilitation counselor must counter the patient's exclusive concern with the physical damage he or she has sustained. To do this, the counselor redirects discussion of physical disabilities to consideration of which functions have been preserved. Given this perspective, the patient can retain his self-esteem. All of the literature and terminology of this body of research must be translated by the vocational specialist into clear functional terms relevant to vocational adjustment. The vocational specialist knowledgeable in behaviors typical of burn patients attempts to alter those behaviors which are incompatible with return to work. When the psychological conditions are understood, a realistic vocational rehabilitation plan can be designed. The specialist should strive to use operational definitions. For instance, "depression" is not very descriptive, but when depression is defined in terms of frequency, intensity, and duration, the term becomes useful in planning for vocational rehabilitation (59).

In assessing the patient's behavior, the rehabilitation counselor can identify residual capacities as well as deficits (64). While a patient's aggressive behavior and anger may be difficult to deal with during the acute phase, such patients can be independent and have powerful emotional resources that can be directed toward recovery. On the other hand, although passive attitudes and lack of affect may be favored by the burn staff in the acute phase of burn treatment that patient may have had a poorly defined self-image before the accident and may need special attention from the psychiatrist as well as the rehabilitation counselor. The rehabilitation counselor must link the severity of the physical injury to the individual's emotional makeup and social adjustment. The latter may be more predictive of successful rehabilitation than level of residual function (64).

VOCATIONAL ASSESSMENT

The fourth element in the vocational rehabilitation model is assessment of the burn patient's vocational potential. Accurate prediction of the patient's vocational functioning potential has always been at the center of professional vocational counseling and evaluation (59). The purpose of a vocational evaluation is to explore systematically and evaluate vocational possibilities in order to determine a feasible vocational objective for the burn victim. The focus of this vocational evaluation is to define the patient's strengths and deficits as they relate to functioning in a job. Advances in recent years in therapeutics for the severely burned patient have given more victims the potential to return to the job. Early intervention is essential if the patient is to achieve this potential; therefore work potential evaluation should begin as soon as possible after the accident (64). The patient and the counselor together should define any functional impairments and deficits that will hamper or preclude return to the former or related job. The counselor must actively direct these discussions toward the patient's assets (perhaps formerly unrecognized) and how they can be used. For example, the patient's job can be identified and the counselor can begin an initial analysis of it; this process in turn details the basic job tasks and their structuring. In a vocational assessment, the rehabilitation counselor should go through the following steps:

Data Collection

The counselor's main job at this stage is to bring together all the data on the patient. This includes the preburn information, the functional limitations caused by the burn injury, and the patient's reaction to the injury and hospitalization. The counselor decides which data are relevant to the vocational rehabilitation task and shares these with the patient. It is likely that the counselor may want some specialized testing such as vocational interest tests, job knowledge tests, and a work evaluation. The results of these tests are explained to the patient in preparation for constructing a "patient profile" specifically related to employability. The profile development should be a joint effort with the counselor and patient. Information at many points in this process will have to be elicited from the patient through a series of interviews.

Assessment of Physical Capabilities

The patient needs to know ahead of time that he has a reasonable expectation of succeeding in a desired job. All job-related tasks, functions, and behaviors need to be studied by the rehabilitation counselor, who can help the patient come to terms with the true extent of his disabilities (64). The counselor balances this painful but necessary realization by the patient of his handicaps by beginning to develop abilities specific to new vocational aspirations long before the patient is physically ready to return to a job. For example, a severely disfigured former receptionist may be helped to manage a telephone physically and to develop a telephone personality, with the aim of running an answering service from his/her home. In addition, this approach develops an understanding of the need for rehabilitative therapies. The use of vocational planning thereby provides the patient undergoing treatment with a reason for therapeutic efforts, i.e., maximizing the patient's ability to function and succeed upon release from the hospital. The rehabilitation counselor determines the extent of vocational handicap based on functional limitations. Physical and occupational therapy programs are thereby augmented to improve physical function, thus increasing the potential to return to work.

Analysis of Current Employment

The rehabilitation counselor and the patient should begin this evaluation by analyzing the job the patient held prior to the burn injury. The job should be analyzed even if it is obvious that the patient will never be able to return to that type of work. The process uncovers the skills, traits, and aptitudes the patient had to perform the job (64). From a patient's answers to questions about tasks involved, the counselor can better assess the patient. The physical demands, working conditions, training time, aptitudes, and personality characteristics needed for the former job are valuable data. The counselor then presents this structured breakdown of the former job to the patient. This information usually helps patients see the full range of their capabilities. For example, the factory worker who has lost physical strength may find unrecognized leadership abilities that could be used in a supervisory position. The approach should be concrete, with the patient himself emphasized less than the job he held. This functional analysis is very helpful to the patient who must make decisions about major life changes (64). Job analysis serves a second purpose of informing the counselor about how a patient's former job might be adapted. Only by conducting an in-depth analysis of the job can the counselor learn the extent of the changes needed and incorporate these changes into an individualized vocational rehabilitation plan.

There are several resources available to aid in the plan once the job has been identified. The most useful is the U.S. Department of Labor's *Dictionary of Occupational Titles*. With this tool, the rehabilitation counselor can, for example, direct a blue collar worker to skills and talents that could be used in a sedentary occupation. Hobbies, community service activities, and other areas of the patient's life before the accident may guide him toward a service occupation. The counselor must be firm and insist on a plan that is both practical and compatible with the patient's redefined goals. The counselor should present the vocational assessment of the patient to the burn team (64). They can help to develop a consistent rehabilitation plan for the patient that should minimize the disabling effects and maximize physical adjustments to the hospitalization and burn injury.

INDIVIDUALIZED VOCATIONAL REHABILITATION PLAN

The fifth element in the vocational rehabilitation model is the individualized vocational rehabilitation plan. This step leads to disability management and job placement. The individualized plan is critical in allowing the burn patient the opportunity to choose a way to make a living. Jobs are more critical to our lives than just a salary. A job determines much else in our lives: our associates both on and off the job; our dress style; our choice of neighborhood; our sleep habits; our travel and time away from home and family; even our health (59).

Burn injuries can impair one or all of the general job-related aptitudes: educational, physical, social, psychological, vocational. When a person's ability is limited in one or more of these five areas, his ability for successful employment is limited. The counselor must analyze residual physical, psychological, social, educational, and/or vocational functioning abilities (Fig. 17.2, four components on left side of arrow) and synthesize the abilities into a viable individualized vocational plan. To assure the program's success, the counselor must allow the patient time to absorb the information and ask questions before proceeding. The patient needs to clearly understand the extent of his disability as well as the breadth of his assets, especially as they relate to his potential for vocational independence.

When the patient has had sufficient opportunity to respond to the vocational data, planning an individualized vocational rehabilitation program should begin (64). Again, this must be a collaborative effort with the patient. The vocational plan must be coordinated with other burn rehabilitative therapies. The rehabilitation counselor consults with other members of the treatment team about splinting, exercises, and functional limitations. Together the counselor and patient integrate these into a vocational rehabilitation plan. The greater the patient's participation in decisions about his life, the stronger will be the gains in treatment. In this individualized plan the patient will explore one of the following possibilities: (1) return to the same job with or without job modifications; (2) career exploration and selecting a new job; (3) retirement—full or partial. These three options will be discussed in the following sections.

Return to the Same Occupation—With or Without Job Modifications

Often persons who are burned on the job initially feel that they cannot return to the same job, especially if the injury is a serious one. This is often a false assumption and this problem should be addressed shortly after hospitalization. Periods of recovery that stretch into weeks and months tend to reinforce a sense of worthlessness. Furthermore, a period between the injury and return to work raises self-doubts: "maybe I really can't do this type of work again." An equally negative consequence of delay is the comfortable feeling one gets from receiving compensation payments. The burn victim may conclude that not working can be just as profitable as returning to work—maybe more so. An alternative to the above is for the burn patient to receive some immediate rehabilitation efforts directed toward vocational adjustment. Early intervention increases the patient's potential for returning to his previous job and being a productive member of society. Preinjury job skills, current level of physical and emotional functioning, tolerance and endurance for work, and a functional analysis of the job task have already been assessed. If the patient will be physically able to return to the former job, the next step is to determine job skills, increase physical tolerance and endurance, improve body mechanics, and begin counseling if needed to remove any psychosocial barriers to employment. Some new skills may need to be learned, the job may need to be modified, or structural changes in the workplace may be called for.

The laws of Workers' Compensation were established as a means to protect workers who were injured through employment. It is important to educate the burn victim, the physician and the employer about the Workers' Compensation laws to assure a smooth transition from rehabilitation to employment. The rehabilitation counselor must be sure the patient is emotionally ready to return to work when the physician releases him/her.

This enables the patient to begin earning wages as soon as his compensation payments are terminated by the insurance company. The employer and insurance company should be informed of the patient's progress and expected date of return to work, patient's progress in rehabilitation, the physician's rating, and final settlement. This process may take years with a burn patient because of the necessary reconstructive procedures.

A major hurdle is convincing the employer to rehire a burn victim. There are many prejudices about hiring the handicapped: will the employer's Workers' Compensation rates be increased? The counselor can intervene and provide accurate information. Since worker compensation rates are based on previous accident rates of the employer's firm, the employer can be assured about holding steady rates. Costs are based on compensation and medical costs rather than the number of disabled workers. Employers should be shown the record of disabled workers; their accident rate matches that of nondisabled workers, but does not exceed it (52). Most states have a second injury law that protects the employer from liability for reinjury. The injured worker will be compensated for the total amount of disability resulting from repeated injury, but the employer is responsible for only the initial injury loss.

Structural changes and job modification to prevent re-injury or allow for placement back on the job need not be costly. They may be as simple as raising a work surface, adding a mechanical aid, changing a container size or allowing periodic changes in position. Employers are reassured when they learn that these practices may help reduce the cost for Workers' Compensation insurance (63). They should also be reminded that it is to their advantage to facilitate recovery and return of the worker to employment as soon as possible. Quick re-employment will also reduce the cost for rehabilitation services as well as the likelihood that injured workers will file liability claims. The vocational specialist can help prevent misunderstandings between the patient and employer as job modifications are being made. The patient will be extremely sensitive to a patronizing attitude, and he or she may feel stigmatized and reject changes.

Employers may express concern regarding a disabled worker's performance. The counselor can remind the employer that comprehensive work evaluation and job placement strategies have been used and these increase the potential for successful placement in competitive employment. Studies on work performance of disabled workers show favorable comparisons with able-bodied workers in production rate, turnover, absenteeism, and accident rate (52). In summary, the counselor's job is to show how both the burn victim and employer stand to gain if an equitable and logical process of rehabilitation is followed.

The following case describes the process of return to the same job after burn injury, and highlights the importance of psychological factors.

Mr. B, a 55-year-old white male, sustained a 14% total body surface burn with second and third degree burns on his left hand and lower extremity. The accident occurred on the job with the State Transportation Department when the hose to an acetaline torch he was using broke. Two weeks after admission, Mr. B underwent tangenital excision and split-thickness skin grafting to his left lower extremity. The patient exhibited a very low tolerance for pain. He was very difficult to handle during tanking and dressing changes.

The vocational counselor was called in for an initial assessment. She learned that Mr. B was divorced and had a grown son. He had an excellent work history in his job of marking highways and painting signs. Based on this evidence and the small extent of the burn, the patient should be able to return to his former job. The counselor, however, recognizing the patient's resistance to treatment, pursued the matter with the patient. During further interviews she learned that the patient was angry with the employer and felt his co-worker, who had been previously cited for carelessness, was to blame for the accident. Mr. B wanted not just recovery, but for a wrong to be made right.

The counselor became an advocate for Mr. B with his employer. After verifying Mr. B's interpretation of the cause, she succeeded in having the accident investigated. Ultimately, a safety feature was installed on the hose of acetaline torches. She also obtained Workers' Compensation early to relieve some of Mr. B's concerns. Throughout these efforts, the counselor carried on systematic desensitization to help Mr. B tolerate the tanking and dressing changes.

The final result of the vocational counseling was that Mr. B chose to return to a different job in the department so that he would not have to work with his former co-worker. The co-worker was put under closer supervision. It became apparent to Mr. B through counseling that these adjustments were more important to him than the slight decrease in salary his new position entailed.

Most of the steps of the vocational rehabilitation counseling process are exemplified with Mr. B's case. It is clear that a number merge together and this clumping pattern varies with each case. The counselor was called in initially because of Mr. B's anger and his refusal to cooperate in his treatment (step 3 in the model). His reaction was unexpected because his treatment had been relatively uncomplicated. In the course of collecting data on the patient's preinjury status, the nature of the burn and the vocational assessment (steps 1, 2, and 4), the counselor learned the source of the patient's emotional distress. She was able to use this knowledge to direct the patient's resources toward recovery and to design an acceptable program for return to a different position within the same job (step 5).

Career Exploration—Selecting a New Job

Residual limitations or other disincentives resulting from the burn injury may preclude return to previous type of employment, making it necessary or desirable to change vocation (23). The task of finding the best job for an individual, especially an injured worker, can be a very complex and difficult endeavor. The task is further compounded when factors such as the laws and regulations pertaining to the employment, benefits of the injured worker, the slowing economy, and the dwindling motivation of some people for work are considered. At the same time, there is a great emphasis on all persons concerned to show cause for their respective actions (e.g., the vocational professional who offers rehabilitation services, the employer who hires or fails to hire the injured worker, etc.). It becomes apparent that the utilization of the knowledge and skills pertaining to job analysis, vocational assessment, and transferability of skills is of critical importance to the burn patient, the rehabilitation counselor, and the employer.

Specific developmental stages in the burn patient's approach to vocational decisions have been identified (43). These can be used to plan vocational rehabilitation interventions. The manner in which the patient interprets and incorporates the meaning of the burn vis-à-vis vocational developmental tasks will dictate the need, the type and the intensity of vocational rehabilitation services. A vocational developmental task is defined as "a work or career task which arises at or about a certain period in the life of an individual. Successful achievement of the task will lead to his or her happiness and success with later tasks" (34). For example, if the age of the burn injured patient falls within the three decades between the ages of 35–65, the counselor can direct his or her work around such important tasks as career advancement, career maintenance, or stabilization and retirement. The patient in this age group worries about money, dependent family, and his/her self-concept as the breadwinner. Thus, the counselor identifies problems and modifies the patient's specific coping styles within vocational environments that may sabotage the eventual return to work.

Career counseling to explore remaining vocational options is indicated if the burn patient cannot return to his or her former job because of functional limitations caused by the burn, or if the patient chooses to explore other options for socioeconomic betterment or emotional reasons. The patient may need help in decision-making skills in order to make a vocational choice. Specific vocational goals need to be considered in light of contingent physical, intellectual, or emotional factors, as the following case history indicates.

Mrs. W, married with two young children, had been on the job just three months when she was severely burned. Previously she had spent several years as a homemaker. She sustained 80% burns and required a long hospitalization and a similar period of rehabilitation, including several surgeries. During the acute phase she experienced ICU psychosis and was convinced her husband was having affairs.

The rehabilitation counselor saw Mrs. W in the first month after the burn. She provided personal counseling for Mrs. W, now severely disfigured, who attached great importance to body image. Her husband had a traditional orientation to sex roles, had opposed his wife's return to work, and had been inordinately proud of his wife's beauty. The counselor, at this early stage, continued to remind Mrs. W that she would help her find a new job when she was ready. She arranged for Workers' Compensation and for a rehabilitation nurse to go home with Mrs. W. She referred Mrs. W to the local vocational rehabilitation office upon return to the community.

At two years after the burn injury Mrs. W continues to see the vocational counselor at each return visit to the Burn Center. Her husband has left her; her sights for economic and personal satisfaction from work are now higher than the assembly line work she formerly did; she still must devote most of her energies to recovery from the burns.

Mrs. W's burn changed her life. She has had to change her values, cope with rejection by her husband, and the economic realities of a single parent. Through this experience Mrs. W has come to recognize her own residual inner strength and her intellectual potential. The vocational counselor's approach has had to change along with Mrs. W. The counselor and Mrs. W have reached the point where she is ready for comprehensive vocational evaluation. Among the many lessons that can be learned from Mrs. W's case, perhaps the most important is that vocational counseling for burn patients can be a long and multifaceted process.

Burn patients like Mrs. W may require additional skills or assistance in finding a new job to meet their goal after discharge. They may need a more intensive vocational evaluation and retraining program financed by most insurance carriers, disability policies and State Vocational Rehabilitation Agencies. Referral to a state agency is dependent upon whether the burn patient has a substantial handicap to employment and whether the patient can achieve gainful employment through rehabilitation services. A comprehensive computerized vocational evaluation may help. There are several systems of computerized vocational evaluation, the Hester and Valpar systems being most prominent. The Hester System consists of a battery of 22 factor-sure vocational tests covering motor, perceptual, and intellectual skills. The Valpar System uses work samples that measure universal traits that are related to a person's success in many occupations with a variety of job characteristics. By matching vocational evaluation with physical, psychosocial, and functional evaluation, a comprehensive plan can be obtained. These computerized evaluations help to clarify the job tasks and functions the patient can perform, and the extent to which he or she could function on a different job. The diagnostic judgment from the evaluation may help the burn victim achieve his potential, provide new options, and ensure prompt settlement of a disability case.

Retirement—Full or Partial

Mr. M is a 62-year-old black male who was injured at home while lighting a barbecue grill. He sustained second and third degree burns over 9% of his body, primarily his right side. During the acute phase he had an episode of hallucinations, and a psychiatric consultation was obtained. Also, early during his recovery, Mr. M was discovered to have cancer of the prostate.

Mr. M was the sole support for his wife, his mother, and an older sister, none of whom were in good health. The psychiatrist diagnosed Mr. M's reaction as a psychosis with paranoid features brought on as a result of stress. He was extremely worried about his family's welfare and future, and he dealt with the news of his cancer by denial. He responded to treatment with Haldol.

The vocational counselor, in working with Mr. M, learned that he had wanted to retire from his job for some time but felt he could not afford to. The job was physically demanding and entailed a 60-mile commute daily. The counselor helped work out a way for Mr. M to retire early and still support his family.

As the above case indicates it may not be best for certain burn patients to return to work. A number of factors may lead to this decision, including decreased functional abilities. There may be too many skill deficits to make it practical and cost-effective to prepare this patient for employment. There may be other legal or economic reasons that prevent the patient from working. Therefore, the patient and family may need help in legitimizing early retirement (23). This situation is more likely to arise in older workers for a number of reasons. These persons may feel they deserve to be relieved of these responsibilities, given long years in the active work force and the fate of the burn accident. Their children may be grown and established in gainful employment. The patients may be eligible for retirement. Apart from these practical realities, older persons usually have more health problems, and can be expected to be more susceptible to complications and other diseases related to the burn injury.

The rehabilitation counselor should play an important role in the recovery of these persons. The patient needs to be taken through an exploration of the meaning the work role held in his or her life. The entire burn team contributes to the patient's developing usefulness and satisfaction through teaching self-care skills. The patient can also be taught how best to participate in normal recreational activities. It is a primary responsibility of the rehabilitation counselor to follow through on informing the patient about and helping him to receive all the social security disability insurance to which he is entitled. This can be a delicate task as concurrent efforts must be made to prevent long-term reliance on these programs, the pattern of deriving secondary gains from the injury.

The Social Security programs are designed to provide for the needs of individuals and families, including the aged and disabled. The largest single program is the Retirement Insurance program. The program which relates most directly to the employer is the Disability Insurance program. Monthly cost benefits are available to the disabled worker. The purpose of these benefits to the disabled burned person is to protect against the loss or reduction in the amount of disability or retirement by providing funds during the period of disability. Benefits to the disabled worker will not be paid if the worker refuses to accept services from the State Vocational Rehabilitation Program. In order to receive disability the patient has to be unable to engage in any substantial gainful activity by reason of any medically determinable physical or mental impairment which can be expected to last for a continuous period of not less than 12 months (59). Some patients, either consciously or unconsciously, remain sick. In the case of a burn injury, patients may not enter wholeheartedly into the therapy program as long as they have the security of some income and personal care. If this process is handled well by the rehabilitation counselor, some patients may change their minds about seeking full or partial retirement. Relieved of legal and economic burdens with the aid of the counselor, a patient may find unexpected capacities in himself as he improves with therapy and reconstructive surgery. His interest may be renewed in vocational objectives, as opposed to retirement planning.

DISABILITY MANAGEMENT

The next step, disability management, is a checkpoint to re-evaluate the patient's progress and to be sure the critical points of adjustment and response have been identified. Patient reliance on psychological and secondary gains are reduced. Some principles of disability management are similar to those necessary for other steps in the vocational rehabilitation process: early intervention, secondary prevention, and attention to the total impact of the burn injury. Disability management is also based on clear identification of secondary gains and of critical points of adjustment and response. The differences between disability management and the usual vocational rehabilitation processes are that (1) services are initiated early; (2) the process is proactive rather than reactive; (3) planning and problem-solving are done collaboratively with the burn rehabilitation team; and (4) the process focuses on the total impact of the disabling events.

The broadly-based orientation has been emphasized in early steps in the model. Here it becomes essential in understanding why a patient wants to stay in the sick role. The "whole man concept" (17) is most comprehensive and, therefore, useful for the purposes of the vocational rehabilitation counselor when approaching the problems of a burned patient. The basic concept is that one does not treat disease and injuries but individuals who are suffering from the effects of such disease and injuries (11). Each of these individuals has a unique set of social, economic, psychological, vocational, marital, and other problems that encroach on the injury-related problems. Thus, personality traits as well as psychological responses to the injury are considered. The whole man concept is based on the belief that many factors influence the return to work of the injured worker, and it guides a successful rehabilitation by requiring an evaluation of the whole man. Coping mechanisms are evaluated in terms of their past expression and present usefulness. On the surface, denial may be a valuable approach to injury in terms of the patient's strong desire to return to work (i.e., normal life, as before the accident). However, when carried too far, denial leads to noncompliance and ultimately more medical problems, leading finally to unemployment. The counselor, adopting the whole man concept, would take the broad view and bring the patient to change behavioral and attitudinal habits that, however comforting initially, will prevent him from moving ahead in his therapy and reconstituted life.

Steger et al. (61) indicated that an individual who suffers an industrial burn injury is at risk to develop psychological post-injury problems relating to return to work. Weak correlations between physical impairments, functional limitations and employment in a number of diseases (28, 46) have led investigators to search for the "psychosocial pathways" by which impairments become limitations on activity and by which these limitations evolve into behavior patterns labeled disability (70). There may even be a negative correlation between receipt of disability payments and recovery rate. While we do not know all the causes of this phenomenon, researchers have most often cited psychological factors. Among these pathogenic mechanisms and behavioral syndromes are accident neurosis (40), secondary gain syndrome (24), the accident process (31–33), acute traumatic neurosis (24, 71) and psychoanalytical explanations (45, 60).

A worker's self-image alters along with changes in physical appearance and functional capacity. Body image has been defined as part of one's self-concept, according to the values and emotions invested in it by the individual (54). Thus, it seems that a burn patient's image of himself as a man physically capable of heavy labor may now be a barrier to his returning to work due to his feelings of self-consciousness, embarrassment, and inadequacy. The counselor cannot circumvent the effects of such feelings by insisting from the start that the patient must accept a less demanding job. To some people it would seem better to have no job at all. The counselor must first deal with these feelings of chronic work disability or significant on-the-job adjustment problems will develop. Employees who have felt rejected by employers in past job experiences may fear more of these encounters (55). Another fear is challenged by loss of vocational identity when one cannot return to his old job or rejoin the work force in any capacity. All of these attitudinal influences are intensified over time. Delay can occur for several reasons: the employer hesitates or refuses to rehire the injured worker; the individual initially wants to receive medical disability; legal issues with slow processing of disability claims; and families may support the patient in the sick role. The patient gets into the habit of having the special social environment meet the needs he once found fulfilled in his job. His inclination is not to return to work (19).

There are other important variables besides the psychological ones that may affect unnecessary extension of disability in a burned person. Policies regarding sick leave, retirement benefits, and disability compensations act as economic disincentives to recovery. How can a person be encouraged to work, under sometimes strained conditions, when his or her salary is no more than disability compensation? Also, when the labor market is tight, opportunities for burned persons—and, in fact, all persons with any disability—are limited. Transportation difficulties and architectural barriers discourage return to work. Limitations in mobility may include difficulties in walking and climbing stairs or barriers to wheelchairs.

Patients who have a clear understanding of their legal rights and limits are less likely to engage in efforts to sabotage or slow their recovery. Rumors and misconceptions abound about the ease and benefits of being classified as disabled. Unrealistic assumptions about automatic lump sum settlements and extended compensation payments (19) may perpetuate the period of disability (55, 57). Educating the burn patient concerning disability laws (57) and the difference between *disability* and *handicap* may be helpful in preventing unnecessary disability claims.

The rehabilitation counselor works with the industry to facilitate an appropriate system of response to the injured worker. The focus on rehabilitation rather than compensation facilitates the utilization of rehabilitation techniques which maintain appropriate levels of employment for burn victims with functional limitations. A rehabilitation orientation within an industry creates a response that emphasizes early intervention of job-related problems, management of physical symptoms, modification of jobs and personnel policies that will facilitate work rather than create a de facto retirement program for the injured worker. Such a proactive policy toward work return provides a positive anticipation of adjustment rather than a "wait and see" or avoidance attitude.

Many industries have established rehabilitation programs within their corporate and plant structures which interact with community resources. Therefore, vocational rehabilitation agencies and facilities must become thoroughly familiar with industry's needs. Currently, a systematic link between industry, burn centers, and rehabilitation programs does not exist. Historically, the medical and rehabilitation services for the injured worker have functioned independently and often in isolation. This independence and isolation can foster divergent and uncoordinated goals, as well as counterproductive efforts by rehabilitation services.

SELECTIVE JOB PLACEMENT

The primary concern of the patient and counselor is placement in a suitable job (52). Most of the means of achieving this goal should already have been done during the hospitalization period; for example, vocational evaluation. Some persons will need job-seeking skills training. Others will require selective placement, and some will need both. Therefore, the type of placement activity depends on the needs of the person.

The selective placement concept "owes its origin to the development of job analysis" (36). Job analysis allows the counselor and patient to focus on the requirements of job, not the patient's limitations regarding a specific job. Each job requires different levels of physical and mental skills. Some need more in one area; some less. Selective job placement implies an individualistic approach to each patient. Return to work for a burned person requires a systematic process of vocational rehabilitation dependent upon early interventions and the development of an individualized rehabilitation program. The result of this process, when successful, should be the same as the patient's vocational objective. The following three steps are essential in selective job placement.

Assessing Employment Potential

Most of the means of making judgments about employability, such as taking the patient's work history and job analysis, should already have been done during the hospitalization period. The counselor needs to keep the patient aware of the barriers he will have to overcome and the adaptations he will have to make in order to succeed in a job. If the patient is planning to return to the type of job he had prior to the accident, the counselor needs to work with the employer, explaining when necessary what can be done at the work site to maximize the employee's productivity. For example, the counselor may wish to provide answers to the employer's questions about the employee's deficits as they apply to the job; provide consultation for job restructuring or modification; facilitate a patient-employer initial meeting to discuss such needs; and provide resources for the employer to aid in his own understanding of burn injuries.

Assessing Job Readiness

Job readiness will depend upon the extent of the residual impairment, the patient's successes in treatment, and the patient's adjustment of the disability. The employer's readiness is also important and must be considered. For example, the employer or a representative should be contacted early so that the patient will see that return is possible and he is still a valued member of the organization. If the impairment is extensive, the patient's return to work should be delayed until he is relatively free of any extensive rehabilitation needs. A premature return to work would leave the patient unable to do the job fully and would lower his chances of success. Therefore, job readiness will hinge upon successful completion of the rehabilitation therapies, any retraining program or job modifications needed, and the development of the patient's ability to cope with his new life and disability.

Assessing Job Seeking Skills

Some patients do not know how to find and follow-up on job leads. They can obtain training in these skills in state vocational rehabilitation programs. A good job-seeking skills program should focus on how and where to seek good job leads, job interview skills, instruction on completing job application forms, and practice in the entire process of looking for work.

EVALUATION OF OUTCOME—SYSTEMATIC FOLLOW-UP

The vocational rehabilitation counselor's job does not end with placement of the burned person since there is a crucial period of adjustment after employment.

The rehabilitation burn specialist should not assume that placement is permanent when a patient returns to work. He should establish a schedule of systematic follow-up (e.g., at one, three, six, and 12 months). Early intervention with former patients having difficulty with transition can prevent their losing the skills they have gained during treatment. A patient might be experiencing difficulty with scar formation that inhibits movement, and yet not know exactly what to do about it, partially because he fears more painful treatment. Early intervention would facilitate the correction of the physical problem, while minimizing any regression due to temporary, common problems. As early as two weeks after employment the rehabilitation counselor should visit the company and talk with the patient's immediate supervisor and co-workers in order to identify additional adjustments that need to be made in the work environment and to gain a first-hand account of how the former patient is progressing. The counselor should see the patient upon each return to the clinic for continued training in disability management and vocational adjustment if needed.

Summary

While future research and testing are needed to establish the effectiveness of the vocational rehabilitation model presented in this chapter, it is clear that the rehabilitation counselor needs more tools and systems to be effective in the overall recovery of burned persons. The vocational counselor's role can be crucial in helping the patient achieve a lasting recovery in this model's context. The counselor should no longer have to depend on subjective evaluations and impressions to plan and carry out rehabilitation programs for this growing group of injured but employable persons.

The problems of burn injured persons will soon capture the attention of health policymakers and lawmakers as these persons become more evident in communities and on the rolls of third-party payment disbursers. Clearly, the best solution for society and for most burned persons is to find ways for them to return to the work force. The burden will be on professionals to accomplish this with an organized and reliable approach. This approach must incorporate among other factors: (1) a comprehensive program; (2) systematic implementation; (3) close involvement of the patient; (4) a whole man view of the patient; and (5) close collaboration with the rest of the burn treatment team.

The model presented here is complex, but testing of it will provide not only information of its validity, but also expanded understanding of the special nature of vocational rehabilitation of burned patients. Thus, trial use of the model can provide early guidelines for professionals who are designing and applying interventions. The ultimate goal of this theoretical work is a human one: to enable burned persons to be competitive in seeking and keeping a job.

REFERENCES

1. Ablon J: Reactions of Somoan burn patients and families to severe burns. *Soc Sci Med* 7:167–178, 1973.
2. Andreasen NJC: Neuropsychiatric complications in burn patients. *Int J Psychiatry Med* 5:161–171, 1974.
3. Andreasen NJC, Norris AS: Long term adjustment and adaptation mechanisms in severely burned adults. *J Nerv Ment Dis* 154:352–362, 1972.
4. Andreasen NJC, Norris AS, Hartford CE: Incidence of long term psychiatric complications in severely burned adults. *Ann Surg* 174:785–793, 1971.
5. Andreasen NJC, Noyes R Jr, Hartford CE: Factors influencing adjustment of burn patients during hospitalization. *Psychosom Med* 34:517–525, 1972.
6. Andreasen NJC, Noyes R Jr, Hartord CE, et al: Management of emotional reactions in seriously burned adults. *N Engl J Med* 286:54–69, 1972.
7. Artz CR, Moncrief JA, Pruitt BA Jr: *Burns: A Team Approach*. Philadelphia, W.B. Saunders and Co., 1979.
8. Avni J: Psychiatric care of burn patients during wartime. *Psychother Psychosom* 26:203–210, 1975.
9. Barnes BA: Mortality of burns at the Massachusetts General Hospital. *Ann Surg* 145:210–222, 1957.
10. Bartlett RH, Wingerson E, Simonton S, et al: Rehabilitation following burn injury. *Surg Clin North Am* 58:1249–1262, 1978.
11. Beals RKJ, Hickman NW: Industrial injuries of the back and extremities. *J Bone Joint Surg* 8:1593–1611, 1972.
12. Bernstein NR: *Emotional Care of the Facially Burned and Disfigured*. Boston, Little Brown and Co., 1976.
13. Blades BC, Jones C, Munster A: Quality of life after major burns. *J Trauma* 19:556–558, 1979.
14. Bowden ML, Feller I: Self esteem of severely burned patients. *Arch Phys Med Rehabil* 61:445–452, 1980.
15. Bowden ML, Jones CA, Feller I: *Psychosocial Aspects of a Severe Burn: A Review of the Literature*. Ann Arbor, National Institute for Burn Medicine, 1979.
16. Bull JP, Fisher AJ: A study of mortality in a burn unit: A revised estimate. *Ann Surg* 139:269–274, 1954.
17. Cameron NA: *The Psychology of Behavior Disorders; A Biosocial Interpretation*. Boston, Houghton Mifflin and Co., 1947.
18. Chang FC, Herzog B: Burn morbidity. A follow-up study of physical and psychological disability. *Ann Surg* 183:34–37, 1976.
19. Eaton MW: Obstacles to the vocational rehabilitation of individuals receiving Workers' Compensation. *J Rehabil* 10:59–63, 1979.

20. Feck G, Baptiste MS, Tate CL Jr: *An Epidemiological Study of Burn Injuries and Strategies for Prevention.* U.S. Dept. H.E.W., Public Health Service, 1978.

21. Feller I, Crane KH, Richards KE: The need for burn care facilities in Michigan. *Mich Med* 71:317–321, 1972.

22. Fisher JC, Wells JA, Fulivider BT, et al: Editorial: Doe we need a burn severity grading system? *J Trauma* 17:252–255, 1977.

23. Fordyce WE: *Behavioral Methods for Chronic Pain and Illness.* St. Louis, C.V. Mosby and Co., 1976.

24. Foster NW, Jr: Neurosis and trauma. *Clin Orthop* 32:54–59, 1964.

25. Goldberg RT: Rehabilitation of the burn patient. *Rehab Lit* 35:73–78, 1974.

26. Goldberg RT: Vocational development of adolescents with burn injury. *Rehabil Counselor Bull* 18:140–146, 1975.

27. Graham WP III, Miller SH, Gottlieb L, et al: Psychological complications of thermal injuries. *Penn Med* 79:58, 1976.

28. Haber LD: Disabling effects of chronic disease and impairment. *J Chron Dis* 24:469–487, 1971.

29. Hamburg DA, Hamburg B, deGaza S: Adaptive problems and mechanisms in severely burned patients. *Psychiatry* 16:1–20, 1953.

30. Helm P, Archterberg J, Peyton S: *Psychosocial Impact of Burn Injury.* Final Report Project No. 240-77-0161, Department of Health and Human Services, Health Services Administration Bureau of Medical Services, Division of Emergency Medical Services, September, 1980.

31. Hirschfeld AH: Some thoughts on disability. *J Occup Med* 6:267–270, 1964.

32. Hirschfeld AH, Behan RC: The accident process: I. Etiological considerations of industrial injuries. *JAMA* 186:193–199, 1963.

33. Hirschfeld AH, Behan RC: The accident process: II. Toward more rational treatment of industrial injuries. *JAMA* 186:300–306, 1963.

34. House J: Job stress and coronary artery disease. In Gentry WP, Williams RB: *Psychological Aspects of Myocardial Infarction and Coronary Care.* St. Louis, C.V. Mosby and Co., 1975.

35. Jorgensen JA, Brophy JJ: Psychiatry treatment of severely burned adults. *Psychosomatics* 14:331–335, 1973.

36. Kessler H. *Rehabilitation of the Physically Handicapped.* New York, University Press, 1935.

37. Kjaer GC: Psychiatric aspects of thermal burns. *Northwest Med* 68:537–541, 1969.

38. Korlof B: Social and economic consequences of deep burns. In Wallace ABS, Wilkinson AW: *Research in Burns.* Edinburgh, E. and S. Livingstone Ltd., 1966.

39. Lewis SR, Goolishian HA, Wolf CW, et al: Psychological studies in burn patients. *Plast Reconstr Surg* 31:323–332, 1963.

40. Matter P, Barclay TL, Konickova Z (Eds): *Research in Burns.* Bern, Hans Huber Publishers, 1971.

41. Miller H: Accident neurosis. *Br Med J* 1:919–925, 1961.

42. Miller WC, Gardner N, Mlott SR: Psychosocial support in the treatment of severely burned patients. *J Trauma* 16:722–725, 1976.

43. Mitchell DK: Principles of vocational rehabilitation: A contemporary view. In Long C: *Prevention and Rehabilitation in Ischemic Heart Disease.* Baltimore, Williams & Wilkins, 1980.

44. Mlott SR, Lira FT, Miller WC: Psychological assessment of the burn patient. *J Clin Psychiatry* 33:425–430, 1977.

45. Moloney JC: The effort syndrome and low back pain. *J Nerv Ment Dis* 108:10–24, 1948.

46. Nagi S: *Disability and Rehabilitation.* Columbus, Ohio State University Press, 1969.

47. National Center for Health Statistics: *Inpatient Utilization of Short-stay Hospitals by Diagnosis: United States, 1975,* Series 13, No. 35. Hyattsville, U.S. Dept. HEW, 1978.

48. Noyes R Jr, Andreasen NJ, Hartford CE: The psychological reaction to severe burns. *Psychology* 12:416–422, 1971.

49. Noyes R Jr, Fry SJ, Slymen DJ, et al: Stressful life events and burn injuries. *J Trauma* 19:141–144, 1979.
50. Pavlovsky P: Occurrence and development of psychopathologic phenomena in burned persons and their relation to severity of burns, age and pre-morbid personality. *Acta Chir Plast* 14:112–119, 1972.
51. Pennisi VR, Deatherage J, Templeton J, et al: The psychogenic dependence of the acute burn patient. In Matter P, Barclay TL, Konickova Z: *Research in Burns*. Bern, Hans Huber Publishers, 1971.
52. Rubin S, Roessler R: *Foundation of Vocational Rehabilitation*. Baltimore, University Park Press, 1978.
53. Rudowski W, Nasilowski W, Zietkiewicz W, et al: *Burn Therapy and Research*. Baltimore, The Johns Hopkins University Press, 1976.
54. Safilias-Rothschild C: *The Sociology and Social Psychology of Disability and Rehabilitation* New York, Random House, 1970.
55. Schlenoff D: Obstacles to the rehabilitation of disability benefits recipients. *J Rehabil* 45:55–58, 1979.
56. Schlichtman KA: Adoptive mechanisms in a selected group of burned patients. *Med Surg Nurs* 259–266, 1968.
57. Seres JL, Newman RI, Yospe LP, et al: Evaluation of chronic pain by nonsurgical means. In Lee J: *Pain Management*. Baltimore, Williams & Wilkins, 1977.
58. Simons RD, Green LC, Malin R, et al: The burn victim: His psychosocial profile and post-injury career. *Burns* 5:97–100, 1978.
59. Sink J, Field T: *Vocational Assessment Planning and Jobs*. Athens, VDRE Service Bureau, 1981.
60. Soloman AP: Low back pain: The psychosomatic view point. *Ind Med* 18:6–12, 1949.
61. Steger HG, Burns AC, Alkiri SK: Psychological impact of Industrial Burns. Presented at the American Psychological Association, Los Angeles, CA, August 1981.
62. Steiner H, Clark WR Jr: Psychiatric complications of burned adults: A classification. *J Trauma* 17:134–143, 1977.
63. Tabor M: Restructuring the science: Back injury. *Occup Health Safety* 2:16–22, 1982.
64. Tate SC, Hollingsworth DK: Vocational rehabilitation counseling in burn treatment. In Newman N, Salisbury R, Dingeldein GP: *Manual of Burn Therapeutics*. Boston, Little Brown and Co., 1983.
65. Waisbren BA, Stern M, Collentine GE: Data for comparative study from a burn center. *Burns* 5:30–35, 1978.
66. Wallace AB, Wilkinson AW (Eds): *Research in Burns*. Edinburgh, E. and S. Livingstone Ltd., 1966.
67. West DA, Shuck JM: Emotional problems of the severely burned patient. *Surg Clin North Am* 58:1189–1204, 1978.
68. Williams BP: Social sequelae of severe burn injury. In Malter P, Barclay TL, Konickova Z: *Research in Burns*. Bern, Hans Huber Publ., 1971.
69. Williams BP: The problems and life-style of severely burned man. In Bergerson BS, Anderson EH, Duffy M, et al: *Current Concepts in Clinical Nursing 11*. St. Louis, C.V. Mosby Co., 1969.
70. Yelin EH, Nevitt MC, Epstein WV: Toward an epidemiology of work disability. *Milbank Mem Fund Quart* 58:387–415, 1980.
71. Yochelson L. Psychiatric aspects of backache. *Curr Pract Orthop Surg* 3:253–272, 1966.
72. Zellweger G, Ganzoni A: Burn mortality and morbidity experience of the burn center in Zurich from 1967–1977. *Helv Chir Acta* 45:753–756, 1979.

18

Disability Determination

STEVEN V. FISHER

Introduction

The rating or evaluation of permanent disability is an important and often a complex task. Inadequate understanding by physicians and others of the scope of medical responsibility in the evaluation of permanent disability and confusion concerning "permanent disability" and "permanent impairment" is not uncommon. With the advances in burn treatment during the last 20 years, an increasing number of burn victims are surviving and returning to work. In addition, Workmen's Compensation laws in the United States have been continuously changing and the frequency of civil negligence cases is increasing. In spite of an increased need for disability determinations for the burn victim, there is little agreement in the medical community as to how these determinations should be made.

It is important for every physician to be aware of the medical role in the evaluation of permanent disability for any private or public program for the disabled and to have the necessary information to assist in competently evaluating a burn victim for a disability determination (1).

One must understand the difference between the terms permanent impairment and permanent disability. The term permanent impairment is a purely medical condition which pertains specifically to an anatomical or functional abnormality or loss after maximal medical rehabilitation has been achieved. This abnormality or loss is considered stable or nonprogressive at the time the evaluation is made. It is the permanent impairment which is the basic consideration in the evaluation of permanent disability (1).

Permanent disability is not a purely medical condition. A patient is permanently disabled when his actual or presumed ability to engage in gainful activity based on multiple psychosocial and economic factors is reduced or absent because of impairment. It is permanent if no fundamental or marked changes can be expected in the future (1).

Therefore, the evaluation or rating of permanent impairment is a physician function and only the physician is competent to perform this evaluation. The evaluation of permanent impairment is an appraisal of the nature and extent of the patient's illness or injury as it affects his personal performance.

The evaluation of disability is an appraisal of the patient's present and future ability to engage in gainful activity as it is affected by factors such as age, sex, education, economics, and social relationships. These are diverse and subjective factors which are difficult to measure. For this reason permanent impairment is, in fact, the major criterion used in arriving at a permanent disability determination. In the final analysis the determination of permanent disability is an administrative decision. However, the determination of permanent impairment is the most important factor in the permanent disability rating (1).

The competent evaluation of permanent impairment requires an adequate and complete medical examination, accurate objective measurements of function, and the avoidance of subjective impressions such as factors of age, sex, or employability (1).

It seems reasonable that unlike disability, permanent impairment can be measured with a reasonable degree of accuracy and uniformity, as it is evidenced by loss of structural integrity, loss of functional capacity, or persistent pain that is substantiated by clinical findings.

The evaluation of the burn victim, however, has some unique features. The necessity to consider such subjective factors as heat and cold intolerance, sensitivity to sunlight, pain, chemical sensitivity and changes in sweating pattern, as well as the more objective considerations of decreased coordination, sensation, strength, and contractures lends itself to a unique evaluation.

Disfigurement and scarring, frequent sequela of burns, may not affect the performance and thereby in and of itself, may cause no impairment. Scarring represents a special type of disfigurement. Again, no percentage of impairment is assigned for the existence of scarring per se. However, if scars affect sweat glands, hair growth, and nail growth and cause pigment changes or contractures, it may well affect the loss of performance and cause impairment. The sensory deficit, pain, or discomfort of scars needs to be evaluated as well as the loss of motion in a scar area.

The impairment due to disfigurement of scarring also may have behavioral or psychological components which subsequently may be rated. The need for intermittent or continuous treatment of the skin with topical agents, compression garments, etc. can impair a person's function and needs to be considered.

The two major areas to discuss are: (1) The medical determination of return to work; and (2) The medical determination of impairment.

Return to Work

It is the physician's ultimate responsibility to decide when a burn victim is medically capable of returning to work. The employee's actual return to work, however, is not a simple matter. Chapter 17 deals in detail with vocational considerations. Medical considerations will be highlighted here.

Some factors which must be considered in determining the patient's employability may include remaining open wounds and their care, skin fragility, cold intolerance, heat intolerance, chemical sensitivity, pain and inattention to job, decreased coordination, visual problems, and the need for continued compression dressings.

OPEN WOUNDS

Employees who deal with food handling obviously should not be allowed to return to employment until all wounds are closed and there is no likelihood of contaminating food from any open wound. In nonfood management areas, if open wounds are aggravated by irritants or dirt in the workplace or by constant friction or pressure, the employee should refrain from all duties which inhibit wound closure.

SKIN FRAGILITY

New immature skin is delicate and blistering is common. Laborers, especially those with hand burns, may cause significant reinjury of freshly burned skin. They should not return to work until the skin can tolerate the work conditions.

COLD INTOLERANCE

Cold intolerance may well keep any employee from returning to work and is an important consideration in cold climates and for those who work in refrigerated areas. Many burn victims, especially those with thermal injuries to their hands, have significant cold intolerance in temperatures of less than 45°F. They may become quite uncomfortable and unable to perform job responsibilities.

HEAT INTOLERANCE

Heat intolerance in persons who have suffered body surface area burns of approximately 50% or greater, may be a problem causing not only discomfort but actual increased body temperature, malaise, fatigue, and heat prostration.

CONTINUED PAIN

If the pain is a continous problem which causes an inability to concentrate fully and if the subject is working in a situation which necessitates continuous concentration, i.e., operating machinery, the inability to attend to the job would cause continued disability.

DECREASED COORDINATION

Decreased coordination, a common initial sequela of burn injury, especially hand burns, can interfere with work and cause danger in a workplace.

COMPRESSION GARMENTS

The use of compression garments especially on the hands may interfere enough to disallow the person to return to work. Compression garments in a dusty or dirty place may cause very significant pruritis which subsequently temporarily disables the subject.

CHEMICAL SENSITIVITY

The use of chemicals at the workplace needs to be evaluated since the likelihood of chemical sensitivity to the new, still immature skin may create a significant problem.

VISUAL PROBLEMS

Cataracts and other visual problems caused by the burn injury would obviously need to be considered in decisions of returning to work.

In summary, the permission or release to work is a medical decision which requires special attention. The actual ability to return to work, however, involves the more complex psychosocial system in which we live.

Impairment Determination

There is a surprising lack of published literature that relates to impairment evaluation of the burn patient. Although there are several texts related to impairment ratings in general (2–5), burns are not dealt with in any specific way. One text discusses disability in burns, but gives no guidelines for the determination of impairment (6). There were two foreign articles on burn ratings but neither one in the English language.

Because physicians are asked for disability evaluations for both Workmen's Compensation cases and common law personal injury cases, clearly, a distinction needs to be made.

In Workmen's Compensation cases, recovery is based on specific permanent injury sustained to a portion of the anatomy. The worker is protected by partial replacement of income loss as a result of the injury incurred during his employment. In common law personal injury cases, the subject is compensated for damages and where negligence and assumption of risk have bearing on the subject's compensation. It is necessary to distinguish personal injury cases from Workmen's Compensation cases because the physician is required to write a different type of medical report in the latter case (3). Although the physician examines the injured person in the same manner for any disability evaluation, emphasis in the medical report for a Workmen's Compensation case is placed on loss of, or loss of use of, a specific body part rather than with reference to the effect of injury on the man in his total existence as in a civil legal proceeding.

The lack of uniformity and the differences that exist in ratings according to the same disability in various states is a major problem. In order to understand this problem, a questionnaire was sent to each of the 50 states asking specifically how permanent partial impairment ratings are determined for burn victims under the Workmen's Compensation laws. Specific questions were asked concerning payment for disfigurement, scarring, and skin changes.

Of the 50 states, thirty-six responded. As expected, laws varied dramatically from one state to another even in the same geographic location. Most states did not mention burns specifically in their Workmen's Compensation laws. Two states, in addition to the usual compensation for loss of a part or loss of function of a part, specifically award permanent partial impairment based on whole man for changes to the skin alone. Seven states offered no extra financial compensation for disfigurement and/or there was no mention of cosmesis in their schedules. Nine states provided compensation for scars if the disfigurement involved the face and head. Six other states gave extra compensation for disfigurement only if it interfered with one's ability to find or maintain employment. Two states paid for disfigurement only if it specifically caused loss of function of a part. Five states paid both for disfigurement as well as impairment from loss of function. Five states mentioned disfigurement in general terms but their schedules provide no specific guidelines for compensation. Obviously the actual compensation for loss of, or loss of use of a body part varied significantly between states.

Many states specifically commented that the American Medical Association's *Guides to the Evaluation of Permanent Impairment* (1) is suggested as an aid to determine impairment ratings.

Because of the confusion which exists among the states, it is obvious that the physician must have some familiarity with the type of case and statute of the state from which the burn victim will be compensated. In general terms, however, the examination of burn victims is the same regardless of whether the compensation is to be through civil law or Workmen's Compensation. Likewise, the impairment examination for any injured person is similar. However, certain specific questions must be asked of the burn patient.

Table 18.1 shows a possible questionnaire worksheet. These include findings on history and physical examination of sensory changes, heat and cold intolerance, sensitivity to sunlight, sensitivity to chemicals, altered perspiration, loss of hair, loss of or malformation of nails, and pigmentation changes. Specific questions of psychological effects that need to be asked include nightmares, depression, agitation, decreased sexual drive or ability, increased fears, and changes in drug use and alcohol consumption. Inquiry about joint pain and skin discomfort are important. Questions regarding the eyes in relation to photophobia, tearing, and changes in visual acuity are important in some cases.

In cases of inhalation injury, changes related to shortness of breath, lack

Table 18.1.
Patient Questionnaire

Decreased sensation	Yes _____	No _____	Areas involved _____
Heat intolerance	Yes _____	No _____	Areas involved _____
Cold intolerance	Yes _____	No _____	Areas involved _____
Sensitivity to sunlight	Yes _____	No _____	Areas involved _____
Sensitivity to chemicals	Yes _____	No _____	Areas involved _____
Altered perspiration	Yes _____	No _____	
Area of increased perspiration _____			
Area of decreased perspiration _____			
Restricted chest motion	Yes _____	No _____	
Restricted abdominal motion	Yes _____	No _____	
Loss of hair	Yes _____	No _____	
Loss of nails or malformed			
nails	Yes _____	No _____	
Dysesthesias	Yes _____	No _____	Where _____
Hypopigmentation	Yes _____	No _____	Where _____
Hyperpigmentation	Yes _____	No _____	Where _____
Psychological effects			
Nightmares	Yes _____	No _____	
Impotence	Yes _____	No _____	
Decreased sexual drive			
or activity	Yes _____	No _____	
Fears	Yes _____	No _____	
Drug use	Yes _____	No _____	
Increased alcohol use	Yes _____	No _____	Amount _____
Donor site scarring	None _____	Minor _____ Moderate _____ Severe _____	
Approximate body surface area of donor _____ %			
Gastric pain	Yes _____	No _____	
Joint pain	Yes _____	No _____	Where _____
Tearing, photophobia	Yes _____	No _____	
Decreased vision	Yes _____	No _____	
Shortness of breath	Yes _____	No _____	FEV_1 _____ FEV_T _____
Lack of endurance	Yes _____	No _____	
Hoarseness or other			
vocal cord problem	Yes _____	No _____	Describe _____

of endurance, and persistent hoarseness or change in vocal quality must be considered. If there is a history of smoke inhalation or complaints of cough and shortness of breath, pulmonary function tests should be performed and an impairment rating determined.

The physical examination of the burned victim is much the same as the disability evaluation for any disabled person. Certain aspects of the examination need to be stressed. Skin changes, specifically those changes relating to loss of function of the skin including neurosensory and aprocrine gland dysfunction should be noted. The scarring, pigment changes, and general disfigurement should be noted in detail. Specific objective testing of proprioception, stereognosis, and two-point discrimination should be performed. The loss of light touch and pain sensation should be mapped and the percentage of body surface area involved with neurosensory dysfunction should be calculated.

Standardized coordination testing and grip strength, lateral pinch, and palmar pinch determination provide objective and functional evaluations of impairment. There are norms developed for standardized coordination testing as well as for strength testing. The data should be compared to those norms in formulating impairment determination.

Contractures can be a major cause of impairment in the burn patient and they may be accurately measured and evaluated. The American Medical Association's *Guides to the Evaluation of Permanent Impairment* (1) contains specific tables from which one may calculate specific impairments based on individual contractures. Table 18.2 shows a sample worksheet which may be utilized for rapid determination of contractures and calculation of impairment ratings while Table 18.3 is a worksheet for functional examination of the hands.

With the information gathered from the history and physical examination and using the tables available in the *Guides to the Evaluation of Permanent Impairment* (1), the physician can arrive at an impairment rating. If decreased strength and/or decreased coordination is present in either the upper or lower extremities using objective testing, further impairment is present and the rating should reflect this increased impairment.

The skin should be considered as an organ system and changes of the skin including neurosensory deficit, changes in apocrine function, as well as sensitivity to sunlight, sensitivity to chemicals, loss of hair, loss of and malformation of nails should be considered. Under the Workmen's Compensation laws of a specific state, disfigurement and scarring may not be considered but loss of function of an organ system should be considered, and therefore, the skin should be given an impairment rating. There are general guidelines available for impairment ratings of the skin in Chapter 12 of the American Medical Association's text (1).

Finally, if permanent psychological or sexual impairment exists according to history and subsequent testing, an impairment rating should be made.

Table 18.2.
Right Upper Extremity

	*(AMA)	**(AAOS)	Range	Lacks	Impairment of Upper Extremity %	Impairment of Whole Man
Shoulder Flexion	(0–150)	(0–180)				
Shoulder Hyperextension	(0–40)	(0–60)				
Shoulder Abduction	(0–180)	(0–180)				
Shoulder Int. Rotation	(0–40)	(0–90)				
Shoulder Ext. Rotation	(0–90)	(0–90)				
Elbow Flexion	(0–150)	(0–150)				
Pronation	(0–80)	(0–90)				
Supination	(0–80)	(0–90)				
Wrist Flexion	(0–70)	(0–80)				
Wrist Extension	(0–60)	(0–70)				
Radial Deviation	(0–20)	(0–20)				
Ulnar Deviation	(0–30)	(0–30)				

THUMB	*(AMA)	**(AAOS)	Range	Lacks	%	Impairment of Thumb	Impairment of Hand
Thumb MP Flexion	(0–60)	(0–50)					
Thumb IP Flexion	(0–80)	(0–80)					
Radial Abduction	(0–45)	(0–50)					
Palmar Opposition		(0–35)					

INDEX	*(AMA)	**(AAOS)	Range	Lacks	%	Impairment of Finger	Impairment of Hand
Index finger MP Flexion	(0–90)	(0–90)					
PIP Flexion	(0–100)	(0–120)					
DIP Flexion	(0–70)	(0–90)					

	*(AMA)	**(AAOS)	Range	Lacks	%	Impairment of Finger	Impairment of Hand
LONG							
Long finger MP Flexion	(0–90)	(0–90)					
PIP Flexion	(0–100)	(0–120)					
DIP Flexion	(0–70)	(0–90)					
RING							
Ring finger MP Flexion	(0–90)	(0–90)					
PIP Flexion	(0–100)	(0–120)					
DIP Flexion	(0–70)	(0–90)					
SMALL							
Small finger MP Flexion	(0–90)	(0–90)					
PIP Flexion	(0–100)	(0–120)					
DIP Flexion	(0–70)	(0–90)					

Total Hand ___

U/E Extremity ___
U/E (above) ___
Total U/E ___

Total Whole Man ___

* ROM of fingers based on American Medical Association.
** ROM of fingers based on American Academy of Orthopedic Surgery.

Table 18.3.
Upper Extremity Sensory, Strength, Coordination Evaluation

LEFT   RIGHT

Proprioception: Instruction:

        L: R:

Shoulder ___ ___   Decreased light touch—
Elbow   ___ ___   color blue
Wrist   ___ ___
Fingers ___ ___   Decreased sharp/dull—
                                            color red

Stereognosis ___ ___

Two-point discrimination:

              L: R:

Fingertips: Thumb ___ ___
         Index   ___ ___
         Middle ___ ___
         Ring   ___ ___
         Little   ___ ___
         Palm   ___ ___

STRENGTH	LEFT	RIGHT
Hand Grasp #		
Lateral Pinch #		
Palmar Pinch (3 pt) #		

Normal for age/sex Age:___

Dominant Hand is_____.

COORDINATION

9-Hole Peg Test   L: R:
(sec/percentile)

Mn. Rate of Manipulation—Two Trials (sec/percentile)

1-Hand Turn & Place   Dominant Hand:
2-Hand Turn & Place   Both Hands:

DATE:_____   THERAPIST: _____

Summary

Disability determination is a difficult and by no means objective procedure. These general guidelines may provide more objectivity than is sometimes utilized in providing a disability impairment rating. It should again be stressed that the final disability determination and compensation is not a medical question but the medical input into the impairment is significant, and in fact is the most important factor in deriving the disability determination.

REFERENCES

1. American Medical Association Committee on Rating of Mental and Physical Impairment: *Guides to the Evaluation of Permanent Impairment*. Chicago, American Medical Association, 1977.
2. Kessler KH: *Disability Determination and Evaluation*. Philadelphia, J.B. Lippincott Co., 1963.
3. Liebenson HA, Miller LF: *Disability Evaluation in Personal Injury Cases*. Mundelein, IL, Callaghan & Co., 1962.
4. Manning GC Jr: *Disability and the Law*. Baltimore, Williams & Wilkins, 1962.
5. McBride ED: *Disability Evaluation and Principles of Treatment of Compensable Injuries*. Philadelphia, J.B. Lippincott Co., 1963.
6. Stolov WC, Clowers MR: *Handbook of Severe Disability*. Washington, DC, U.S. Government Printing Office, 1981.

Index

Page numbers in italics denote figures; those followed by t or f denote tables or footnotes, respectively.

413